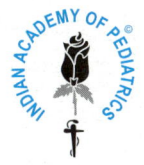

INDIAN ACADEMY OF PEDIATRICS

W0230649

IAP
Guidebook on
Immunization

Disclaimer

'IAP ACVIP' has formulated these guidelines on the most optimum way of using available licensed vaccines in the country to provide best possible protection to an individual child in an office practice setting. However, members may use their own discretion while using them in a given situation within the framework suggested. They may not necessarily be construed as the Academy's approval of the particular product for wider, mass use in national/sub-national large-scale programs.

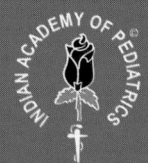

IAP
Guidebook on
Immunization

By
Advisory Committee on Vaccines and Immunization Practices (ACVIP)

Editors ———————

Vipin M. Vashishtha
Panna Choudhury
C.P. Bansal
Vijay N. Yewale
Rohit Agarwal

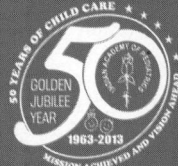

Students' Edition

Published by

IAP National Publication House, Gwalior
Indian Academy of Pediatrics

CBS Publishers & Distributors Pvt Ltd

IAP Guidebook on Immunization

© Indian Academy of Pediatrics 2014

ISBN: 978-81-239-2454-0
First Edition: 2014
CBS Reprint: 2014
CBS Reprint: 2018

Address for correspondence:
Indian Academy of Pediatrics
Kailas Darshan, Kennedy Bridge, Near Nana Chowk, Mumbai, India 400 007.
Tel: +91-22-23889565   e-mail: centraloffice@iapindia.org   Website: www.iapindia.org

Published by
IAP National Publication House, Gwalior
Indian Academy of Pediatrics
Published by Satish Kumar Jain and Produced by Varun Jain for
CBS Publishers & Distributors Pvt Ltd
4819/XI Prahlad Street, 24 Ansari Road, Daryaganj, New Delhi 110 002, India.
Ph: 23289259, 23266861, 23266867   Website: www.cbspd.com
Fax: 011-23243014   e-mail: delhi@cbspd.com; cbspubs@airtelmail.in

Corporate Office: 204 FIE, Industrial Area, Patparganj, Delhi 110 092, India
Ph: 4934 4934   Fax: 4934 4935   e-mail: publishing@cbspd.com; publicity@cbspd.com

Branches

- **Bengaluru:** Seema House 2975, 17th Cross, K.R. Road, Banasankari 2nd Stage, Bengaluru 560 070, Karnataka
  Ph: +91-80-26771678/79   Fax: +91-80-26771680   e-mail: bangalore@cbspd.com
- **Chennai:** 7, Subbaraya Street, Shenoy Nagar, Chennai 600 030, Tamil Nadu
  Ph: +91-44-26260666, 26208620   Fax: +91-44-42032115   e-mail: chennai@cbspd.com
- **Kochi:** Ashana House, No. 39/1904, AM Thomas Road, Valanjambalam, Ernakulam 682 016, Kochi, Kerala
  Ph: +91-484-4059061-65   Fax: +91-484-4059065   e-mail: kochi@cbspd.com
- **Kolkata:** No. 6/B, Ground Floor, Rameswar Shaw Road, Kolkata-700014 (West Bengal)
  Ph: +91-33-2289-1126, 2289-1127, 2289-1128   e-mail: kolkata@cbspd.com
- **Mumbai:** 83-C, Dr E Moses Road, Worli, Mumbai-400018, Maharashtra
  Ph: +91-22-24902340/41   Fax: +91-22-24902342   e-mail: mumbai@cbspd.com

Representatives

- **Hyderabad** 0-9885175004
- **Jharkhand** 0-9811541605
- **Nagpur** 0-9021734563
- **Patna** 0-9334159340
- **Pune** 0-9623451994
- **Uttarakhand** 0-9716462459

Printed At : Goyal Offset Printers

From the IAP Office

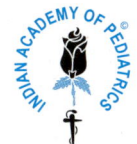

"Vaccines are the tugboats of preventive health".

– William Foege

Childhood vaccines are one of the great triumphs of modern medicine. They are undoubtedly the most cost-effective healthcare interventions. We often fail to realize that rupees spent on a childhood vaccination not only helps save a life, but also greatly reduces spending on future healthcare. The success of smallpox eradication and now of polio eradication programs in the country are testimony to this. IAP has always accorded highest priority to vaccines and vaccination issues. In fact, a separate subcommittee with complete autonomy has been assigned the task of framing recommendations on childhood vaccines and dealing with other issues pertaining to pediatric immunization.

The IAP recommendations on immunization are the most sought after publication of the Academy. Not only IAP members and pediatricians follow them religiously, but also public health experts, vaccine industry people, policy makers, and healthcare professional dealing with preventive medicine, need to consult them at some point of time. Considering the huge stakes, the academy tries its level best to ensure that these guidelines are evidence-based, transparent, rational and ethical. Still there is criticism of the recommendations, often labeled as 'biased', 'unfair', or 'influenced' by different quarters on many occasions in the past. The constitution of the new committee on immunization, IAP Advisory Committee on Vaccines and Immunization Practices (ACVIP) must be seen as an earnest attempt to avoid all these speculative controversies.

IAP now has a basket of publications related to immunization. 'IAP Immunization Timetable' is revised every year, the detailed recommendations are published in a booklet form, 'IAP Guidebook on Immunization' every two year, and a comprehensive discourse on almost every aspect related to immunization with details is contained in a book form, 'IAP Textbook of Vaccines'. The academy has now empowered individual pediatrician and health professional to access IAP's immunization guidelines on their own mobile sets with facility to customize their patients' vaccination schedule or set vaccine reminders for them with the launch of interactive 'Mobile Apps'. However, the Guidebook on Immunization still remains the most premium publication. We are thankful to the editors and to all the committee members for revising and bringing this publication in a new, much more improved form. It would be our endeavor to make this prestigious publication available to each member of the academy at free of cost.

C.P. Bansal
(President 2013)

Rohit Agarwal
(President 2012)

Vijay N. Yewale
(President 2014)

Sailesh Gupta
(Hon. Secretary General, 2011–13)

Preface

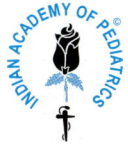

"…..So it's an absolute lie that has killed thousands of kids. Because the mothers who heard that lie, many of them didn't have their kids take either pertussis or measles vaccine, and their children are dead today. And so the people who go and engage in those anti-vaccine efforts -- you know, they, they kill children. It's a very sad thing, because these vaccines are important."

-Bill Gates commenting on the paper by Dr. Wakefield, published in Lancet using fraudulent data

Vaccination scene in India has been at crossroads as newer vaccines are being regularly licensed in the country but public sector catering to vast number of beneficiaries is extremely slow to absorb it. Private sector is the main user of newer vaccines but caters to only small section of well-to-do populations. Controversies are plenty and financial motive is the buzzword in vaccination practices. Many vaccination policies are openly criticized by the media and handful of disbelievers able to block the propagation of newer vaccines. This is despite clear benefits of vaccination in eradication of smallpox, near eradication of polio and significant reduction of many diseases including measles-related deaths through vaccination. Main reasons for this situation are lack of awareness and demand for vaccines from the within, absence of hard-core evidence, inability to present the evidence in a structured format, lack of transparency including dealing with conflict of interest issues while formulating immunization policies, etc. Further there is exaggeration of adverse events associated with new vaccines in the lay media and each serious event is blamed to the vaccine. James A. Shannon, former director of the NIH had once stated, "The only safe vaccine is a vaccine that is never used". Candidly, all vaccines do have inherent risk of AEFI, but the benefits are undoubtedly immense, and clearly outweigh the risks.

Recognizing the need of creditability, IAP constituted 'Advisory Committee on Immunization Practices'(ACVIP) through a completely transparent and democratic process and put in place very strict code of conduct to take care of conflict of interest issues.

Process involved for framing this guidebook involved an exhaustive review of published literature including standard textbooks, vaccine trials, recommendations of various international health agencies, World Health Organization (WHO) position papers on vaccines, literature from the vaccine industry, post-marketing surveillance reports, cost-effective analysis, epidemiology of disease in India and if available Indian studies on vaccine efficacy, immunogenicity and safety. The current committee has tried its level best to issue recommendations based entirely on available indigenous data on the vaccine preventable diseases and vaccines as far as possible. The committee met in person to discuss many issues. At this meeting, the members of the Committee and some invited experts discussed the issues related to vaccines in exhaustive detail. Decisions are taken on crucial matters through a democratic process and the minutes of every meeting are recorded. Efforts are made to issue guidelines based on consensus decisions, however if unanimity is not achieved, voting is resorted on specific recommendations. The Academy is committed to base its recommendation on 'evidence-based process' and started this process by providing Rotavirus disease burden based on a systematic review supported by IAP. In this edition, we have tried to split all our recommendations in two sections, individual use and public health perspectives. The key recommendations are provided in the end of the chapter as boxed items.

It is to be recognized that recommendations in this book are the 'best individual practice guidelines' on available vaccines in the Indian market for a given child and at variance from the Universal Immunization Schedule of the Government of India, which is meant for the public at large. However, core message remains that no child should be denied vaccination and that licensed newer vaccine should be made affordable and available to needy children in equitable manner. The text has been extensively referenced for the first time for a guidebook to instill confidence in statements made and provide readers with an opportunity to cross-check the facts mentioned. We hope that this updated guidebook will empower the pediatricians and vaccine providers in their immunization practices immensely in most situations. Reviewers need to be acknowledged for putting hard work and making possible to publish the book in time. We do sincerely hope that publication of these guidelines of the Academy shall empower not only the pediatricians but also all healthcare professionals to practice vaccination in a more confident and rational ways to shrink the huge burden of VPDs in the country.

Vipin M. Vashishtha
Panna Choudhury
C.P. Bansal
Vijay N. Yewale
Rohit Agarwal

Acknowledgments

The editors are thankful to the dedicated team IAP National Publication House, Gwalior particularly to Dr. Ashok Banga, Dr. Mukul Tiwari, Dr. Rashmi Gupta, Dr. Ajay Gaur and Dr. Suhas Dhonde for their help in proofreading and layout of the book.

The assistance and support provided by the publishers Nandini Graphics for their untiring efforts that culminated in publication of this book is also appreciated.

IAP Committee on Immunization (IAPCOI) 2011–13

Chairpersons
Dr. Rohit C. Agrawal
Dr. T.U. Sukumaran

Convener
Dr. Vipin M. Vashishtha

Members
Dr. Amarjeet Chitkara
Dr. Manjori Mitra
Dr. S. Sanjay
Dr. S.G. Kasi
Dr. Suhas V. Prabhu

Advisors
Dr. Nitin K. Shah
Dr. Raju C. Shah
Dr. Naveen Thacker
Dr. A. Parthasarathy

Ex-officio
Dr. Panna Choudhury
Chairman, IAPCOI, 2009–11

Dr. Vijay N. Yewale
Convener, IAPCOI, 2009–11

Dr. Sailesh Gupta,
Hon Secretary General, IAP

Dr. Ritabrata Kundu,
Chairperson, Infectious Diseases Chapter of IAP

Dr. Abhaya Shah,
Secretary, Infectious Diseases Chapter of IAP

IAP Advisory Committee of Vaccines and Immunization Practices (ACVIP) 2013–14

Chairperson
Dr. C.P. Bansal

Co-chairpersons
Dr. Rohit Agarwal,
Dr. Vijay Yewale

Convener
Dr. Vipin Vashistha

IAP Coordinator (HSG)
Dr. Sailesh Gupta

Members
Dr. Shashi Vani
Dr. Anuradha Bose
Dr. Ajay Kalra
Dr. A.K. Patwari
Dr. Surjit Singh

Consultants
Dr. N.K. Arora
Dr. Naveen Thacker
Dr. Rajesh Kumar
Dr. Ajay Gambhir
Dr. V.G. Ramchandran
Dr. H.P. Sachdev

Rapporteur
Dr. Panna Choudhury

Contents

SECTION IV

Vaccination of Special Groups

ANNEXURE

SECTION
I

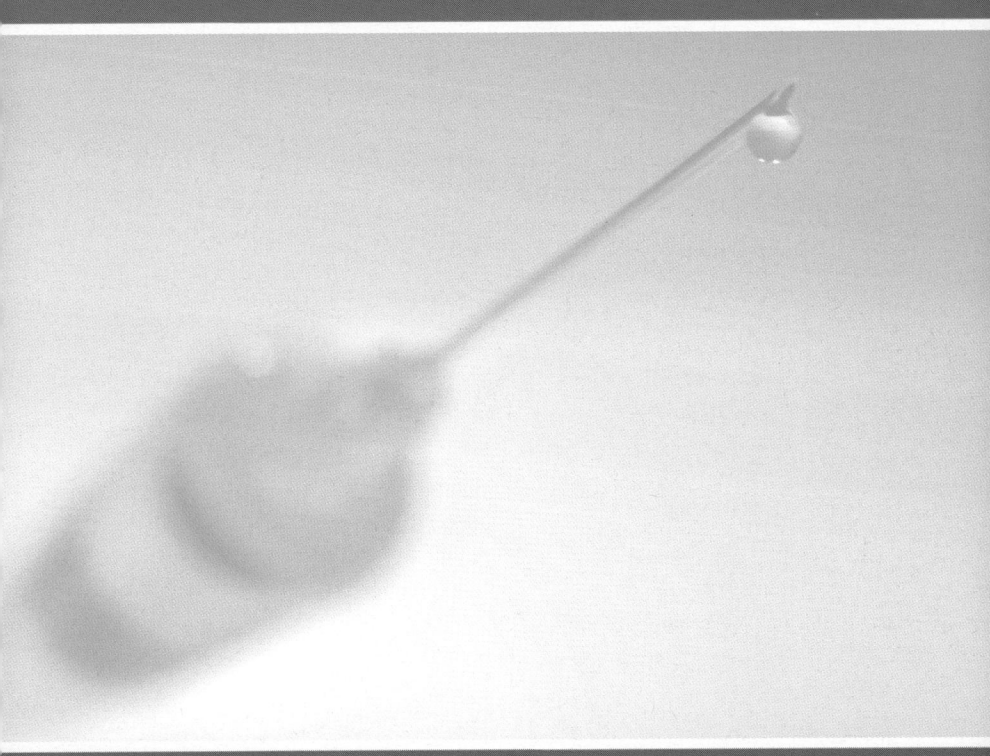

Background
and Process

Immunization in India — *Past, Present and Future*

Reviewed by
Rajesh Kumar

Immunization is a proven tool for controlling and even eradicating disease. An immunization campaign, carried out by the World Health Organization (WHO) from 1967 to 1977, eradicated smallpox. Eradication of poliomyelitis is within reach. Since Global Polio Eradication Initiative in 1988, infections have fallen by 99%, and some five million people have escaped paralysis. Although international agencies such as the World Health Organization (WHO) and the United Nations International Children's Emergency Fund (UNICEF) and now Global Alliance for Vaccines and Immunization (GAVI) provide extensive support for immunization activities, the success of an immunization programme in any country depends more upon local realities and national policies. A successful immunization program is of particular relevance to India, as the country contributes to one-fifth of global under five mortality with a significant number of deaths attributable to vaccine preventable diseases. There is no doubt that substantial progress has been achieved in India with wider use of vaccines, resulting in prevention of several diseases. However, lot remains to be done and in some situations, progress has not been sustained (Table 1).

Table 1: Vaccine preventable diseases: India reported cases (Year wise)

Diseases	1980	1985	1990	1995	2000	2005	2010	2012
Diphtheria	39,231	15,685	8,425	2,123	5,125	10,231	3,123	2,525
Measles	114,036	161,216	89,612	37,494	38,835	52,454	29,808	18,668
Pertussis	320,109	184,368	112,416	4,073	31,431	13,955	38,493	44,154
Polio	18,975	22,570	10,408	3,263	265	66	43	0
Neonatal Tetanus	-	-	9,313	1,783	3,287	891	373	588
Total Tetanus	45,948	37,647	23,356	-	8,997	3,543	1,574	2,404

Source: WHO vaccine-preventable diseases: monitoring system 2013 global summary.[1]

Successful immunization strategy for the country goes beyond vaccine coverage in that self-reliance in vaccine production, creating epidemiological database for infectious diseases and developing surveillance system are also integral parts of the system. It is apparent that the present strategy focuses on mere vaccine coverage.

The history of vaccine research and production in India is almost as old as the history of vaccines themselves. During the latter half of the 19th century, when institutions for vaccine development and production were taking root in the Western world, the British rulers in India promoted research and established about fifteen vaccine institutes beginning in the 1890s. Prior to the establishment of these institutions, there were no dedicated organizations for medical research in India. Haffkine's development of the world's first plague vaccine in 1897 (which he developed at the Plague Laboratory, Mumbai, India, later named the Haffkine Institute) and Manson's development of an indigenous Cholera vaccine at Kolkata during the same period bear testimony to the benefits of the early institutionalization of vaccine research and development in India. Soon, Indian vaccine institutes were also producing Tetanus toxoid (TT), Diphtheria toxoid (DT), and Diphtheria, Pertussis, and Tetanus toxoid (DPT). By the time Indians inherited the leadership of the above institutions in the early 20th century, research and technological innovation were sidelined as demands for routine vaccine production took priority. However, after independence, it took three decades for India to articulate its first official policy for childhood vaccination, a policy that was in alignment with the WHO's policy of "Health for All by 2000" (famously announced in 1978 at Alma Atta, Kazakhstan). The WHO's policy recommended universal immunization of all children to reduce child mortality under its Expanded Programme of Immunization (EPI).

In line with Health for All by 2000, in 1978 India introduced six childhood vaccines (BCG, TT, DPT, DT, Polio, and Typhoid) in its EPI. Measles vaccine was added much later, in 1985, when the Indian government launched the Universal Immunization Programme (UIP) and a mission to achieve immunization coverage of all children and pregnant women by the 1990s. Even though successive governments have adopted self-reliance in vaccine technology and self-sufficiency in vaccine production as policy objectives in theory, the growing gap between demand and supply meant that in practice, India had to increasingly resort to imports. In fact, Government of India had withdrawn indigenous production facilities for oral polio vaccine that existed earlier in Conoor, Tamil Nadu and at Haffkine's Institute in Mumbai for trivial reasons. At Conoor after making several batches of good quality OPV, one batch of OPV had failed to pass the neuro-virulence test. This happens with all manufacturers, and if a facility has to be closed down for such reason, there would have been no OPV in the world today. Thus, oral polio vaccine has been imported in India for last several years. Similarly decision of production of inactivated polio vaccine in the country was revoked more than two decades ago for no known reasons. Many vaccine manufacturing units have suspended production or closing down in recent years for minor reasons. One wonders who is benefitting by the closure of facilities for manufacturing vaccines in public sector.

The vaccination coverage at present with EPI vaccines is far from complete despite the long-standing commitment to universal coverage. Though the reported vaccination coverage has always been higher than evaluated coverage, the average vaccination coverage has shown a consistent increase over the last two decades as shown in Figure 1. While gains in coverage proved to be rapid throughout the 1980s, taking off from a below 20% coverage to about 60% coverage for some VPDs, subsequent gains have been limited (Figure 1). Estimates from the 2009 Coverage Evaluation Survey (CES 2009) indicate that only 61% of children aged 12–23 months were fully vaccinated (received BCG, measles, and 3 doses of DPT and polio vaccines), and 7.6% had received no vaccinations at all.[2] Given an annual birth cohort of 26.6 million, and an under 5 year child mortality rate of 59/1000, this results in over 9.5 million under-immunized children each year.

There is also a tremendous, heterogeneity in state and district levels immunization coverage in India. In the recent District Level Health Survey-3 (2007–08) full immunization coverage of children varies from 30% in Uttar Pradesh, 41% in Bihar, 62% in Orissa to 90% in Goa. Tamil Nadu, Kerala, Punjab and Pondicherry have above 80% coverage (Table 2).[3]

Table 2: Percent of children age 12–23 months (born during 3 years prior to the survey) who received full vaccination, BCG, three doses of DPT, three doses of polio and measles in DLHS-3 survey (2007–08).

State	Full vaccination	BCG	Three doses of DPT vaccine	Three doses of polio vaccine	Measles vaccine
Andhra Pradesh	67.1	97.5	79.0	82.1	88.6
Bihar	41.4	81.5	54.4	53.1	54.2
Chhattisgarh	59.3	94.8	71.4	69.7	79.9
Goa	89.8	98.4	91.5	94.1	94.1
Jharkhand	54.1	85	62.6	64.4	70.5
Karnataka	76.7	96.9	84.8	90.3	85.2
Kerala	79.5	99.1	87.1	86.6	87.9
Madhya Pradesh	36.2	84.2	47.4	55.1	57.7
Orissa	62.4	94.2	74.3	78.8	81.1
Pondicherry	80.4	96.6	88.3	88.3	91.1
Rajasthan	48.8	82.8	55.6	63.9	67.5
Sikkim	77.8	98.4	88.7	86.5	92.5
Tamil Nadu	82.6	99.6	90.5	91.1	95.5
Uttar Pradesh	30.3	73.4	38.9	40.4	47.0
West Bengal	75.8	96.2	83.6	83.6	82.8

In CES 2009, the reasons for poor immunization coverage have been found to be: Did not feel the need (28.2%), not knowing about vaccines (26.3%), not knowing where to go for vaccination (10.8%), time not convenient (8.9%), fear of side effects (8.1%), do not have time (6%), wrong advice by someone (3%), cannot afford cost (1.2%), vaccine not available (6.2%), place not convenient (3.8%),

ANM absent (3.9%), long waiting time (2.1%), place too far (2.1%), services not available (2.1%), others (11.8%).[2]

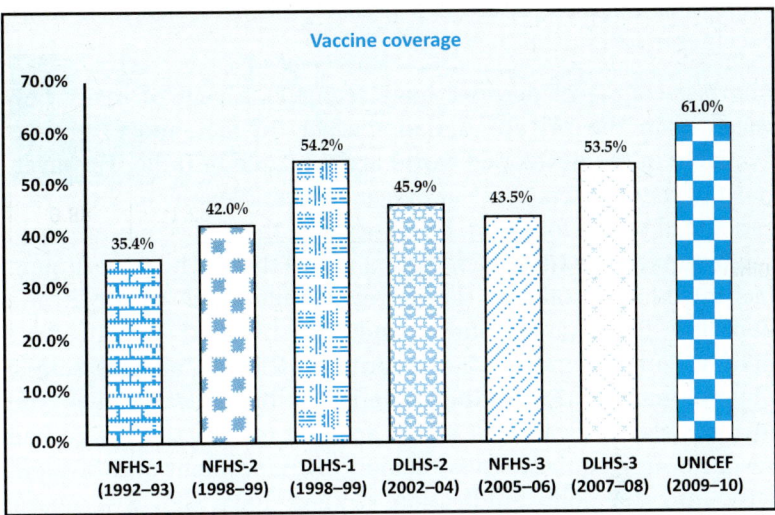

Figure 1: Trends in vaccination coverage over the last twenty years as shown in different surveys

(Source: Multi Year Strategic Plan 2013–17, Universal Immunization Program, Department of Family Welfare, Ministry of Health & Family Welfare, Government of India)

An urgent need at present is to strengthen routine immunization coverage in the country with EPI vaccines. India is self sufficient in production of vaccines used in UIP. As such the availability of the vaccine is not an issue. For improving coverage, immunization needs to be brought closer to the communities. There is need to improve immunization practices at fixed sites along with better monitoring and supervision. Effective behavior change communication would increase the demand for vaccination. There is certainly a need for introducing innovative methods and practices. In Bihar, 'Muskan ek Abhiyan' an innovative initiative started in 2007 is a good example, where a partnership of Government organization, agencies and highly motivated social workers has paid rich dividends. Full vaccination coverage, a mere 19% in 2005 but zoomed to 49% in 2009.[4]

Globally, new vaccines have been introduced with significant results, including the first vaccine to help prevent liver cancer, hepatitis B vaccine, which is now routinely given to infants in many countries. Rapid progress in the development of new vaccines means protection being available against a wider range of serious infectious diseases. There is a pressing need to introduce more vaccines in EPI.

The last couple of decades have seen the advent of many new vaccines in the private Indian market. In fact, most vaccines available in the developed world are available in India. However, most of these vaccines are at present accessible only to those who can afford to pay for them. Paradoxically, these vaccines are most often required by those that cannot afford them. The Government has introduced some of the newer vaccines such as MMR and hepatitis B in some states and has planned to introduce pentavalent vaccine (DPT+Hepatitis B+Hib) in all states in a phased manner. Expanding coverage with these vaccines and introducing new vaccines which are cost effective in the Indian scenario are required. Introduction of monovalent and bivalent OPV into the polio eradication strategy have shown dramatic results with no polio cases being reported since 13 January 2011. Now concerted efforts are underway to eliminate measles, introduction of second dose of measles is a step in that direction.

Several areas in the national immunization program need a revamp. Vaccine production by indigenous manufacturers needs to be encouraged to bring down the costs, reduce dependence on imports and ensure availability of vaccines specifically needed by India (e.g. typhoid) and custom made to Indian requirements (Rotavirus and pneumococcal vaccines). The recent vaccination related deaths signal a need for improving immunization safety and accountability and strengthening of an adverse event following immunization (AEFI) monitoring system. Finally setting up a system for monitoring the incidence of vaccine preventable diseases and conducting an appropriate epidemiological studies is necessary to make evidence-based decisions on incorporation of vaccines in the national schedule and study impact of vaccines on disease incidence, serotype replacement, epidemiologic shift, etc.

Several of the abovementioned issues have been addressed by National Vaccine Policy[5] and mechanism such as National Technical Advisory Group on Immunization (NTAGI) is likely to facilitate evidence-based decisions on new vaccines. Global

Vaccine Action Plan (GAVP)[6] signed by 144 member countries of the WHO has also given a call to achieve the Decade of Vaccines vision by delivering universal access to immunization. The GVAP mission is to improve health by extending by 2020 and beyond the full benefits of immunization to all people, regardless of where they are born, who they are or where they live. It has also called for development and introduction of new and improved vaccines and technologies.

Immunization is considered among the most cost-effective of health investments. In the United States, cost-benefit analysis indicates that every dollar invested in a vaccine dose saves US$ 2 to US$ 27 in health expenses.[7] There has been improvement in last few years: Introduction of newer antigens in UIP (hepatitis B, 2nd dose of measles, Japanese encephalitis and pentavalent vaccine in many states), framing of National Vaccine Policy, support to indigenous vaccine industry, and acknowledging the need to intensify RI are steps in right direction.[8] We now need to step up our efforts to strengthen all components of UIP (vaccination schedule, delivery and monitoring, and VPD/AEFI surveillance), overcome all barriers (geographical, politico-social and technical) and invest heavily in Research & Development to achieve immunization's full potential and a healthier Nation.

References

1. WHO Vaccine-Preventable Diseases: Monitoring System 2013 Global Summary. Available at http://apps.who.int/ immunization_monitoring/ globalsummary/countries?countrycriteria%5Bcountry%5D%5B%5D=IND& commit=OK. (Accessed on 27 October 2013)

2. 2009 Coverage Evaluation Survey: All India Report. New Delhi: The United Nations Children's Fund; 2010. Available at http://www.unicef.org/india/ health_5578.htm. (Accessed on 27 October 2013)

3. International Institute of Population Sciences (IIPS). District Level Household and Facility Survey(DLHS-3) 2007–08: India. Mumbai: IIPS; 2010. Available at http://www.rchiips.org/pdf/ INDIA_REPORT_DLHS-3.pdf. (Accessed on 27 October 2013)

4. Goel S, Dogra V, Gupta SK, Lakshmi PV, Varkey S, Pradhan N, Krishna G, Kumar R. Effectiveness of Muskaan Ek Abhiyan (the smile campaign) for strengthening routine immunization in Bihar, India. Indian Pediatr 2012; 49: 103–108.

5. National Vaccine Policy. New Delhi: Ministry of Health and Family Welfare, Government of India; 2011. Available at http://mohfw.nic.in/

WriteReadData/l892s/1084811197NATIONAL%20VACCINE%20POLICY%20BOOK.pdf. (Accessed on 27 October 2013)

6. Global Action Plan 2011–2020. Geneva: World Health Organization; 2013. Available at http://www.who.int/immunization/ global_vaccine_action_plan/ GVAP_doc_2011_2020/en/index.html. (Accessed on 27 October 2013)

7. World Health Organization. Fact Sheet WHO/288, March 2005. Available at http://whqlibdoc.who.int/fact_sheet/ 2005/ FS_288.pdf. (Accessed on 27 October 2013)

8. Vashishtha VM, Kumar P. 50 years of immunization in India: Progress and future. Indian Pediatr 2013; 50: 111–118.

■ ■ ■ ■ ■ ■

PROCESS OF ISSUING IAP ACVIP'S RECOMMENDATIONS AND EVIDENCE-BASED RESEARCH

Reviewed by
A.K. Patwari

Indian Academy of Pediatrics (IAP) Advisory Committee on Vaccines & Immunization Practices (ACVIP), set up as a special subcommittee of the academy, has been entrusted with the responsibility to frame recommendations for IAP members as well as for the benefit of general public.

Aims and Objectives

The main objective of the sub-committee is to frame recommendations in two broad heads:

i. For the members of the academy about the usage of available licensed vaccines in the country— primary responsibility

ii. For the public or mass use of a particular vaccine, i.e. public health perspectives of a particular vaccine

The committee also devises an annual IAP Immunization Timetable on a yearly named basis.

The committee's recommendations are an attempt to formulate guidelines on the most optimum way of using available licensed vaccines in the country to provide best possible protection to an individual child in an office practice setting. They may not necessarily be construed as the Academy's approval of a particular product for wider, mass use in national/sub-national large scale immunization programs. Members may use their own discretion while using them in a given situation and there is no compulsion to use the recommended vaccines/ schedule in every single child.

The Current Process for Issuing Recommendations

The process involves review of recent published literature including standard textbooks, vaccine trials, recommendations of reputed international bodies like ACIP of CDC, World Health Organization (WHO) etc, post-marketing surveillance reports from industry, cost-effective analysis, etc. More reliance is given to studies emanating from India, especially on disease epidemiology, and vaccines' immunogenicity, efficacy, and safety studies. If knowledge gaps are present, then expert opinion is sought to fill the gaps. The existing national immunization schedule and government policies are also taken into account while drafting recommendations.[1]

The IAP ACVIP meets in person to discuss these matters. At this meeting, the members of the Committee and some invited experts discuss the issues related to vaccines in exhaustive detail. Decisions are taken about all the matters and recorded. Following the meeting, the recommendations are circulated among the members, and any inaccuracies are removed at this stage. The recommendations are then sent to the Executive Board of the Academy for their approval, following which they are published.

The IAP Guidebook on Immunization contains the Academy's official recommendations in some detail. The guidebook is published regularly at every two-year's interval. Interim recommendations, changes in earlier published recommend-ations, and related matters are published in the official journal, Indian Pediatrics.

The recommendations of IAP ACVIP are primarily for pediatricians in office practice. In addition, the committee also submits its position on incorporation of various new vaccines in the national immunization schedule.

New revised process for issuing recommendations

It is decided to develop a uniform approach to making explicit the evidence base for IAP ACVIP recommendations. The committee will adopt a new evidence-based methodology, e.g. GRADE (Grades of Recommendation Assessment, Development and Evaluation), for issuing not only the future recommendations but to apply to existing recommendations also, especially on newer vaccines. A subcommittee is also constituted that will devise a new model based entirely on evidence to grade the available evidences and on its basis decide the strength of recommendations in 2–3 different categories. The main focus will be on scientific evidence and transparency so that the system can be reproducible and can also be reviewed by other experts.

The committee has also decided to prepare position papers on important vaccines and vaccine preventable diseases highlighting the committee's stand on various issues on the format of WHO position papers. The ACVIP has already published position papers on measles, influenza, and pertussis vaccines[2-4] and also on AEFI.[5]

WHO and Vaccine Recommendations

Vaccines are one of the most successful public-health interventions of all time, and millions of lives have been saved and disability averted due to the advent of critical vaccines. However, availability of the products does not ensure their appropriate use. The World Health Organization (WHO) is tasked to provide leadership in global health, to shape research agendas, provide guidance and standards for public-health practice, and to provide support to country programs. Since 1998, WHO has published vaccine position papers with global recommendations for vaccine use.[6] Each position paper is specific to a vaccine-preventable disease and displays the WHO position on optimal vaccine use specifically for public use of that particular vaccine. The Strategic Group of Advisory Experts on immunization (SAGE) is an independent advisory committee with a mandate to advise the WHO on the development of policy related to vaccines and immunization. Since past few years, the WHO has also adopted the GRADE process of issuing its recommendations and special web tables, 'Grading of scientific evidence' are published along with a position paper on vaccine.[6]

Need for Evidence-based Information to Frame Recommendations for Immunization

A careful review and consideration of the scientific evidence is a necessary step in the development of recommendations and guidelines. The results of the full range of studies on a given topic need to be carefully considered to identify trends in magnitude, geographic variability, and other factors that are important for assessing impact and generalizability. In developing the most appropriate recommendations, committee weigh the desirable and undesirable consequences based on the best available evidence and take into account social values and preferences. While the evidence reviewed is the result of scientific endeavors, evaluating the quality of the evidence and making recommendations are activities that require expert interpretation and judgment in addition to rigorous scientific review.

In addition to the results of studies themselves, consideration needs to be given to the methodology and study design used to conduct such studies. It is generally accepted that randomized controlled trials (RCTs) are the gold standard to minimize various forms of bias when investigating associations between interventions and health outcomes, but there are many characteristics of RCTs or observational studies that determine their quality and relevance. In some cases, faulty randomization or blinding may reduce the quality of an RCT below that of a well-designed observational study. Hence, a review of the potential risks for bias and other aspects of study design quality is crucial when drawing conclusions from a study of any type. The quality of evidence reflects the extent to which confidence in the estimation of effect is adequate to support a particular decision or recommendation.

What is Evidence-based Research?

Evidence-based research (EBR) means that the information we are using or intend to use, as professionals, is based on sound research, not someone's opinion. The published article (in printed journals or in electronic form) is assessed to review actual research results so that one can understand the methodology used, carefully look at the data presented and interpreted by the researcher, assess how the conclusions were reached and decide how the presented data supports the conclusion. EBR is a process of turning clinical problems into questions and then systematically locating, appraising, and using contemporaneous research findings as the basis for making decisions and developing guidelines.

In order to locate the best published research work on the topic under enquiry, the hierarchy of levels of scientific evidence is followed in the descending order, i.e. large randomized trials with clear-cut results (and low risk of error), small randomized trials with uncertain results (and moderate to high risk of error), non-randomized trials with concurrent or contemporaneous controls, nonrandomized trials with historical controls, and case series with no controls (Figure 1).

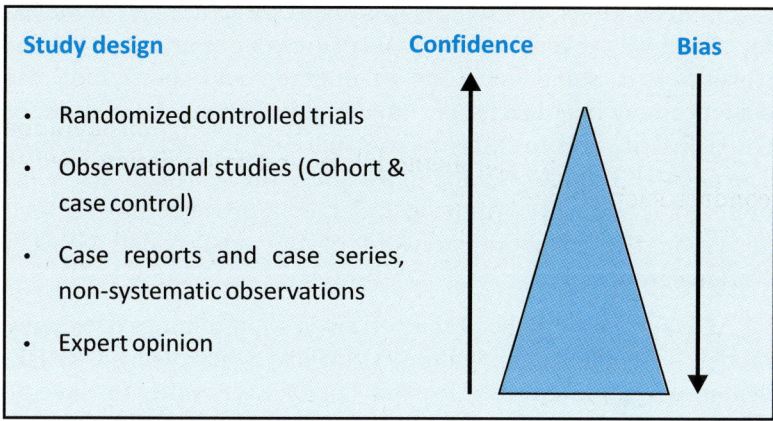

Study design

- Randomized controlled trials

- Observational studies (Cohort & case control)

- Case reports and case series, non-systematic observations

- Expert opinion

Confidence

Bias

Figure 1: Hierarchy of evidence

Process of using EBR in Formulating Recommendations for Immunization

Guidelines for evidence-based review on vaccine-related recommendations are available from Advisory Committee on Immunization Practice (ACIP), SAGE, European Center for Disease Control (ECDC) and WHO. These guidelines for immunizations serve as the basic evidence-based resource material which are adapted by the countries as per the local epidemiological situation and programmatic needs. The Centers for Disease Control and Prevention (CDC) Advisory Committee on Immunization Practices (ACIP) recommends adoption of the Grading of Recommendations, Assessment, Development and Evaluation (GRADE) approach for developing evidence-based recommendations.[7]

The GRADE Approach[8]

Quality of the evidence for assessing strength of recommendations are based on a grading system which provides an important component in evidence-based medicine. Grades of Recommendation, Assessment, Development and Evaluation (GRADE) working group scoring is one of many frameworks developed over the years to assess the quality of evidence, and it has been adopted by WHO and over 50 other organizations. The GRADE framework is a systematic and explicit approach to making judgments about quality of evidence and strength of recommendations. It attempts to provide structure and guidance for objectively reviewing the quality of evidence and risk of bias. Nevertheless, some decisions to upgrade and downgrade the evidence may be a matter of individual judgment. A hallmark of GRADE is its aim to improve transparency in decision-making. The GRADE framework, and particularly the scoring process has undergone, and will continue to undergo, improvements over time based on the collaborative work of the open-ended GRADE working group.

GRADE addresses many of the perceived shortcomings of existing models of evidence evaluation. Crucially, when using GRADE, evidence is not rated study by study, but across studies for specific clinical outcomes. The GRADE approach specifically assesses following:

- Methodological flaws within the component studies
- Consistency of results across different studies
- Generalizability of research results to the wider patient base
- How effective the treatments/ interventions have been shown to be

In the GRADE process questions of importance related to a recommendation are identified, a systematic literature review is conducted to identify the evidence available to answer the question(s), and the quality of relevant evidence is reviewed and rated. **Five criteria** (limitations in study design commensurate with the type of study, inconsistency, indirectness, imprecision and publication bias) are used to downgrade the quality of evidence when studies do not meet the published standards, and **three criteria** (magnitude of the effect, dose-response gradient, and ability of the study to limit biases and control for confounding) are used to upgrade the quality of evidence when study results increase confidence in their validity. Based on this rating, as well as other factors (balance between benefits and risks, social values and preferences, and cost and resources), recommendations are made and rated as strong or weak. A strong recommendation can still be made with low or very low quality evidence. It is the net result of how all the other factors come into play that is important.

GRADE tables are only applied to issues regarding the effectiveness and safety of vaccines and are generally created for overall vaccine efficacy/effectiveness and safety such as the duration of protection, schedule considerations, and use in subpopulations, such as specific age or risk groups or HIV-infected populations.

Active participation of the Working Groups (WGs) is essential to ensure that the most appropriate studies are utilized and that the results are carefully considered. In addition to formulating the questions for GRADE, the WGs review the evidence and the resulting GRADE tables considering following important aspects:

- Categorization of studies
- GRADE quality assessment criteria
- Quality of evidence rating
- Application of GRADE to recommendations
- Presentation of GRADE tables

GRADE Score[9]

Grade scoring is based on : (i) type of evidence (e.g. systematic reviews, RCTs, observational studies), (ii) quality points (e.g. sparse data, follow-up, withdrawals, blinding, allocation concealment, incomplete reporting of results, etc.), (iii) consistency (e.g. in heterogenous studies a point is deducted for inconsistent results among studies, or a point added for evidence of a dose response), (iv) directness (points deducted for issues that may limit the generalizability of the reported results to the specified population of interest) and (v) effect size (add points for relative risk or odds ratio).

An overall GRADE score (from 4 to 0) is assigned based on the assessment of the overall quality of evidence for that outcome. The final GRADE score consists of 4 categories of evidence quality based on the GRADE scores for each comparison: High (at least 4 points), moderate (3 points), low (2 points), and very low (one or less).

SAGE process for reviewing the evidence

Over the past few years, SAGE expressed concern about the use of the GRADE scoring scheme and more specifically how it was applied to vaccines, as important data of particular relevance to population-based immunization programs were sometimes excluded. At times, the GRADE scoring ranked the quality of evidence as low or moderate, which may not have adequately reflected the quality of the overall evidence base. This was particularly true for traditional vaccines for which, despite many years of successful field use and impact demonstrated through many observational studies, or population impact demonstrated by rigorous surveillance, the evidence quality level could not be upgraded appropriately. These rankings present a potential problem for communicating the basis for a recommendation to use a vaccine. As a result, SAGE is working towards refining the methodology to ensure its relevance to immunization public-health policy. Complex issues are routinely examined in careful detail by SAGE working groups, though in some instances, it builds on specific reviews of the data or data collection tools done by other technical advisory group (e.g. The Global Advisory Committee on Vaccine Safety for vaccine risk assessment and the Quantitative Immunization and Vaccine Research Advisory Committee for disease burden and cost-effectiveness data).

Discussions with other national technical advisory groups and the GRADE working group have resulted in some improvements to the scoring scheme itself. Working groups review the evidence pertaining to a given topic and present proposals for recommendations to SAGE, which in turn then discusses, deliberates and ultimately provides its recommendations to WHO. Thus, the initial review of the evidence occurs in working groups. In addition to recommendations for vaccine usage, SAGE also makes strategic recommendations regarding public-health programs and research priorities which do not undergo formal GRADE scoring. However, SAGE recommendations and vaccine position papers are evidence based and follow the GRADE approach.

Rating of the quality of evidence

SAGE has optimized the GRADE methodology[10] and fine-tuned it to strengthen its relevance and facilitate its use for immunization.

IAP Guidebook on Immunization 2013–14

Many of the adjustments to the more traditional presentation of the GRADE tables are an attempt to clarify its application to vaccines/vaccination recommendations without changing the intent. The adjustments ensure that the many types of data available for immunizations are adequately taken into consideration in the decision-making process.

The key activities involved in creating evidence-based recommendations are as follows:

1. Definition of the questions to inform recommendations.

2. Identification of the critical questions for which an in-depth review of evidence is needed.

3. Conducting systematic review of the literature with or without meta-analysis.

4. Review the quality of the evidence, in particular through assessment of the risk of bias and confounding.

5. Scoring of the quality of the evidence (using the GRADE approach for data on safety and effectiveness).

6. Discussion, deliberation and formulation of recommendation by IAP -ACVIP.

7. Submission of recommendation of IAP-ACVIP to IAP Executive Board.

8. EBR committee can identify the process of EBR (WHO model as decided by the committee), decide on prioritization of VPD/Vaccine and could broadly prepare definition of questions.

The guiding principles of the review process are that careful review and consideration of the evidence should precede development of recommendations, and that the entire process should be transparent, robust and reproducible.

Throughout the evidence review process (steps 1–8), expert opinion is critical in the assessment of these factors and their importance to the question under consideration. The application of the GRADE criteria, and the inferences that may be drawn from the studies relating to the question under consideration are inherently subjective, and rely on the judgment of skilled and experienced public-health professionals.

Vaccine recommendation development — beyond rating the evidence

Much work goes into information-gathering and synthesis that forms the basis of vaccine recommendations and guidance. Even recommendations that do not utilize a formal GRADE evaluation are the product of data review, evaluation of data quality, discussion and deliberation. In addition to the scientific evidence base, other factors are important to the final recommendation including:[11] (i) disease epidemiology and clinical profile, (ii) vaccine and immunization characteristics (efficacy, effectiveness and population impact, safety, cold chain and logistics, availability, schedules, schedule's social and programmatic acceptability, ability to reach the target populations, ability to monitor programme impact), (iii) economic considerations, (iv) health-system opportunities, and (v) interaction with other existing intervention and control strategies.

In addition, updating recommendations from time to time is essential as the evidence and/or other factors do change, and recommendations need to reflect the best data available.

All important public health decisions that may lead to the savings of many lives are in fact a matter of urgency in themselves, but there are situations that require more rapid decisions. When outbreaks, natural disasters or humanitarian emergencies occur, lack of time and context-specific data may necessitate a modified process for development of recommendations. Quick decisions may be needed that rely on indirect data interpreted using expert judgment. In such situations, recommendations may be issued quickly and revised as the context changes and/or additional data are available.

References

1. Indian Academy of Pediatrics Committee on Immunization (IAPCOI). Consensus recommendations on immunization and IAP immunization timetable 2012. Indian Pediatr 2012 Jul; 49(7): 549–564.

2. Vashishtha VM, Choudhury P, Bansal CP, Gupta SG. Measles control strategies in India: Position paper of Indian Academy of Pediatrics. Indian Pediatr 2013 Jun 8; 50(6): 561–564.

3. Vashishtha VM, Kalra A, Choudhury P. Influenza vaccination in India position paper of Indian Academy of Pediatrics, 2013. Indian Pediatr 2013 Sep 8; 50(9): 867–874.

4. Chitkara AJ, Thacker N, Vashishtha VM, Bansal CP, Gupta SG. Adverse Event Following Immunization (AEFI) surveillance in India, position paper of Indian Academy of Pediatrics,2013. Indian Pediatr 2013 Aug; 50(8): 739–741.

5. Vashishtha VM, Bansal CP, Gupta SG. Pertussis Vaccines: Position Paper of Indian Academy of Pediatrics (IAP). Indian Pediatr 2013; 50: 1001–1009.

6. http://www.who.int/immunization/position_papers/en/

7. Ahmad F. U.S. Advisory Committee on Immunization Practices (ACIP) Handbook for Developing Evidence-based Recommendations. Version 1.1, National Center for Immunization and Respiratory Diseases Centers for Disease Control and Prevention (CDC) Atlanta, GA, USA. March 1, 2012. 1–46.

8. Guyatt GH et al. for the GRADE Working Group. Rating quality of evidence and strength of recommendations GRADE: An emerging consensus on rating quality of evidence and strength of recommendations. British Medical Journal, 2008, 336: 924–926.

9. http://clinicalevidence.bmj.com/x/set/static/ebm/ learn/665072.html

10. Balshema H et al. GRADE Guidelines: Rating the quality of evidence. Journal of Clinical Epidemiology, 2011, 64: 401–406.

11. A World Health Organization. Guidance for the development of evidence-based vaccine related recommendations. WHO, version 2, 8 March 2012, pp 1–32.

■ ■ ■ ■ ■ ■

CONFLICT OF INTEREST ISSUES AND ACVIP RECOMMENDATIONS

A.K. Patwari

A stringent requirement for preventing and mitigating a conflict of interest (COI) in discharging duties and fulfilling assigned responsibilities by individuals, groups and organizations is increasingly gaining ground with ever-increasing demand for transparency and model code of conduct. There is always a possibility when an individual or an organization is involved in multiple interests, one of which could possibly corrupt the motivation for an act in another. The presence of a conflict of interest is independent from the execution of impropriety. Therefore, a COI can be discovered and voluntarily defused before any corruption occurs. A common understanding of COI is "A set of circumstances that creates a risk that professional judgment or actions regarding a primary interest will be unduly influenced by a secondary interest." Primary interest refers to the principal goals of the profession or activity, such as the protection of clients, the health of patients, the integrity of research, and the duties of public office. Secondary interest includes not only financial gain but also such motives as the desire for professional advancement and the wish to do favors for family and friends. But COI rules usually focus on financial relationships because they are relatively more objective, tradable, and quantifiable. The secondary interests are not treated as wrong in themselves, but become objectionable when they are believed to have greater weight than the primary interests. The conflict in a COI exists whether or not a particular individual or a group is actually influenced by the secondary interest. It exists if the circumstances are reasonably believed (on the basis of past experience and objective evidence) to create a risk that decisions may be unduly influenced by secondary interests.

Definition of Conflict of Interest

The legal definition of COI is "A term used to describe the situation in which a public official or fiduciary who, contrary to the

IAP Guidebook on Immunization 2013–14 | 23

obligation and absolute duty to act for the benefit of the public or a designated individual, exploits the relationship for personal benefit, typically pecuniary".[1] The other, expressions used is "A situation where a professional, or a corporation, has a vested interest which may make them an unreliable source. The interest could be money, status, knowledge or reputation, for example. When such a situation arises, the party is usually asked to remove themselves, and it is often legally required of them."[2] COI can also be ascribed to "A situation that has the potential to undermine the impartiality of a person because of the possibility of a clash between the person's self-interest and professional interest or public interest".[3]

A COI in research exists when the individual has interests in the outcome of the research that may lead to a personal advantage and that might therefore, in actuality or appearance compromise the integrity of the research.[4] The term COI in research "refers to situations in which financial or other personal considerations may compromise, or have the appearance of compromising, an investigator's professional judgment in conducting or reporting research. A conflict of interest depends on the situation, and not on the actions or character of an individual investigator."[5]

Types of conflicts of interests[6]

- **Self-dealing:** An official who controls an organization causes it to enter into a transaction with another official, or with another organization that benefits the official. The official is on both sides of the "deal".

- **Outside employment:** The interests of one job contradict another.

- **Family interests:** A spouse, child, or other close relative is employed (or applies for employment) or where goods or services are purchased from such a relative or a firm controlled by a relative. For this reason, many employment applications ask if one is related to a current employee. If this is the case, the relative could then recluse from any hiring decisions. Abuse of this type of conflict of interest is called *Nepotism*.

- **Gifts:** Gifts from friends who also do business with the person receiving the gifts (including non-tangible things of value such as transportation and lodging).

- **Pump and dump:** A stockbroker who owns a security artificially inflates the price by "upgrading" it or spreading rumors, sells the security and adds short position (selling securities or other financial instruments that are not currently owned, with the intention of subsequently repurchasing them at a lower price), then "downgrades" the security or spreads negative rumors to push the price down.

Other improper acts that are sometimes classified as COI are: Accepting bribes is corruption, and use of Government or corporate property or assets for personal use is fraud. However, unlike COI, there is no inherent conflict of roles for these improper acts. COI is sometimes termed "competition of interest" rather than "conflict", emphasizing a connotation of natural competition between valid interests rather than violent conflict with its connotation of victimhood and unfair aggression. Nevertheless, denotatively, there is too much overlap between the terms to make any objective differentiation.

Pharmaceutical Industry and COI

Over the years the influence of the pharmaceutical industry on medical research has been a major cause for concern. In 2009 a study found that "a number of academic institutions" do not have clear guidelines for relationships between Institutional Review Boards and industry.[7] Due to repeated accusations and findings that some clinical trials conducted or funded by pharmaceutical companies may report only positive results for the preferred medication/vaccine, the industry has been looked at much more closely by independent groups and government agencies. Drug researchers not directly employed by pharmaceutical companies often look to companies for grants, and companies often look to researchers for studies that will make their products look favorable. Sponsored researchers are rewarded by drug companies, for example, with support for their conference/symposium costs, etc. Lecture scripts and even journal articles presented by academic researchers may actually be "ghost-written" by pharmaceutical companies.[8]

Conflicts of interest in vaccine safety research

Vaccines are a multi-billion dollar industry internationally and for many pharmaceutical companies, it is the fastest-growing segment of their business. COIs cloud vaccine safety research because sponsors of research have competing interests that may impede the objective study of vaccine side effects. Vaccine manufacturers, health officials, and medical journals may have financial and bureaucratic reasons for not wanting to acknowledge the risks of vaccines. Conversely, some advocacy groups may have legislative and financial reasons to sponsor research that finds risks in vaccines. Minimizing COIs in vaccine safety research could reduce research bias and restore greater trust in the vaccine program.[9] Medical journal authors' ties to vaccine manufacturers are pervasive, as revealed in a review of authors of vaccine safety articles published in top journals. Even on the peer-reviewed side of things, it has been said that the journals are the marketing arm of the pharmaceutical industry. [10]

Ways to prevent /mitigate conflicts of interests

Generally, COIs should be eliminated. Often, however, the specifics can be controversial. Codes of ethics help to minimize problems with COIs because they can spell out the extent to which such conflicts should be avoided, and what the parties should do where such conflicts are permitted by a code of ethics. Thus, professionals cannot claim that they were unaware that their improper behavior was unethical. As importantly, the threat of disciplinary action helps to minimize unacceptable conflicts or improper acts when a conflict is unavoidable. Various ways to prevent or mitigate COI are:

Disclosure: Commonly members of the technical committee are required to disclose their COI pertaining to receiving any remuneration/ honorarium/ travel grant/ research support from a commercial entity with an interest related to the subject of the meeting or work for at least preceding 4 years. In some instances, the failure to provide full disclosure is considered a crime.

Recusal: Those with a COI are expected to recuse themselves from (i.e., abstain from) decisions where such a conflict exists. The imperative for recusal varies depending upon the circumstance and profession, either as common sense ethics, codified ethics, or by statute. Recusal may be limited to abstaining only from 'voting' or from a particular meeting/ committee itself.

Removal: The best way to handle COIs is to avoid them entirely. For example, someone nominated/ elected to a technical committee may break all relations with the pharmaceutical industry and resign from all such positions which have a potential of COI just before taking over the membership of the committee. Such a member may preferably not be allowed to continue as a member.

How IAP ACVIP is addressing the issue of COI ?

IAP Advisory Committee on Vaccines & Immunization Practices (ACVIP) has been entrusted with the responsibility to serve as a source of evidence-based information pertaining to vaccination in children, to inform and update the members of IAP as well as educate and benefit public at large. This unique responsibility demands that ACVIP members have integrity of the highest order, particularly those members who are empowered with the right of voting for important decisions made by ACVIP, which have far reaching consequences and impact on child health. In order to ensure professional integrity and public confidence in the activities and recommendations made by ACVIP, each member is expected to voluntarily declare any potential conflict of interest (i.e. any interest that may effect, or may reasonably be perceived to effect, the member's objectivity, independence and judgment) while discharging his/her professional duties as a member. The potential conflict of interest also includes relevant interest of the immediate family members of ACVIP member.

Each member/office bearer/advisor of ACVIP is needed to sign a strict "Code of Conduct". He/she is asked to abide by all the conditions enlisted in the code. Utmost precaution is taken to avoid any violation in letter and spirit. Any violation/complaint is reviewed by the ACVIP secretariat/IAP Executive Board to take necessary remedial action. All the potentially significant interests are disclosed to the ACVIP Secretariat at least one month before the meeting and updated for any recent change /endorsed before the start of the meeting. Self-declaration forms of each member, submitted at least one month before the meeting, are scrutinized by a sub-committee constituted by ACVIP. The declaration forms are scrutinized based on the information provided by the members.

If any member discloses a conflict of interest or is unable or unwilling to disclose the details of an interest that may pose a real or perceived conflict in member's objectivity, independence or judgment, the ACVIP Secretariat may decide to ask him/her to totally recluse from the meeting. In the event of discovering later on that the declaration was incorrect or some facts have been suppressed, ACVIP Secretariat will refer the matter to IAP Executive Board for appropriate action that have the option of banning the member from the committee for three years.

References

1. Conflict of interest. The Free Dictionary by Farlex: http://legal dictionary. thefreedictionary.com /conflict+of+interest

2. Definition of Conflict Of Interest. Investopedia: http://www.investopedia. com/terms/c/conflict-of-interest.asp

3. Conflict of interest. Business Dictionary: http://www.businessdictionary .com/definition/conflict-of-interest.html

4. Teaching the responsible conduct research in humans (RCRH). Chapter 4 (Conflict of Interest): http://ori.hhs.gov/education/products/ucla/ chapter4/default.htm

5. UCLA. Guidance and Procedure: Investigator Financial Conflict of Interest. Office of the Human Protection Program: http://ora.research.ucla.edu/ OHRPP/Documents/Policy/10/Investigator_COI.pdf

6. Conflict of Interest: http://en.wikipedia.org/wiki /Conflict_of_interest

7. Policies regarding IRB members' industry relationships often lacking. Massachusetts General Hospital: http://www.eurekalert.org / pub_releases/2009–03/mgh-pri032309.php

8. Barnet A. Revealed: How drug firms 'hoodwink' medical journals: http://www.theguardian.com /society/2003/dec/07/health. businessofresearch

9. DeLong G. Conflicts of Interest in Vaccine Safety Research, Accountability in Research. 2012, 19: 65–88.

10. House of Commons Science and Technology Committee. Peer review in scientific publications: Eighth report of session 2010–12, The Parliamentary Bookshop, London, 2011, pp 1–25.

SECTION
II

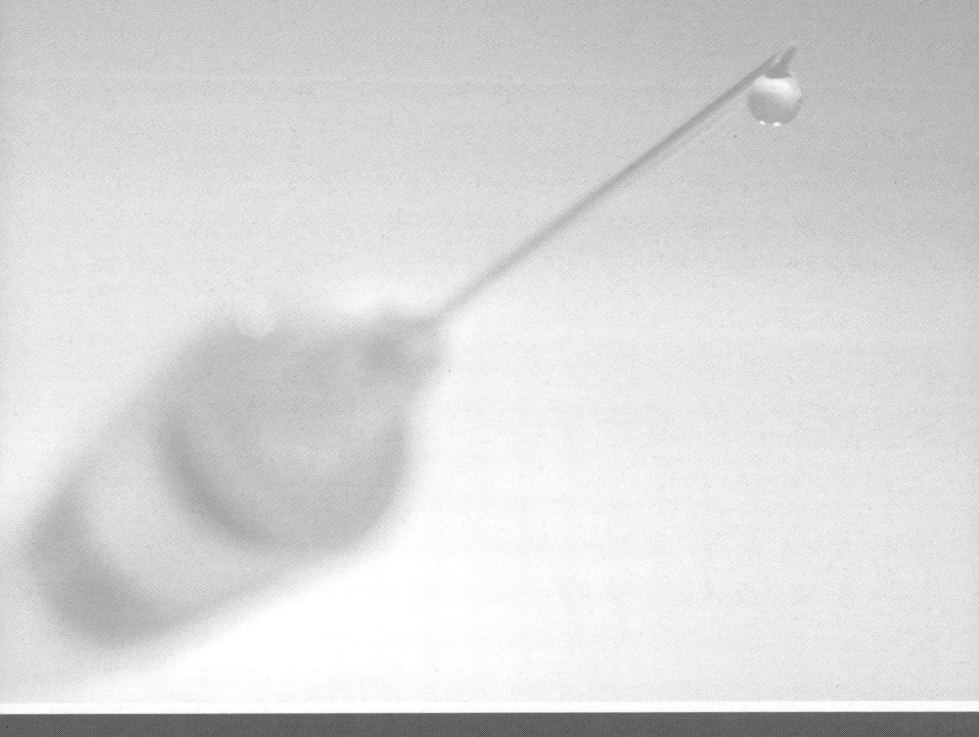

General Aspects
of Vaccination

BASIC IMMUNOLOGY

2.1

Reviewed by
A. J. Chitkara, Panna Choudhury

Immunology of Vaccination

Innate and adaptive immune responses:

Immunity may be broadly classified as innate and adaptive immunity. Innate immunity comprises the skin and mucosal barriers, phagocytes (neutrophils, monocytes and macrophages) and the natural killer (NK) cells. It comes into play immediately on entry of the pathogen and is non-specific. Adaptive immunity is provided by the B lymphocytes (humoral/antibody-mediated immunity) and T lymphocytes (cellular/cell-mediated immunity). The innate immune system triggers the development of adaptive immunity by presenting antigens to the B lymphocytes and T lymphocytes. Vaccines that stimulate innate immunity effectively are better immunogens. This can be achieved by live vaccines, adjuvants, TLR agonists, live vectors and DNA vaccines. Adaptive immunity takes time to evolve and is pathogen-specific (Table 1 and Figure 1).[1]

Table 1: Differentiating features between innate and adaptive immunity

Innate Immunity	Adaptive Immunity
Its response is antigen-independent.	Its response is antigen-dependent.
There is immediate response.	There is a lag time between exposure and maximal response.
It is not antigen-specific.	It is antigen-specific.
Exposure does not result in induction of memory cells.	Exposure result in induction of memory cells.
Some of its cellular components or their products may aid specific immunity	Some of its products may aid specific immunity

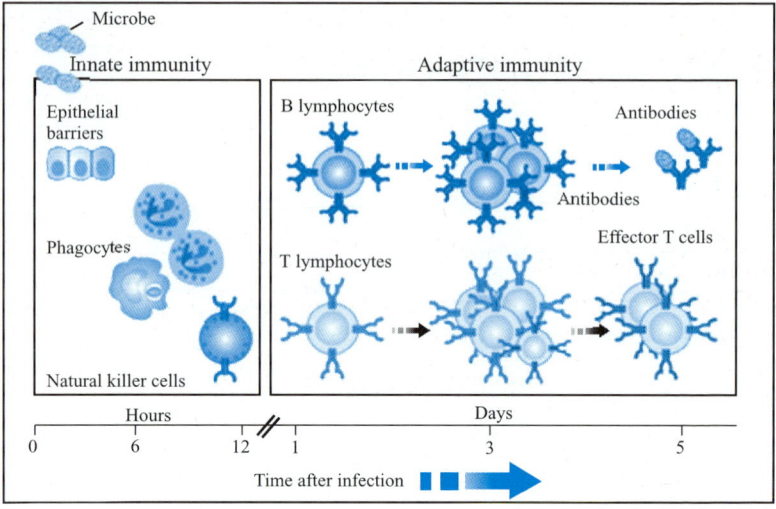

Figure 1: Innate and adaptive immunity (Adapted from Ref. 1)

Humoral Vs Cell-mediated Immunity

Humoral immunity is the principal defence mechanism against extracellular microbes and their toxins.[2] B lymphocytes secrete antibodies that act by neutralization, complement activation or by promoting opsonophagocytosis which results in early reduction of pathogen load and clearance of extracellular pathogens. Also humoral antibodies prevent colonization, being the first step in pathogenesis by encapsulated organisms like Hib, pneumococcal, meningococcal and organisms like diphtheria and pertussis. Antibodies are of several different types (IgG, IgM, IgA, IgD and IgE) and they differ in their structure, half life, and site of action and mechanism of action.

Cell-mediated immunity (CMI) is the principal defense mechanism against intracellular microbes. The effectors of CMI, the T cells, are of two types. The helper T cells secrete proteins called cytokines that stimulate the proliferation and differentiation of T cells as well as other cells including B lymphocytes, macrophages and NK cells. The cytotoxic T cells act by lysing infected cells. Cellular immunity is essential for clearance of intracellular pathogens. BCG is the only currently used human vaccine for which there is conclusive evidence that T cells are the main effectors. The T cell responses are more robust, long lasting and more cross protective than humoral responses, hence modern vaccinology is being directed in this direction. The inherent T cell mediated immune regulatory mechanisms prevent any vaccines causing autoimmune diseases.[3]

Active Vs Passive Immunity

Active immunity is acquired through natural infection/ immunization and is long lasting. Passive immunity is conferred by maternal antibodies or immunoglobulin preparations and is short lasting.

Type of Vaccines

Vaccines may be broadly classified as live attenuated vaccines and killed/inactivated vaccines. Commonly used live attenuated vaccines include BCG, oral polio, measles, MMR and chickenpox vaccines. Killed vaccines may be inactivated toxins/ toxoids (diphtheria/ tetanus toxoids), killed organisms (whole cell pertussis vaccines) or most commonly subunit vaccines (Hib, hepatitis B, hepatitis A, typhoid, meningococcal, influenza). Subunit vaccines comprising only of the polysaccharide antigens are called unconjugated vaccines. Conjugation of the polysaccharide with a protein carrier (Glycoconjugates) significantly improves the immune response as discussed later.

How do vaccines work?

Early protective efficacy of currently available vaccines is primarily conferred by the induction of antigen-specific antibodies that are capable of binding specifically to a toxin or a pathogen.

The role of cell-mediated immunity in currently used vaccines (that have T cell dependent antigens) is mainly by supporting antibody production. Other important mechanisms by which cell-mediated immunity works is by cytotoxic CD8+ T lymphocytes (CTL) that may limit the spread of infectious agents by recognizing and killing infected cells or secreting specific antiviral cytokines. T cell independent antigens (e.g. polysaccharides) do not stimulate cell-mediated immunity and therefore do not produce long lasting immunity. T cell independent antigens can be converted to T cell dependent antigens by conjugating them with proteins.

First step after immunization

Following injection, the vaccine antigens attract local and systemic dendritic cells, monocytes and neutrophils. Innate immune responses activate these cells by changing their surface receptors and migrate along lymphatic vessels, to the draining lymph nodes where the activation of T and B lymphocytes takes place.

In case of killed vaccines, there is only local and unilateral lymph node activation. Conversely for live vaccines, there is multifocal lymph node activation due to microbial replication and dissemination. Consequently the immunogenicity of killed vaccines is lower than the live vaccines; killed vaccines require adjuvants which improve the immune response by producing local inflammation and recruiting higher number of dendritic cells/ monocytes to the injection site. Secondly, the site of administration of killed vaccines is of importance; the intramuscular route which is well vascularised and has a large number of patrolling dendritic cells is preferred over the subcutaneous route. Intradermal route recruits the abundant dendritic cells in the skin and offers the advantage of antigen sparing and early and effective protection but the GMT's are lower than that achieved with IM and may wane faster. The site of administration is usually of little significance for live vaccines. Finally due to focal lymph node activation, multiple killed vaccines may be administered at different sites with a little immunologic interference. Immunologic interference may occur with multiple live vaccines unless they are given on the same day or at least 4 weeks apart or by different routes.

Immune responses to vaccines

I. Immune response to polysaccharide antigens

Bacterial (*S. pneumoniae, N. meningitidis, H. influenzae, S. typhi*) polysaccharide (PS) antigens are T cell independent antigens. On being released from the injection site, they reach the marginal zone of the spleen / nodes and bind to the specific Ig surface receptors of B cells. In the absence of antigen-specific T cell help, B cells activate, proliferate and differentiate in plasma cells without undergoing affinity maturation in germinal centers. The antibody response sets in 2–4 weeks following immunization, is predominantly IgM with low titers of low affinity IgG. The half life of the plasma cells is short and antibody titers decline rapidly.

Additionally the PS antigens are unable to evoke an immune response in those aged less than 2 years due to immaturity of the marginal zones. As PS antigens do not induce germinal centers, bonafide memory B cells are not elicited. Consequently, subsequent re-exposure to the same PS results in a repeat primary response that follows the same kinetics in previously vaccinated as in naïve individuals.

Revaccination with certain bacterial PS, of which Group C meningococcus is a prototype, may even induce lower antibody responses than the first immunization, a phenomenon referred to as hyporesponsiveness. Due to this phenomenon, only a single booster of either pneumococcal or meningococcal polysaccharide vaccine is recommended even in patients who require lifelong protection.[4, 5]

II. Immune response to protein antigens or T cell dependent antigens

Protein antigens which include pure proteins (hepatitis B, hepatitis A, HPV, toxoids) or conjugation of PS antigens with a protein carrier (Hib, Meningo, Pneumo) are T cell dependent antigens. The initial response to these antigens is similar to PS antigens. However, the antigen-specific helper T cells that have been activated by antigen bearing dendritic cells trigger some antigen-specific B cells to migrate towards follicular dendritic cells (FDC's), initiating the Germinal Center (GC) reaction. In GC's, B cells receive additional signals from follicular dendritic cells (FDC) and follicular T helper cells and undergo massive clonal proliferation, switch from IgM towards IgG/ IgA, undergo affinity maturation and differentiate into plasma cells secreting large amounts of antigen-specific antibodies. Most of the plasma cells die at the end of germinal center reaction and thus decline in antibody levels is noted 4–8 weeks after vaccination. However, a few plasma cells exit nodes/spleen and migrate to survival niches mostly located in the bone marrow, where they survive through signals provided by supporting stromal cells and this results in prolonged persistence of antibodies in the serum. Memory B cells are generated in response to T-dependent antigens, during the GC reaction, in parallel to plasma cells. They persist there as resting cells until reexposed to their specific antigens when they readily proliferate and differentiate into plasma cells, secreting large amounts of high-affinity antibodies that may be detected in the serum within a few days after boosting.[3, 6]

III. Immune response to live vaccines

The live vaccines induce an immune response similar to that seen with protein vaccines. However, the take of live vaccines is not 100% with the first dose (primary failure). Hence, more than 1 dose is recommended with most live vaccines. Once the vaccine has been taken up, immunity is robust and lifelong or at least for several decades. This is because of continuous replication of the organism that is a constant source of the antigen. The second dose of the vaccine is therefore mostly for primary vaccine failures (no uptake of vaccine) and not for secondary vaccine failures (decline in antibodies over time). However, varicella and mumps do not follow this general principles and have waning antibody levels demonstrated therefore need second dose.[2, 7]

Primary Versus Secondary Immune Responses

In primary immune response, the antigen exposure elicits an extrafollicular response that results in the rapid appearance of low IgG antibody titers. As B cells proliferate in GCs and differentiate into plasma cells, IgG antibody titers increase up to a peak value usually reached 4 weeks after immunization. The short life span of these plasma cells results in a rapid decline of antibody titers, which eventually return to baseline levels.[3]

In secondary immune responses, booster exposure to antigen reactivates immune memory (memory B cells) and results in a rapid (< 7 days) increase of IgG antibody titer by a rapid proliferation of memory B cells and their evolution into abundant antibody secreting plasma cells. Short-lived plasma cells maintain peak Ab levels during a few weeks—after which serum antibody titers decline initially with the same rapid kinetics as following primary immunization. Long-lived plasma cells that have reached survival niches in the bone marrow continue to produce antigen-specific antibodies, which then decline with slower kinetics. This generic pattern may not apply to live vaccines triggering long-term IgG antibodies for extended periods of time.[3]

Determinants of Intensity and Duration of Immune Responses

I. Primary response

Primary immune responses after vaccination depend on various factors such as vaccine type, nature of antigen, vaccination schedule, genetic and environmental factors and age at immunization.

a. Vaccine type

Live vs inactivated: Higher intensity of innate responses, higher antigen content following replication and more prolonged antigen persistence generally result into higher antibodies (Ab) responses to live than inactivated vaccines.

Protein vs polysaccharide: Recruitment of T cell help and induction of germinal centers (GCs) results into higher antibody responses to protein or glycoconjugate than to polysaccharide vaccines. Hence, broadly speaking live vaccines are superior (exception BCG, OPV) to protein antigens which in turn are superior to polysaccharide vaccines.

Adjuvants: Adjuvants improve immune responses to inactivated vaccines by either modulation of antigen delivery and persistence (depot or slow-release formulations) or enhancement of Th responses (immunomodulator) which may support or limit antibody responses.[3]

b. Antigen nature

Polysaccharide antigens: Failure to induce GCs limit immunogenicity.

Protein antigens: Inclusion of epitopes readily recognized by B cells (B cell repertoire), inclusion of epitopes readily recognized by follicular helper T cells, elicitation of efficient follicular T cell help and the capacity of antigen to associate/persist in association to follicular dendritic cells (FDCs) result into higher antibody responses.

Antigen dose: As a rule, higher antigen doses increase the availability of antigen for B/T cell binding and activation, as well as for association with FDCs, however, there is a limiting dose for each.

c. Vaccination schedule

Interval between doses: The immune response improves with proper spacing of vaccine doses.

Traditionally, '0-1-6' month schedule (prime & boost) is considered as a more immunogenic schedule than 6-10-14 week or 2-3-5 month or 2-4-6 month schedules for non-live T-cell dependent vaccines like hepatitis-B vaccine. This is mainly due to adequate time interval between first few doses which act by inducing immune responses and last dose that works as boosters. Since, affinity maturation of B-cells in GCs and formation of memory-B cells take at least 4–6 months, this schedule quite well fulfills these requirements.

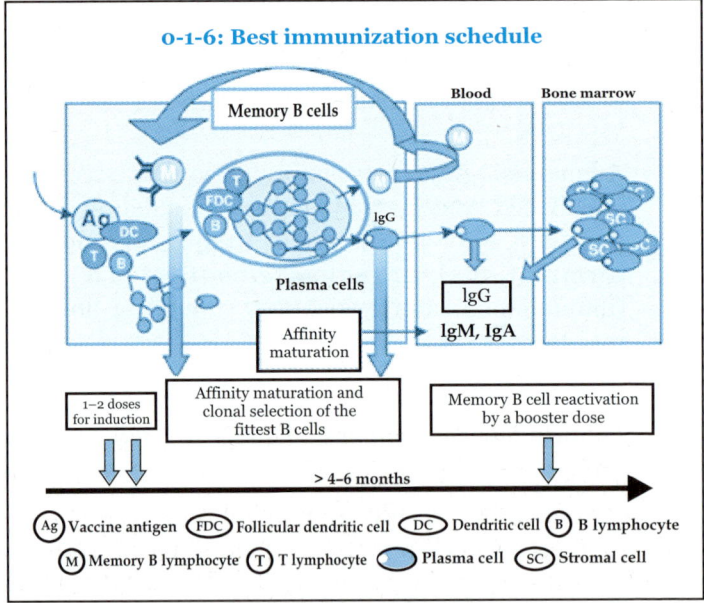

Figure 2: Schematic presentation of various components of 0-1-6 month immunization schedule at cellular level. Ag–Vaccine antigen, B–B lymphocyte, T–T lymphocyte, DC–Dendritic cell, M–Memory B lymphocyte, FDC–Follicular dendritic cell, SC=Stromal cells (in bone marrow) (Adapted from Ref. 1)

More than one dose is needed for better induction and recruitment of more number of GCs in young age considering young age limitations of immune system. A four week minimal interval between primary doses avoids competition between successive waves of primary responses.[2,3]

d. Other factors

Genetic factors: The capacity of antigen epitopes to associate to a large panel of MHC molecules increases the likelihood of responses in the population. MHC restriction may limit T cell responses. Gene polymorphisms in molecules critical for B and T cell activation/differentiation are likely to affect Ab responses. T cell responses differ markedly between individuals and populations because of genetic variability of MHC molecules (HLA A2).

Environmental factors: Mostly yet to be identified.

Age at immunization: Early life immune immaturity or age-associated immune senescence impairs immune responses to an administered vaccine.[3]

II. Secondary immune responses

Many factors that determine primary immune responses after immunization also affects secondary immune responses.

Live vs inactivated: Live vaccines generally induce more sustained antibody responses, presumably through prolonged antigen persistence within the host. Secondary responses with inactivated vaccines are highly pronounced (anamanestic response). However, secondary responses are usually blunted with live viral vaccines as pre-existing antibody neutralizes the vaccine virus.

Polysaccharide antigens: Failure to generate GCs limits the induction of memory responses and of high-affinity long-lived plasma cells.

Interval between primary doses: A minimal interval of 4 weeks between primary doses allows development of successive waves of antigen-specific primary responses without interference.

Interval before boosting: A minimal interval of 4 months between priming and boosting allows affinity maturation of memory B cells, and thus higher secondary responses.

Age at immunization: Early life immune immaturity and age-associated immunosenescence limit the induction/persistence of long-live plasma cells.[3]

Immune Memory and Need for Boosters

Immune memory is seen with live vaccines/ protein antigens due to generation of memory B cells which are activated on repeat vaccination/natural exposure. Immune memory allows one to complete an interrupted vaccine schedule without restarting the schedule. Activation of immune memory and generation of protective antibodies usually takes 4–7 days. Diseases which have incubation periods shorter than this period such as Hib, tetanus, diphtheria and pertussis require regular boosters to maintain protective antibody levels. However, diseases such as hepatitis A, hepatitis B do not need regular boosters as the long incubation period of the disease allows for activation of immune memory cells.

Immune responses during early life immunization

Limitations of young age immunization
The two important factors negatively affect immune responses during young age: Maternal antibodies, and immaturity of immune system.

Young age limits antibody responses to most vaccine antigens since maternal antibodies inhibit antibodies responses but not T cell response, and due to limitation of B cell responses.[8,9]

IgG antibodies are actively transferred through the placenta, via the FcRn receptor, from the maternal to the fetal circulation. Upon immunization, maternal antibodies bind to their specific epitopes at the antigen surface, competing with infant B cells and thus limiting B cell activation, proliferation and differentiation. The inhibitory influence of maternal antibodies on infant B cell responses affects all vaccine types, although its influence is more marked for live attenuated viral vaccines that may be neutralized by even minute amounts of passive antibodies. Hence, antibody responses elicited in early life are short lasting. However, even during early life, induction of B memory cells is not limited which is mediated through Th (CD4). The extent and duration of the inhibitory influence of maternal antibodies increase with gestational age, e.g. with the amount of transferred immunoglobulins, and declines with post-natal age as maternal antibodies wane.[3, 10]

Early life immune responses are characterized by age-dependent limitations of the magnitude of responses to all vaccines. Antibody responses to most PS antigens are not elicited during the first two years of life, which is likely to reflect numerous factors including: The slow maturation of the spleen marginal zone; limited expression of CD21 on B cells; and limited availability of the complement factors. Although this may be circumvented in part by the use of glycoconjugate vaccines, even the most potent glycoconjugate vaccines elicit markedly lower primary IgG responses in young infants.

Although maternal antibodies interfere with the induction of infant antibody responses, they may allow a certain degree of priming, i.e. of induction of memory B cells. This likely reflects the fact that limited amount of unmasked vaccine antigens may be sufficient for priming of memory B cells but not for full-blown GC activation, although direct evidence is lacking. Importantly, however, antibodies of maternal origin do not exert their inhibitory influence on infant T cell responses, which remain largely unaffected or even enhanced.[11]

Limitations of young age immunization can be countered to a certain extent by increasing the number of a vaccine doses for better induction, use of adjuvants to improve immunogenicity of vaccines, and by use of boosters at later age when immune system has shown more maturity than at the time of induction. Increasing the dose of vaccine antigen may also be sufficient to circumvent the inhibitory influence of maternal antibodies, as illustrated for hepatitis A or measles vaccines.

Impact of young age limitations on immunization schedules

Disease epidemiology of vaccine-preventable diseases (VPDs) in a country often determines a particular vaccination schedule. Since, majority of childhood infectious diseases cause morbidity and mortality at an early age in developing countries, there is need to protect the children at the earliest opportunity through immunizations. This is the reason why early and accelerated schedules are practiced in developing countries despite the known limitations of young age immunization.

Immunization schedules commencing at 2 months and having 2 months spacing between the doses are considered technically appropriate. However, for operational reasons and for early completion of immunization the 6-10-14 week's schedule is chosen in developing countries. Such a schedule has shown to give adequate protection in recipients. However, with the availability of newer vaccines, an immunologically superior schedule of 2, 4 and 6 months may have to be considered for future.

For killed vaccines such as DPT, Hib, pneumococcal and hepatitis B which are administered as early as birth / 6 weeks, the first dose acts only as a priming dose while subsequent doses provide an immune response even in presence of maternal antibodies. However, a booster at 15–18 months is required for durable immunity. As the age of commencement of vaccination advances, the number of doses reduces (2 doses at 6–12 months followed by a booster dose and 1–2 doses between 12 and 23 months for Hib and pneumococcal vaccines).

Live vaccines are even more susceptible to maternal antibodies as compared to killed vaccines. However, BCG may be given as the maternal antibodies actually enhance T cell responses. OPV may be given as there are no maternal IgA in the gut to neutralize the virus. Furthermore, measles vaccine if given at the age of 6 months (in an outbreak situation) may work by inducing T cell immunity.[3]

Correlates of vaccine-mediated immunity

A given marker that is measurable, whether the antibody or a cellular component elicited in response to a vaccine that confers protection against a disease is termed a "correlate of protection".[12] Conventionally due to a relative ease of measurement, it's a specific antibody in the serum of a vaccine. Measurement of cellular components is difficult, invasive and highly cost intensive. The correlate can be absolute, e.g. Hib (0.15 mcg/ml), hepatitis B (10 mIU/ml) which are directly protective or surrogates (indirect markers), e.g. Varicella (gp elisa units), ROTA (IgA). Diseases like pertussis and HPV, however, have no established correlates till now. Correlates of protection are important to confirm immunity, compare vaccines and therefore need to be standardized and replicable.

References

1. FAQ on Vaccines and Immunization Practices, Eds. Vashishtha VM, Kalra A, Thacker N. New Delhi, Jaypee Brothers 2011.

2. Plotkin SA. Vaccination against the major infectious diseases. C.R. AcadSci III. 1999, 322: 943–951.

3. Siegrist CA. Vaccine Immunology. In Vaccines Ed. Plotkin SA, Orenstein W, Offit, P. Saunders Elsevier, 5th Edition, 2008.

4. Lee CJ, Lee LH, Lu Cs et al. Bacterial Polysaccharides as vaccine-immunity and chemical characterization. AdvExp Med Biol. 2001, 491: 453–471.

5. Kobrynski LJ, Sousa AO, Nahmias AJ, et al. Cutting edge: Antibody production to pneumococcal polysaccharides requires CD1 molecules and CD8+ T cells. J Immunol. 2005, 174: 1787–1790.

6. MacLennan IC, Toellner KM, Cunningham AF, et al. Extrafollicular antibody responses. Immunol Rev. 2003, 194: 8–18.

7. Comparative trial of live attenuated measles vaccine in Hong Kong by intramuscular and intradermal injection. Bull World Health Organ. 1967, 36: 375–384.

8. Timens W, Boes A, Rozeboom-Uiterwijk T, et al. Immaturity of the human splenic marginal zone in infancy. Possible contribution to the deficient infant immune response. J Immunol.1989, 143: 3200– 3206.

9. Siegrist CA. Neonatal and early life vaccinology. Vaccine. 2001, 19: 3331–3346.

10. Siegrist CA. Mechanisms by which maternal antibodies influence infant vaccine responses: Review of hypotheses and definition of main determinants. Vaccine.2003, 21: 3406–3412.

11. Rowe J, Poolman JT, Macaubas C, et al. Enhancement of vaccine-specific cellular immunity in infants by passively acquired maternal antibody. Vaccine. 2004, 22: 3986–3992.

12. Kamat D, Madhur A. Vaccine Immunology. In: IAP Textbook of Vaccines. Ed. Vashishtha VM, Jaypee Bros, New Delhi, 2013.

ELEMENTARY EPIDEMIOLOGY

Reviewed by
A.J. Chitkara, Panna Choudhury

Epidemiology of Vaccination

Basics of epidemiology

Epidemiology is the study of the distribution and determinants of disease frequency in man.[1] It is the foundation science of public health. It provides insights for applying intervention. It informs if intervention is succeeding. It is the systematic study of the pathogen amplification and transmission systems. Epidemiology can often pin-point the weak links in the chains of the source and transmission pathways of the pathogen so that interventions can be directed at those points. Vaccination is one such intervention.

Impact of vaccinology on disease epidemiology

Vaccinolgy often perturbs the epidemiology of infectious diseases. From vaccinology perspective, there are three reasons to learn epidemiology. They include the rational choice of vaccines for vaccination programs, to design appropriate intervention program including vaccinations, and to monitor and measure the progress and impact of any vaccination program.

Knowledge of epidemiology helps in choosing the appropriate vaccines for inclusion in public health programs after carefully assessing disease burden and economic factors. It also helps in designing disease-specific control/elimination/eradication strategies after acquiring exact epidemiological data on prevalence, incidence, and transmission characteristics of target pathogens, and their transmission pathways. In the last, it also helps in monitoring intervention success/failure in order to improve performance/efficiency of the vaccination programs.[2]

Incidence and Prevalence of Diseases

Basic measures of disease frequency are done by incidence and prevalence. Incidence relates to the number of new cases of the disease which occur during a particular period of time (e.g. new TB cases). Prevalence relates to total number of cases of a disease in a specified period of time (includes both old and new cases) usually during a survey. Often it is expressed as a rate which is a misnomer and it is actually a proportion. In the long run, incidence should be more than the deaths and recoveries, for prevalence to accumulate. Prevalence of various diseases is a good indicator of the load on health services.[3]

Force of Transmission and Basic Reproductive Number (Ro)

The key determinant of incidence and prevalence of infection depends on force of transmission which is determined by 'Reproductive Rate'. Reproductive rate is a simple concept in disease epidemiology. Incidence and prevalence of infection depends on reproductive rate.

'Basic reproductive number' (Ro) measures the average number of secondary cases generated by one primary case in a susceptible population. Suppose all others were susceptible—then how many will be infected? That is Ro. Since population is a mix of susceptible and immune persons, one case must attempt to infect more than one person.[4]

In the long term, pathogen can survive only if one "case" reproduces another "case" (effective reproductive rate, Ro = 1). If Ro < 1, the disease is declining (e.g. herd effect). If Ro > 1, an outbreak is occurring. For endemic diseases with periodic fluctuations, Ro may swing from <1 to >1 but in the long-term the average may remain 1. Pathogen can survive if it reproduces. For all endemic infectious diseases (IDs), Ro = 1 for steady state or for long-term endemicity. The community benefit of a vaccination program is to reduce Ro to <1 and sustain it for long periods. Such beneficial effect, measured as the degree of disease reduction due to a vaccination programme is sometimes called vaccine effectiveness to distinguish it from vaccine efficacy, which refers to only the direct benefit of immunity in vaccinated individuals. Ro is not a static entity and changes according to different time periods even at a same geographic region.

IAP Guidebook on Immunization 2013–14

The magnitude of Ro varies according to location and population. It is strongly influenced by birth rate, population density and behavioral factors. The magnitude of Ro can be ascertained by cross sectional surveys. Eradication is difficult when Ro is large and population density plus net birth rate are high.

'Endemic', 'epidemic' and 'pandemic' patterns of diseases

'Endemic' refers to normal occurrence of disease in defined population, e.g. cholera, malaria, TB, etc. Outbreaks/epidemics are the occurrence of more cases of disease than expected in a given area or among a specific group of people over a particular period of time, e.g. measles, influenza, meningococcal disease. During epidemics, the disease spreads rapidly and extensively by infection and affects many individuals in an area at the same time. The difference between epidemic and outbreak is arbitrary. The terms epidemic and outbreaks are often used similarly; however, former usually indicates higher intensity, for example, epidemic of Japanese encephalitis in a district or region and outbreak of Salmonella in a neonatal unit. A community-based outbreak meningococcal disease is defined as the occurrence of >3 cases in <3 months in the same area who are not close contacts of each other with a primary disease attack rate of >10 primary cases/100,000 persons. In terms of the flu, the difference between an outbreak and an epidemic is the percentage of overall deaths caused by the disease. 'Pandemic' is a global epidemic. Disease originates in one country and then spreads to a number of countries, e.g. AIDS, H1N1, etc.[5]

Vaccine characteristics and development

Vaccine immunogenicity

This is the ability of a vaccine to induce antibodies. These antibodies may be protective or may not be protective to the vaccine. The protective threshold for most vaccines is defined. However, there is often controversy about the cutoffs (pneumococcus/Hib). Levels below the limits may be protective due to other reasons such as immune memory/ T cell immunity. 'Bridging studies' are those that look at vaccine immunogenicity but not efficacy.[6]

Vaccine efficacy

This is the ability of the vaccine to protect an individual. It can be assessed through clinical trials, cohort studies or case control studies. It is calculated as

$$VE = \frac{ARU - ARV}{ARU} \times 100$$

(VE= Vaccine Efficacy, ARU = Attack Rate in Unvaccinated Population, ARV = Attack Rate in Vaccinated Population)

Vaccine effectiveness

This is the ability of the vaccine to protect the community and is a sum of the vaccine efficacy and herd effect. It is revealed after a vaccine is introduced in a program.

Cost effectiveness

This is a method of economic evaluation which is carried out by mathematical modeling usually prior to introduction of a vaccine in a national program. It is expressed as cost per infections/ deaths/ hospitalizations prevented/ life years gained.

Phases in vaccine development

Phase 1 trials are conducted on small number of healthy human volunteers for assessing vaccine immunogenicity and safety.

Phase 2 trials are conducted with a similar objective in larger number of subjects.

Phase 3 trials are randomized controlled trials in large number of subjects for assessing vaccine efficacy and safety.

Cost effectiveness analysis is conducted prior to introduction of vaccines in a national program. Data on vaccine effectiveness and more data on safety emerge following use of vaccines on a widespread basis in programs.

'Herd immunity', 'herd effect', 'herd protection' and 'contact immunity'

The "herd immunity" refers to "the proportion of subjects with immunity in a given population" or, in other words, it reflects the "immunity of a population or a community" reflecting the literal meaning of the word.[7] It should not be confused with 'herd effect' which is defined as "the reduction of infection or disease in the unimmunized segment as a result of immunizing a proportion of the population". Both 'herd immunity' and 'herd effect' can be measured either by testing a sample of the population for the presence of the chosen immune parameter, in the former or by quantifying the decline in incidence in the unimmunized segment of a population in which an immunization program is instituted, in the latter. Herd effect is due to reduced carriage of the causative microorganism by the vaccinated cohort and thus is seen only with vaccines against those diseases where humans are the only source. An effective vaccine is a prerequisite for good herd effect; tetanus and BCG vaccines have no herd effect. Conjugated pneumococcal and Hib vaccines have good herd effect.[8]

Conventionally, "herd immunity" theory suggests that, in contagious diseases that are transmitted from individual to individual, chains of infection are likely to be disrupted when a large number of population are immune or less susceptible to the disease. For example, in Finland when coverage with 3 doses IPV reached 51%, the poliomyelitis disappeared from the country. The greater the proportion of individuals who are resistant, the smaller the probability that a susceptible individual will come into contact with an infectious individual. However, it does not apply to diseases such as tetanus (which is infectious, but is not contagious), where the vaccine protects only the vaccinated person from disease.

'Herd immunity' should not be confused with 'contact immunity', a related concept wherein a vaccinated individual can 'pass on' the vaccine to another individual through contact. Not all vaccines possess this virtue which is mainly the quality of certain live, attenuated vaccines that shed very efficiently either through gut or nasal mucosa though still producing 'herd effect' and contributing in generation of 'herd immunity'. OPV has got this unique quality and provides efficient 'contact immunization'. Other live oral vaccine like rotavirus vaccines may theoretically also exhibit this phenomenon, however, the evidence is lacking. On the other hand, IPV despite providing 'herd immunity' and 'herd effect', do not provide 'contact immunity'. The greater the transmissibility, the higher the contact immunization.

'Herd protection' is another term often used to describe a group of unimmunized individuals that remain protected in a herd by virtue of protection rendered by immunized individuals in a herd or population. However, when this group of individuals moves out of that group/population, they again become susceptible. In this situation, the unvaccinated individuals are indirectly protected by vaccinated individuals, as the latter will not contract and transmit the disease between infected and susceptible individuals.

Herd immunity applies to immunization or infection, human to human transmitted or otherwise. On the other hand, herd effect applies to immunization or other health interventions which reduce the probability of transmission, confined to infections transmitted human to human, directly or via vector.

Epidemiologic shift

This refers to an upward shift in age of infection/disease in communities with partial immunization coverage. Owing to vaccination, the natural circulation of the pathogen decreases and the age of acquisition of infection advances. This is especially important for diseases like rubella, varicella and hepatitis A, wherein severity of disease worsens with advancing age.

References

1. Last JM. Dictionary of public health. Am J Prev Med. 2002; 23(3): 235.

2. Dowdle WR. The principles of disease elimination and eradication. Bull World Health Organ. 1998; 76 Suppl 2: 23–25.

3. Park K. Park's Textbook of Preventive and Social Medicine. 21st ed. Jabalpur: Banarsidas Bhanot Publishers; 2011.

4. K. Dietz. The estimation of the basic reproduction number for infectious diseases. Stat Methods Med Res. 1993; 2(1): 23–41.

5. Porta M, Greenland S, Last JM, editors. A Dictionary of Epidemiology. 5th ed. New York: Oxford University Press; 2008.

6. Weinberg GA, Szilagyi PG. Vaccine epidemiology: Efficacy, effectiveness, and the translational research roadmap. J Infect Dis. 2010; 201: 1607–1610.

7. Fine P . "Herd immunity: history, theory, practice". Epidemiol Rev 1993; 15 (2): 265–273.

8. John TJ, Samuel R. Herd immunity and herd effect: New insights and definitions. Eur J Epidemiol. 2000; 16: 601–606.

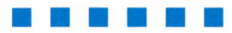

VPD SURVEILLANCE AND IDSURV

2.3

Reviewed by
Deep Thacker, Vipin M. Vashishtha

Background

Disease surveillance is an important component of public health programme. The key objectives of an efficient surveillance system include, first to assess burden of a disease in the community, second, to monitor the progress of any ongoing interventions for disease reduction including the impact on disease epidemiology, and finally, early detection of outbreaks in order to initiate investigations and control measures. Surveillance of vaccine preventable diseases (VPDs) acquires a higher significance than all other surveillance systems like surveillance of non-communicable illnesses since most of the infectious diseases are now being prevented by highly effective vaccines. The number of effective vaccines is going to go up further in coming time considering the rapid advancement in the field of vaccinology today.

Why VPD surveillance is necessary?

The goals of an effective disease surveillance system should serve the following functions:

- To define epidemiology of a disease;

- To identify high-risk populations and regions having high transmission of the disease;

- To monitor progress of a disease control program;

- To specify and monitor molecular epidemiology of an infectious disease including identification of circulating strains of the pathogen responsible for the infectious disease;

- To monitor impact of the vaccination program on overall disease (VPD) epidemiology.

Surveillance: Terminologies

Before we go further and understand the implications of a good VPD surveillance system, we should first understand a few common terminologies employed in describing surveillance.

- Active surveillance, which is done actively by designated persons at any health institutions or community. For example, AFP surveillance done by NPSP.

- Passive surveillance, where suspected or confirmed cases of a disease are reported routinely and passively from identified health facilities, such as IDSP, IDSurv, etc.

- Sentinel surveillance, where clinical syndromes after lab confirmation are reported from selected health institutions, such as Rotavirus (IRSN), Hib-surveillance, etc.

- Population based surveillance is conducted for selected groups with active diseases in a well-defined area/populations.

- Outbreak surveillance, where notification is done only whenever there is cluster of cases as per predefined norms, such as measles surveillance and diseases reported through IDSP.

- Case-based surveillance where any suspected case is immediately notified for further investigations like AFP and AES surveillance.

- Zero reporting means reporting even when there is no case found like AFP surveillance.

Current status of VPD surveillance in India

Vaccine preventable diseases (VPDs) are still responsible for over 500,000 deaths annually in India.[1] There is lack of disease burden data on many important VPDs in India that results in the perception that the disease is not important public health problem. Further, there is scarcity of diagnostic tools for certain VPDs. Lack of baseline surveillance data also is a bottleneck in introduction of many new vaccines in the national immunization program (NIP) and also in monitoring the impact of vaccination provided through UIP.[2]

VPD Surveillance systems in India

Following is the synopsis of available key surveillance systems in India:

IDSP (Integrated Disease Surveillance Project)

Nationwide outbreak surveillance system.

Including measles, diphtheria, pertussis, AFP, hepatitis and AES.

CBHI/SBHI (Central and State Bureaus of Health Intelligence)

Nation-wide passive reporting system of suspected cases.

Measles: ICMR

Selected practitioners and institutions provide clinical samples to NIV-Pune for measles virus isolation and genotyping **(Measles NetIndia)**.

A type of case-based surveillance system.

AES/JE: NVBDCP and ICMR

Facility based surveillance for acute encephalitis syndrome in endemic areas.

It is run by Government of India under National vector-borne diseases control program.

Multicentre Pneumonia and Meningitis surveillance

Established in preparation for Hib vaccine probe study

A type of case-based surveillance.

WHO-NPSP supported surveillance systems

Three different models for three different VPDs.

i. **AFP and lab surveillance for poliovirus:** Global eradication program.

ii. **Fever and rash for measles/rubella:** National mortality reduction target; may be scaled up to a regional elimination goal.

iii. Acute Encephalitis Syndrome (AES) for JE: Control program for endemic districts.

IDSurv— An Innovative Project to Report Infectious Diseases

Background

Indian Academy of Pediatrics (IAP), in collaboration with its Kutch branch, has started an Infectious Disease Surveillance and AEFI (Adverse Event Following Immunization) reporting system for reporting serious AEFI, known as IDSurv.org.[3]

The "standard case definitions" for all the diseases covered under this project are provided at the website.[3] All the cases reported through various methods are collected in a single database in real time and reports are sent to all users on weekly basis. In case a disease outbreak is recorded on the system, email and SMS alert are sent to all users instantaneously.

The idea of IDsurv was conceived by IAP's Kutch Branch and was designed only for Kutch district. However, after interest shown in this project by IAP's committee on Immunization and central IAP, a MoU was signed between IAP Kutch Branch and central IAP to make this project available nationwide for all IAP members. Initially only nine infectious diseases were included for surveillance and hepatitis surveillance was added later on. More recently, surveillance for serious AEFI on the IDsurv platform was also added with the support of GoI.

Objectives

The main objectives of the program are:[3]

*   To generate data on burden of key vaccine preventable diseases in India

*   To develop an early warning system for pediatric vaccine preventable diseases in India

*   To sensitize pediatricians about serious AEFIs and generate data on serious AEFI in India

Infectious diseases covered under IDSurv project

At present only ten key infectious diseases are targeted for surveillance under this project and they include:

1.	Acute bacterial meningitis	6.	Measles
2.	Chickenpox	7.	Mumps
3.	Diphtheria	8.	Pertussis
4.	Dengue	9.	Pneumonia
5.	Enteric fever	10.	Hepatitis

How to join IDsurv network?

To join IDsurv project, you need to open IDsurv website www.idsurv.org and register yourself.

The administrator will validate your account and password will be sent to you by SMS and email. You need to mention your IAP membership number/MCI registration number. If you are already registered user, login from the 'Member's Login' area.[3]

How to report a new infectious disease case?

One can report a case by various ways such as

1. through website idsurv.org, after logging into your account.

2. by sending a SMS to 57333 through your registered mobile number.

3. through mobile website m.idsurv.org

4. by calling IVR system on 02653090533

1. Reporting a case through website

First, one should go to the site www.idsurv.org and click on login and a panel will open. Enter your Username and Password. You will be redirected to your account. Click on 'Report a Case'. Select the diagnosis. Enter patient's details including all other details and click on submit.[3] A reference number will be generated for the patient and given to you.

2. Reporting a case through sms

Type'IT' space 'IDS' space 4-letter 'code of the disease' space 'age' in months space 'sex' space 'severity of disease' space 'microbial diagnosis established' space 'immunization status' space 'outcome' and send it to 57333. The details about SMS codes are provided on the website.[3]

3. Reporting case through mobile website

Log in to your account on m.idsurv.org. Click on report a case and fill up the form and click on submit.[3]

4. Reporting a case through IVR

To report a case using IVR system, call 02653090533 using your registered mobile number and follow the instructions. It usually takes less than 2 minutes to register the case. You can enter the details later.

How to report an Adverse Event Following Immunization (AEFI)?

An AEFI is defined as "a medical incident that takes place after an immunization, causes concern and is believed to be caused by immunization". Only serious AEFI that includes deaths, hospitalization, clustering of cases, and disability is reported to the system.

To report serious AEFI cases click on "report an AEFI" and fill in all the fields regarding patient, AEFI and the vaccine, and then click on "save". One can view the AEFI cases reported by clicking on 'View/ Update AEFI cases reported by me'. You can have a customized search from the search bar also. You can also update the AEFI cases reported by you similar to update an ID case by clicking on "Update this".[3] Once a serious AEFI reported through this system, automated e-mail intimation is sent to the designated government authority for further necessary actions.

Who can see the cases reported by me?

Anybody who opens idsurv.org can see the cases reported on the platform. But the identity of the doctor and patient is kept confidential and provided only to Government authorities if requested by them.

How to view surveillance data available at IDSurv?

The data can be viewed either on a map, in tabular form and in charts. The compiled data of last three months is displayed on a Google map showing total number of cases along with break-up of the cases reported from a particular district. The charts display the total number of all the ten ID cases reported so far along with data on different diseases.[3] However, an option for the customized search is also available.

Early warning system/IDsurv alerts

An early warning system (IDsurv alerts) is being introduced on the site wherein if the system detects unusually high number of cases being reported of a particular disease in a geographical area in a short period of time, an automatic (SMS and Email) alert is sent to all the registered users and government authorities in that area and same is also reflected on the website.

Current status of IDSurv

The IDSurv has a great potential in fulfilling the need of infectious disease surveillance of the country. It can provide impetus to the overall VPD reporting in the country especially amongst the practicing pediatricians. The user-friendly interface and appealing display of the data should provide motivation to pediatricians hitherto neglected by the government-based programs. So far, as of Nov. 2013, **10,146** cases of all the ten IDs are reported through this project from all over the country as shown in Figure 1.[3] Water borne infectious diseases like enteric fever and hepatitis are topping the chart (Figure 1). The total number of registered users is only 602 that represent around 3% of total membership of IAP in the country. The majority of cases either had no immunization or were only partially immunized.

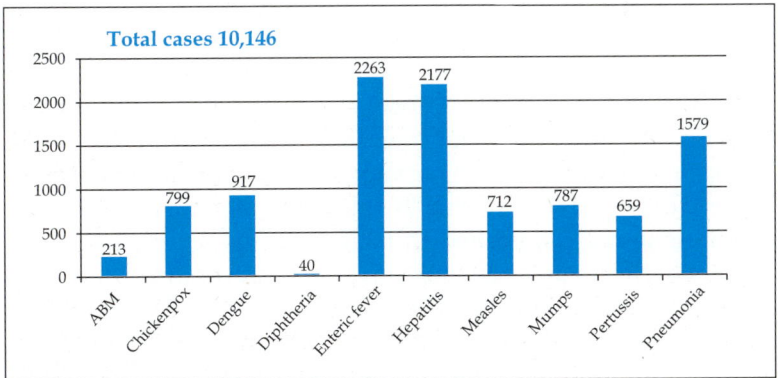

Figure 1: Distribution of total cases of 10 Infectious disease cases reported through IDsurv (data till 17th November, 2013.)

Conclusions and the need of the hour

The burning need of the hour is to develop and establish well functioning, coordinated and all-inclusive infectious disease surveillance in the country. Universal Immunization Program (UIP) can seize the opportunity and establish a competent surveillance system for all important childhood infectious diseases. As has been demonstrated by the success of AFP surveillance network, efficient surveillance systems can be established, even in resource-poor settings, at quite low cost relative to the cost of the intervention itself.[2] Where appropriate, this network should serve as the platform both for an integrated disease surveillance system that provides epidemiological data on other communicable diseases, and for detection and response to emerging infectious disease threats.[4] The NPSP under the instructions of Global Polio Eradication Initiative has started following this approach, but the need is to expand it to cover the entire country so that nationally representative data on common infectious diseases can be obtained. Integrated Disease Surveillance Project (IDSP)—a state-based decentralized passive surveillance program in the country launched by Ministry of Health and Family Welfare, GoI in November 2004 is a laudable effort in this regard. However, it also needs upgradation and consolidation.

As discussed above, the great potential of IDSurv is not fully exploited so far. The site is operational now for more than two years, yet the number of registered and more importantly, actively participating members are very low considering the large membership of the academy. The reported number of ID cases represents only a tip of the iceberg since large part of the country remains unrepresented, and even those districts from where the regular reporting is done have very few reporting units. Another aspect that needs bolstering is lab component. The microbial diagnosis is not established in majority of the cases; hence the validity of these cases remains suspect. However, this is partially offset by the fact that the diagnosis is made by IAP members, a group of highly qualified pediatricians. There is a need of involving a few more key diseases like malaria, diarrhea, AES (Acute Encephalitis Syndrome), etc. Furthermore, there is need of regular analysis and sharing of reported data by periodic publications.

In the last, there is need of having a functional real-time AEFI and post-marketing surveillance system in the country.[4] This will help in generating national data and will also provide sound basis for decisions to modify/abandon certain vaccine preparation based on reactogenicity profile, should the need arise.

References

1. World Health Organization (Regional Office for South-East Asia). Available online: http://www.searo.who.int/en/Section1226/Section2715.htm. (Accessed on June 20, 2013).

2. Vashishtha VM, Kumar P. 50 years of immunization in India: Progress and future. Indian Pediatr 2013 Jan 8; 50(1): 111–118.

3. IDsurv. Available online: www.idsurv.org. (Accessed on June 20, 2013)

4. Vashishtha VM. Status of immunization and need for intensification of routine immunization in India. Indian Pediatr 2012 May; 49(5): 357–361.

■ ■ ■ ■ ■ ■

PRACTICAL ASPECTS OF IMMUNIZATION

Reviewed by
Panna Choudhury, Vipin M. Vashishtha

Communicating with parents/care givers

With several newer vaccines available in open market, it is an arduous task for pediatricians to offer ideal advice to parents regarding pros and cons of each vaccine. Most of these vaccines are included in the IAP COI recommendations necessitating one to one discussion. Thus, pediatricians are required to communicate properly with clarity and appropriate information that should help parents to make their own decision in favor or against each of these vaccines. Ideally we need to offer a balanced scientific view without appearing to suggest one way or another. Unfortunately, most of the educated parents would leave the choice to their pediatricians and it is quite unfair to take responsibility of making a choice for parents.

Prerequisite of one to one discussion is commitment on the part of pediatrician to inform relevant facts about disease and vaccine. It takes very little time if one uses structured format covering important aspects in simple language. Following points need to be discussed regarding each vaccine.

1. Risk of developing disease—it is not possible to evaluate risk of disease in an individual child, but figures from literature may be quoted, e.g. the risk of Invasive Pneumococcal Disease (IPD) in a healthy child aged less than 1 year is roughly 200 per 100,000 (as per Western data). Some general statements are also helpful. Water or food-borne infections are preventable to some extent but not airborne droplet infections. Risk of complications of disease is higher in infants and younger children and in undernourished population. Age prevalence of disease decides appropriate age of vaccination as per the standard recommendations.

2. Efficacy of vaccine—no vaccine provides 100% protection though most of the vaccines do offer high degree of protection. Vaccines significantly decrease chance of disease and even partial protection is useful to prevent complications. Occasional failure of vaccine protection is no reason to consider against its use.

3. Safety of vaccine—vaccines are very safe and serious adverse reactions are extremely rare. Media outbursts of fatal reactions to vaccines are mostly due to human error of administration and not due to vaccine itself. Thus benefits of vaccines outweigh the risk of side effects caused by vaccines.

4. Cost of vaccine—decision of affordability should be left to parents. It is important to reiterate facts that all vaccines are equally efficacious even though they may differ in their cost. For example, DTwP and DTaP are equally efficacious though differ in reactogenicity. Similarly, vaccines from different manufacturers are equally effective and indigenously manufactured vaccines are usually as good as imported ones.

5. Finally, it is important to emphasize that above discussion is based on the current understanding of vaccine and its present place in prevention of disease. With increasing experience over time, there can be a change in the recommendations of individual vaccine and it is necessary to adapt to such changes. For example, second dose of MMR is now recommended.

Many new vaccines are likely to be introduced over the next few years. It would be a challenge for pediatricians to develop communication skills to discuss pros and cons of all these vaccines. But far more relevant is the need to keep updated on issues related to vaccines and disease prevention. It is only then that "one to one discussion" will become more meaningful.[1,2]

Injection procedure

Sterile technique and injection safety

Hands should be washed with soap and water for 2 minutes using WHO's 6 steps technique. Alternately, alcohol-based waterless antiseptic hand rub can be used. Gloves need not be worn when administering vaccinations, unless the person administering the vaccine has open lesions on hands or is likely to come in contact with potentially infectious body fluids. Needles used for injections must be sterile and preferably disposable. Auto disable (AD) syringes are single use, self-locking syringes designed in such a way that these are rendered unusable after single use. Thus they prevent immediate/ downstream reuse and their use is being promoted in the national immunization program. A separate needle and syringe should be used for each injection. Changing needles between drawing vaccine from a vial and injecting it into a recipient is not necessary.

If multi-dose vials are used, the septum should be swabbed with alcohol prior to each withdrawal and the needle should not be left in the stopper in between uses. Different vaccines should never be mixed in the same syringe unless specifically licensed for such use, and no attempt should be made to transfer between syringes. Pre-filling of syringes should not be done because of the potential for administration errors as the majority of vaccines have a similar appearance after being drawn into a syringe. Thus vaccine doses should not be drawn into a syringe until immediately before administration. To prevent inadvertent needle-stick injury or reuse, needles and syringes should be discarded immediately after use in labeled, puncture-proof containers located in the same room where the vaccine is administered. Needles should not be recapped before being discarded.[3-5] Box 1 summarizes a few key recommendations on practical aspect of vaccination of a child.

Injection route, site, method and needle length

With the exception of BCG and sometimes rabies, all parenteral vaccines are given by either intramuscular (IM) or subcutaneous (SC) route. The SC route is recommended for measles, MMR, varicella, meningococcal polysaccharide, JE, Yellow fever vaccines; either SC or IM route may be used for pneumococcal polysaccharide vaccines, IPV; the rest of the vaccines should be given intramuscularly. Generally speaking, there is no harm done if SC vaccines are given IM. However, vaccines designated to be given IM should not be given SC due to risk of side effects (as seen with aluminium adjuvanted vaccines) or reduced efficacy (due to reduced blood supply in SC tissue and hence reduced immunogenicity). The gluteal region should never be used for administration of IM injections due to risk of sciatic nerve injury and reduced efficacy (rabies and hepatitis B vaccines). When used at the recommended sites where no large blood vessels exist, pulling back of the syringe to check for blood is not recommended. The needle should be withdrawn a few seconds after finishing administration of the vaccine (to prevent backflow of vaccine into the needle track) following which the injection site should be pressed firmly for a few seconds with dry cotton. The injection site should not be rubbed following injection.[6,7]

Box 1: General instructions on immunization

General instructions

- Vaccination at birth means as early as possible within 24 to 72 hours after birth or at least not later than one week after birth.
- Whenever multiple vaccinations are to be given simultaneously, they should be given within 24 hours if simultaneous administration is not feasible due to some reasons.
- The recommended age in weeks/months/years mean completed weeks/months/years.
- Any dose not administered at the recommended age should be administered at a subsequent visit, when indicated and feasible.
- The use of a combination vaccine generally is preferred over separate injections of its equivalent component vaccines.
- When two or more live parenteral/intranasal vaccines are not administered on the same day, they should be given at least 28 days (4 weeks) apart; this rule does not apply to live oral vaccines.
- If given <4 weeks apart, the vaccine given 2nd should be repeated.
- The minimum interval between 2 doses of inactivated vaccines is usually 4 weeks (exception rabies).
- Vaccine doses administered up to 4 days before the minimum interval or age can be counted as valid (exception rabies). If the vaccine is administered > 5 days before minimum period, it is counted as invalid dose.

- Any number of antigens can be given on the same day.
- Changing needles between drawing vaccine into the syringe and injecting it into the child is not necessary.
- Different vaccines should not be mixed in the same syringe unless specifically licensed and labeled for such use.
- Patients should be observed for an allergic reaction for 15 to 20 minutes after receiving immunization(s).
- When necessary, 2 vaccines can be given in the same limb at a single visit.
- The anterolateral aspect of the thigh is the preferred site for 2 simultaneous IM injections because of its greater muscle mass.
- The distance separating the 2 injections is arbitrary but should be at least 1 inch so that local reactions are unlikely to overlap.
- Although most experts recommend "aspiration" by gently pulling back on the syringe before the injection is given, there are no data to document the necessity for this procedure. If blood appears after negative pressure, the needle should be withdrawn and another site should be selected using a new needle.
- A previous immunization with a dose that was less than the standard dose or one administered by a nonstandard route should not be counted, and the person should be re-immunized as appropriate for age.

If multiple vaccines are administered at a single visit, administration of each preparation at a different anatomic site is desirable. For infants and younger children, if more than two vaccines must be injected in a single limb, the thigh is the preferred site because of the greater muscle mass; the injections should be sufficiently separated (i.e., 1 inch or more if possible) so that any local reactions can be differentiated. For older children and adults, the deltoid muscle can be used for more than one intramuscular injection (Table 1). If a vaccine and an immune globulin preparation are administered simultaneously (e.g., Td/Tdap and tetanus immune globulin [TIG], hepatitis B and hepatitis B immunoglobulin [HBIG]), separate anatomic sites should be used

Table 1: Injection site, type of needle and technique

	Site	Type of needle	Comments
Intramuscular injections (needle should enter at a 90° angle)			
Preterms and neonates	Anterolateral thigh (junction of middle and lower third)	22–25 gauge, 5/8 inch	Skin should be stretched between thumb and forefinger
Infants (1 to < 12 months)	Anterolateral thigh	22–25 gauge, 1 inch	Bunch the skin subcutaneous tissue and muscle to prevent striking the bone
Toddlers and older children (12 months– 10 years)	Deltoid or	22–25 guage, 5/8 inch	Skin should be stretched between thumb and forefinger
	Anterolateral thigh	22–25 gauge, 1 inch	Bunch the skin, subcutaneous tissue and muscle
Adolesocents and adults (11 yrs onwards)	Deltoid or anterolateral thigh	< 60 kg 1 inch > 60 kg 1.5 inch	
Intramuscular injections (needle should enter at a 45° to the skin)			
Infants	Thigh	22–25 G, 5/8 inch	
> 12 months	Outer triceps	22–25 G, 5/8 inch	
Intradermal injections			
All ages	Left deltoid	26/27 G, 0.5 inch	A 5 mm wheal should be raised

for each injection. The location of each injection should be documented in the patients' medical record (Figures 1–4).

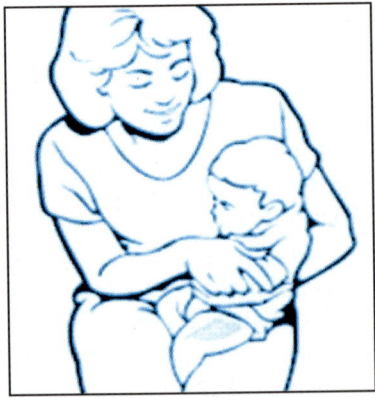

Figure 1: Intramuscular/ subcutaneous site for administration: Anterolateral thigh

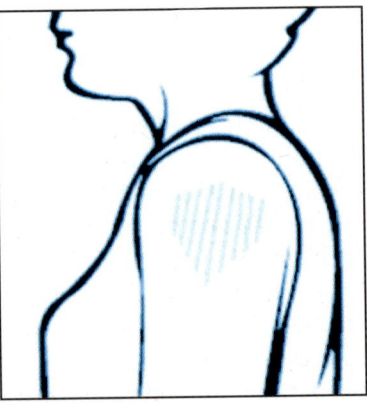

Figure 2: Intramuscular site for administration: Deltoid muscle at upper arm

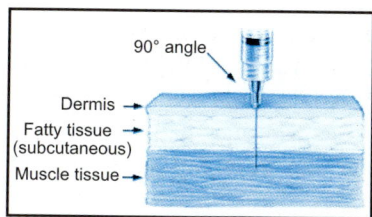

Figure 3: Intramuscular needle insertion

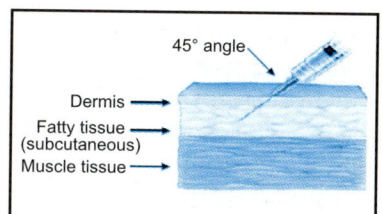

Figure 4: Subcutaneous needle insertion

Alleviation of pain associated with injections

Comfort measures, such as distraction (e.g., playing music or pretending to blow away the pain), ingestion of sweet liquids, breastfeeding, cooling of the injection site, and topical or oral analgesia, can help infants or children cope with the discomfort associated with vaccination. Pretreatment (30–60 minutes before injection) with 5% topical lidocaine-prilocaine emulsion can decrease the pain of vaccination by causing superficial anesthesia. Topical lidocaine-prilocaine emulsion should not be used on infants aged <12 months who are receiving treatment with methemoglobin-inducing agents because of the possible development of methemoglobinemia. Use of a topical refrigerant (vapocoolant) spray immediately before vaccination can reduce the short-term pain associated with injections and can be as effective as lidocaine prilocaine cream. Acetaminophen may be used immediately following DTP vaccination @ 15 mg/kg/dose to reduce the discomfort and fever.[7]

Contraindication and Precautions

Contraindication: A condition in a recipient that greatly increases the chance of a serious adverse reaction.[7] It is a condition in the recipient of the vaccine, not with the vaccine per se. If the vaccine were given in the presence of that condition, the resulting adverse reaction could seriously harm the recipient.

For instance, administering influenza vaccine to a person with a true anaphylactic allergy to egg could cause serious illness or death in the recipient. In general, vaccines should not be administered when a contraindication condition is present.

The most common animal protein allergen is egg protein found in vaccines prepared using embryonated chicken eggs (e.g., yellow fever and influenza vaccines). Ordinarily, a person who can eat eggs or egg products can receive vaccines that contain egg; persons with histories of anaphylactic or anaphylactic-like allergy to eggs or egg proteins should not. Asking persons whether they can eat eggs without adverse effects is a reasonable way to screen for those who might be at risk from receiving yellow fever and influenza vaccines.

True contraindications are very few. Only three permanent contraindications are:

- Severe allergic reaction to a vaccine component or following a prior dose of a vaccine;

- Encephalopathy occurring within 7 days of pertussis vaccination;

- Severe combined immunodeficiency (SCID) as a contraindication to rotavirus vaccine (Figure 5).

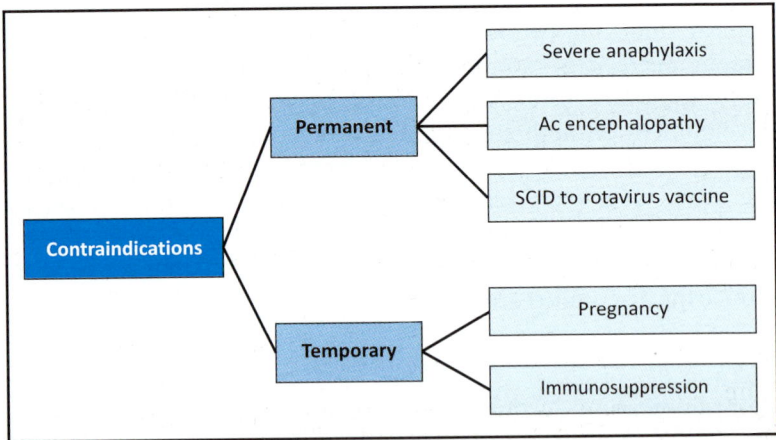

Figure 5: Contraindications—permanent and temporary

Precautions: It is similar to a contraindication. A precaution is a condition in a recipient that might increase the chance or severity of a serious adverse reaction, or that might compromise the ability of the vaccine to produce immunity (such as administering measles vaccine to a person with passive immunity to measles from a blood transfusion). Injury could result, but the chance of this happening is less than with a contraindication.[7] In general, vaccines are deferred when a precaution condition is present (Figure 6).

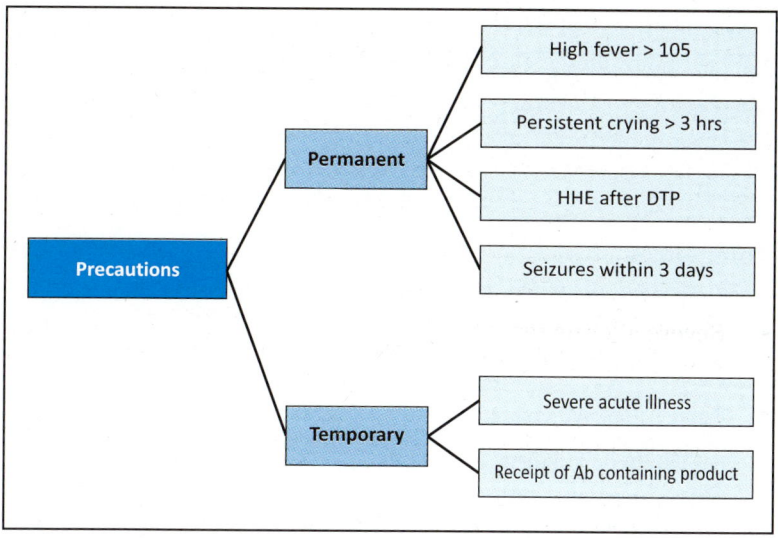

Figure 6: Precautions— permanent and temporary

Record keeping

The vaccine administrator must record the type of vaccine, brand name and date of administration of the vaccine in the patient's file/ immunization record. In addition, recording of the batch number of the vaccine is also recommended. Record keeping is very important as guidelines issued for reporting of AEFI are also applicable to the private practitioners.[8]

Medicolegal aspects

The vaccine administrator must explain in detail the characteristics and anticipated side effects of the vaccine in reasonable detail to the caregivers prior to immunization. A verbal consent is usually adequate. In any case, the recipient must be observed for any allergic effects for at least 15 minutes after vaccination and all resuscitative equipment must be kept standby for possible anaphylaxis. The care givers should also be counseled about possible side effects, their management and danger signs before the vaccine is sent home.[8, 9] Box 2 provides the list of bare minimum equipment and drugs needed to take care of any immediate adverse events following immunization, particularly any hypersensitivity reaction to vaccine.

Box 2: Minimum resuscitative equipment

Airway, ambu bag, mask, IV access (scalp vein, venflon), oxygen cylinder

Injection adrenaline (1: 1000 solution)

IV hydrocortisone

Normal saline

References

1. Kimmel SR, Wolfe RM. Communicating the benefits and risks of vaccines. J Family Practice. 2005; 54: S51–57.

2. Healy MC, Pickering LK. How to communicate with vaccine –hesitant parents. Pediatrics 2011; 127: S127–133.

3. Hutin Y, Hauri A, ChiarelloL, Catlin M, Stilwell B, Ghebrehiwet T et al. Best infection control practices for intradermal, subcutaneous, and intramuscular needle injections. Bull World Health Organization 2003; 81: 491–500.

4. WHO best practices for injections and related procedures toolkit. March 2010. WHO/EHT/10.02 accessed from http://whqlibdoc.who.int/publications/2010/9789241599252_eng.pdf

5. Atkinson WL, Kroger A L, Pickering LK. General immunization practices. In:Plotkin SA, Orenstein WA, Offit PA (Eds). Vaccines. 5th edition. Saunders Elsevier 2008: pp 83–109.

6. Nicoll LH, Hesby A. IM injection: An integrative research review and guideline for evidence based practice. Appl Nurs Res 2000; 16: 149–162.

7. General Recommendations on Immunization, Recommendations of the Advisory Committee on Immunization Practices (ACIP), MMWR; Recommendations and Reports / Vol. 60 / No. 2 January 28, 2011.

8. AEFI Surveillance and Response-Operational Guidelines. Ministry of Health and Family Welfare, 2010 accessed from http://www.cdsco.nic.in/ AEFI %20 Guidelines% 20 Print %20ready%202010.pdf

9. Rajput M, Sharma L. Informed consent in vaccination in India: Medicolegal aspects. Hum Vaccin. 2011; 7: 723–737.

■ ■ ■ ■ ■ ■

COLD CHAIN AND STORAGE OF VACCINES

Reviewed by
Pravin J. Mehta, Panna Choudhury

Introduction

The system of transporting, storing and distributing vaccines in a potent state at the recommended temperature from the point of manufacture to the point of use is the cold chain. Vaccine potency once lost cannot be restored. The cold chain remains a highly vulnerable point for both National Immunization Programs and office practice in developing countries with tropical climates. Hence presently there is no substitute to rigorous maintenance of cold chain.[1]

The essential components of a cold chain include

1. Personnel responsible for vaccine distribution
2. Appropriate equipment to store and transport vaccines
3. Appropriate transport facilities
4. Maintenance of equipment
5. Monitoring

Temperature and light sensitivity of vaccines

The correct temperature is the most important factor in maintaining the potency of vaccines. Unlike popular belief vaccines are damaged by excessive cold in addition to heat.[2]

Sensitivity of vaccines to heat

Each exposure to ambient temperature causes some degradation of the vaccine and subsequent exposures lead to cumulative impact. Vaccine potency cannot be restored after placing back at recommended temperatures. All vaccines are sensitive to heat but to different degrees. Live vaccines are more susceptible and in decreasing order of sensitivity include two brands of varicella and MMRV (Varivax TM, ProQuadTM, currently not available in India), live attenuated influenza vaccine, OPV, measles, MMR, BCG, yellow fever, rotavirus and other brands of varicella/ MMRV vaccines.

Sensitivity of vaccines to freezing

Cold injury is more common than assumed. Vaccines susceptible to damage by freezing include mainly all aluminium adjuvanted vaccines (DTwP, DTaP, TT, DT, Td, TT, hepatitis B, combination vaccines, hepatitis A, HPV, PCV 7) but also other vaccines including IPV, PPV 23, inactivated influenza vaccines, meningococcal vaccines, rotavirus vaccines, typhoid vaccines, Hib and brands of varicella vaccines except Varivax TM. Vaccines that can be frozen without harm include OPV (vial must not be frozen and thawed repeatedly), and lyophilized measles, MMR, BCG vaccines, LAIV, certain brands of varicella and MMRV (Varivax TM, Proquad TM).

Sensitivity of vaccines to light

Lyophilized and reconstituted BCG, measles, MMR, varicella, rotavirus, human papilloma virus, most DTaP containing vaccines are particularly susceptible to light and need protection from strong light, sunlight, ultraviolet and fluorescent neon lights.

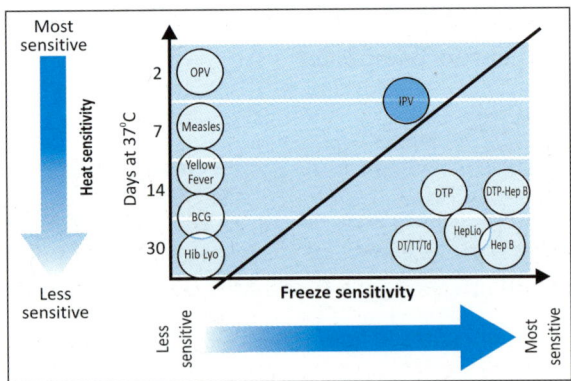

Figure 1: Graphic depiction of heat and freeze sensitivity of commonly used vaccines

To ensure that we maintain desired optimum temperature, we need to use vaccine monitoring tools.

Vaccine Monitoring Tools

Box 1: Vaccine monitoring tools

Indicators:
  Freeze Watch Indicators: e.g. Freeze-Tag®
  Vaccine Vial Monitors (VVMs)

Thermometers:
  Dial, stem, max/min, electronic

Vaccine Vial Monitors

The Vaccine Vial Monitor (VVM) is a time and temperature sensitive colored label that provides an indication of the cumulative heat to which the vial has been exposed. VVMs were first introduced on OPV vials supplied to UNICEF and WHO in 1996. The VVM warns the end user when exposure to heat is likely to have degraded the vaccine beyond an acceptable level. It is used especially for temperature monitoring of OPV, which is the most thermo labile of all vaccines. The VVM is applied to the outside of a vaccine vial, and it applies only to that vial. It cannot be taken as a surrogate marker for the potency of the vaccine in other vials of the same lot or in the same storage facility.[3]

VVMs consist of a temperature sensitive material, which changes color gradually on being exposed to heat. This change of color is irreversible, and thus corresponds to the heat induced damage to the vaccine inside the vial. VVM's do not give any information on cold injury to vaccines. There are different types of VVMs available, to be used according to the heat stability characteristics of different vaccines.

Interpretation of the color change of VVM is as follows:

1. Inner square is white, or lighter than outer circle: If the expiry date has not passed, vaccine can be used.

2. Inner square matches color of outer circle or is darker than outer circle: Vaccine should be discarded, regardless of the expiry date.

The vaccines can be used as long as the VVM has not changed color to the "discard" level. This is of tremendous help in outreach programs, where vaccine has to be carried to far away places, or given door to door. Now VVMs are available for all vaccines and should be demanded from all manufacturers. VVMs are thus a low cost tool for assessing the adequacy and finding the weak links in the cold chain. They save children from receiving impotent, ineffective vaccines and avoid vaccine wastage.

Box 2: Freeze watch indicators

A freeze watch indicator consists of a small vial of red liquid attached to a white card and covered in plastic. The vial breaks if the temperature where the indicator is located drops below 0° C for more than one hour.

These are very useful for cold sensitive vaccines like DTwP, DTaP, TT, DT, Td, TT, hepatitis B.

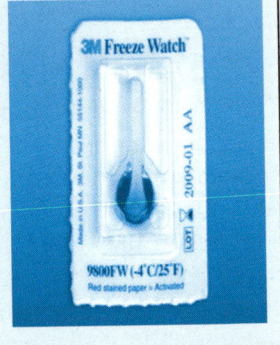

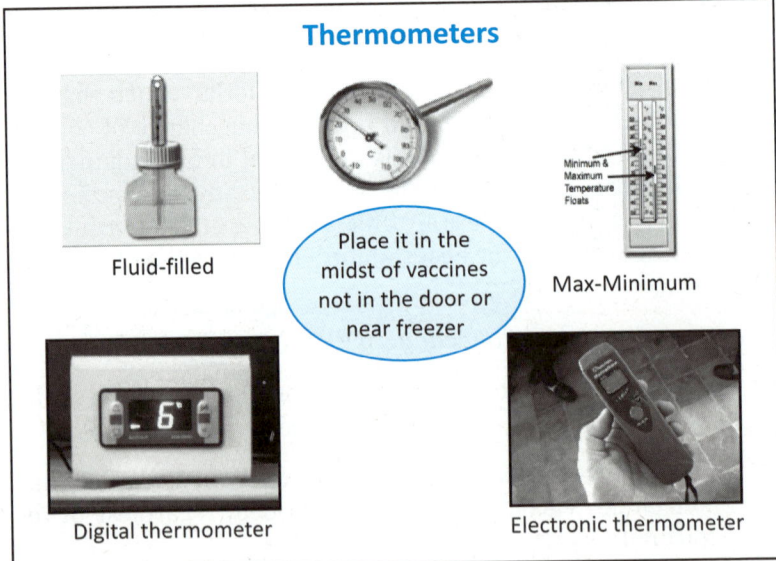

Figure 2: Different types of thermometers used in monitoring temperature of vaccines

CDC recommends using a continuous, certified and calibrated thermometer.

- Continuous means having no gaps, holes or breaks. Logging temperatures only twice a day gives you just a snap shot of what happened, creating uncertainty about the temperatures the rest of the time.

- Calibration is the process of making a device accurate. If someone tells you the time of day, how do you know they are correct? Is their watch running correctly, or it is running slow or fast? This same theory applies to a temperature device. Calibrated lets you know this instrument has been compared to a higher standard that is deemed the most accurate instrument to which all other units are compared.

- Certified gives you the assurance of the calibration. It is a document that officially confirms the accuracy of the instrument. The CDC recommends that thermometers be certified by an appropriate agency.

Box 3: The VFC70 thermometer, it is one of the brands which comply with the CDC-recommended continuous and calibrated thermometers for vaccine storage monitoring. It has a 4" (101mm) Chart-Jumbo Display; it operates on a single AA Battery and displays temperature in Fahrenheit or Celsius.

CDC recommends using a continuous, calibrated and certified chart recording thermometer

Continuous ⟶ Records without break

Calibration ⟶ Accurate reading

Certified ⟶ Assured of proper calibration

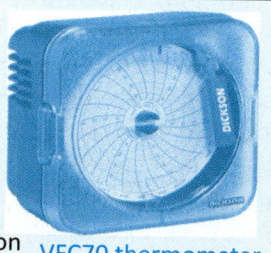

VFC70 thermometer

Box 4: Typical causes of freezing

- Storage of T series vaccines in ILR
- Transport with frozen ice packs
- Belief that colder is better
- Low awareness and understanding
- Incorrect thermostat adjustments

Cold chain equipment

The cold chain involves two complementary aspects: 1) the set chain represented by the walk-in cold rooms, deep freezers and refrigerators and 2) the mobile chain represented by isothermic boxes and vaccine carriers.[2,3]

Walk in cold rooms (WIC) and walk- in freezers (WIF) are used for bulk storage of vaccines at the manufacturer site, or at major distribution points. They have two cooling units and standby generator sets, and are fitted with temperature recorders and alarm systems. Deep freezers are used for long term storage of OPV/ measles / MMR vaccines. They are also used for making ice-packs for use in outreach programs. Ice lined refrigerators (ILR) are used where the power supply is intermittent. Most of the space is taken up by water which is frozen when electricity is available. Appropriate temperatures can be maintained for several hours.

Cold chain equipment commonly used in office practice including domestic refrigerators, cold boxes and vaccine carriers are discussed further in detail.

Domestic refrigerator

The main compartment should have a temperature of 2 to 8°C, and the freezer compartment should maintain a temperature of −5 to −15°C. It should be large enough to store the largest inventory of a month and should be CFC free. Ideally, a double door refrigerator should be used. It is impossible to maintain optimum temperatures unless the refrigerator has two separate external doors for the two compartments. Without separate doors, either the freezer will be too warm, or the vaccines in the main compartment will suffer freezing damage. The doors should close snugly, be free of leakages of water and coolant, quiet and have features such as auto defrost and auto door closure. Bar and dormitory fridges should not be used. A voltage stabilizer is mandatory when voltage fluctuations are many and power cuts are frequent. A good well calibrated thermometer is a must; options include a stem thermometer, dial thermometer, digital thermometer, max/min thermometer or a data logger. The thermometer should be placed in both the freezer and the main compartment in the center and away from the walls, door, air vent or frozen packs and never in the door.

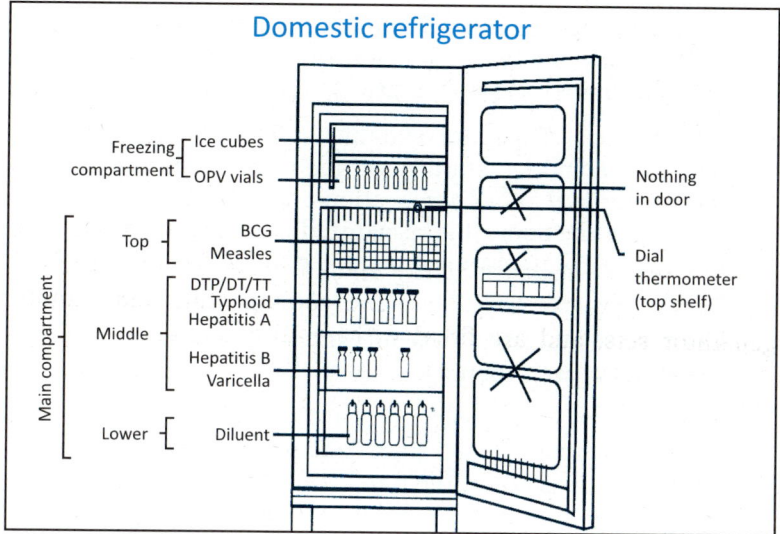

Figure 3: Recommended placement of different vaccines in different compartments of a domestic refrigerator

The vaccines can be placed as follows:

- Freezer compartment: OPV.

- Top shelf: BCG, measles and MMR.

- Middle shelf: DTwP, DTaP, DT, TT, Tdap, combination vaccines, IPV, HPV, typhoid, hepatitis A, Hib, PCV7, influenza, rotavirus vaccines.

- Lower shelf: Hepatitis B and varicella

- Crispator: Diluents

- Baffle tray: Should be kept empty. No vaccines should be stored in the door.

The following measures are recommended to maintain appropriate temperatures and ensure vaccine potency in domestic refrigerators.

- Temperatures should be recorded at least twice a day and a temperature log maintained regardless of temperature alarm, a chart recorder thermometer, or a digital data logger. Fast action should be taken in case of out of range temperatures. The log helps to identify recurring problems and loss of function in ageing units. Temperatures should be monitored twice a day for a week prior to using a new/ repaired refrigerator for vaccine storage.

- The vaccine refrigerator should not be used for any other purpose including storage of food, beverages, pathology specimens and other medications. This will minimize the opening of the door. It is recognized that opening of the door can increase temperatures much as 2 to 5°C for as long as 2 to 8 minutes.

- The door should have a warning sticker in order to discourage unnecessary door opening.

- Access to the vaccine refrigerator should be restricted to anyone else than trained staff. A map of inside content of the refrigerator pasted on the outside of the door can minimize opened-door time while searching vaccine inside.

- Ice packs and jars/ bottles of non drinkable water should be kept in the freezer and the door of the main compartment and the lowest part (baffle tray) respectively. This increases the cool mass of the refrigerator and helps maintain temperature during power failures and cuts for at least 3 to 4 hours, and minimizes temperature fluctuations during door opening. The thermostat should be reset according to the ambient temperatures; e.g. to coolest during summers.

- The refrigerator should be kept at least 10 cm away from the floor and the walls so as to allow good air circulation.

- The vaccines should be kept in transparent labeled boxes that will help in minimizing time required for retrieving the vaccines. Each vaccine pack/ vial must be labeled with the expiry date and the principle of FEFO (first expired first out) and FIFO (First in first out) followed.

- The refrigerator should not be overloaded and overstocked so as to allow good air circulation around the vaccines.

- The refrigerator should be checked regularly daily for door closure, monthly for coils, door seals, hinges and leveling and undergo maintenance on a periodic basis.

- In non-frost free refrigerators regular cleaning and defrosting should be done weekly or whenever ice layer of more than 4 mm forms in the freezer. Thicker ice layer will hamper proper functioning of the unit. Vaccines should be transferred to a safe place during defrosting and cleaning.

- The power supply should be secured. The plug should have a sticker saying "Do Not Unplug". Staff must be trained never to turn off the refrigerator that holds vaccines.

- If power cuts are frequent, an alternative power source should be available capable for running for at least 72 hours.

- Rapid action should be taken in case of power failure or refrigerator malfunction. A plan must be in place for dealing with power failure. For short intervals, such as 2–3 hours, it is appropriate to just keep the refrigerator door closed, to maintain the temperature inside. For longer power cuts, it is necessary to move the vaccines, in a vaccine carrier, to a place where a working refrigerator is available. Refrigerator malfunctions need to be dealt with similarly. If the temperature inside is not within the acceptable range, the vaccines must be moved to another refrigerator, in a vaccine carrier. Regular training of staff and audit of practices should be done. Assign duties to specific trained staff to be held responsible for the vaccine storage and identify back up staff. But all the staff should be versed with the plan to handle power failures and out of range temperatures.

- IAP ACVIP strongly recommends use of purpose-built refrigerator because of the several advantages.

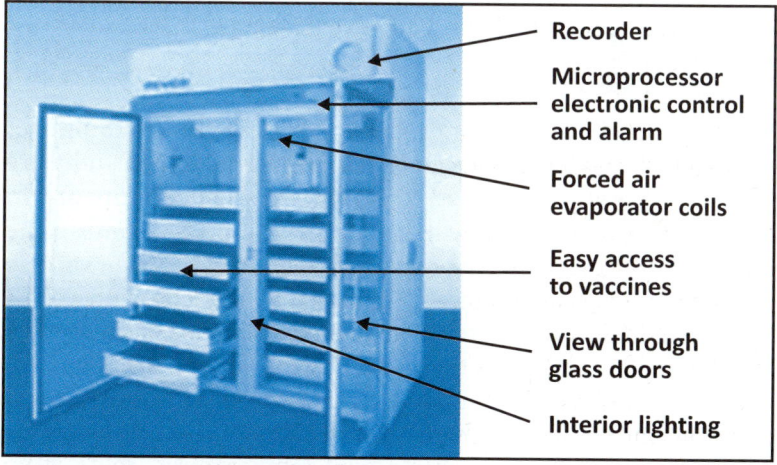

Figure 4: Purpose built refrigerator

Cold box / Vaccine carriers

These are used for transport of vaccines. They should have frozen ice packs lining the sides. To prevent cold injury, conditioned icepacks should be used rather than frozen packs. The vaccine pack should not be placed in direct contact with the icepacks but should have an intervening layer of plastic/ bubble wrap/ styroform peanuts. A thermometer should be placed in the cold box/ vaccine carrier for recording temperatures. For keeping vaccines for longer durations the walls of the thermocol box should be 2 inches thick and have a snugly fitting lid.

Box 5: Advantages of purpose built refrigerators

Purpose-built refrigerators

- Management is simpler.
- Temperatures are maintained in the 2 to 8°C range.
- Minimizes the risk of vaccines being stored outside the recommended temperature.
- Good temperature recovery after a door has been opened.
- There is more usable space for storing vaccines.
- External temperature display with mini & max
- Alarm when minimum or maximum temperatures are breached.
- Will automatically defrost, whilst maintaining a 2 to 8°C range.
- Have a lockable door and are of glass.
- Will meet medical accreditation requirements.

Storage of Vaccines

Vaccines should be kept in original packaging till use to protect from light exposure. All vaccines currently available in India are safe at temperatures between 2 and 8°C. At a temperature of 2 to 8°C, most of these vaccines have a shelf life of 24 months. The manufacturer's instructions regarding shelf life of a given vaccine must be rigorously followed. BCG, OPV, measles and MMR vaccines should be preferably kept frozen for long term storage (shelf life of 2 years). Even these vaccines, however, can be kept at 2 to 8°C for shorter periods, e.g. 6 to 12 months for OPV and 18 to 24 months for measles. Though vaccines may retain potency for variable amounts of time at ambient temperatures, there is no simple and cheap method that can be used in the field to assess whether a vaccine exposed to ambient temperature has retained at least the minimum required potency. Hence such vaccines are best discarded.[1,4]

Box 6: Various steps involved in loading a vaccine carrier

Loading a vaccine carrier

- Put conditioned ice-packs against each of the 4 sides of the vaccine carrier

- Take required vaccines and place them inside a plastic bag and place bag

- In vaccine carriers, place a foam pad on top of the conditioned ice-packs.

- Close the cold box or carrier lid tightly

- Keep thermometer inside

- Wall should be minimum 2"

Aluminium adjuvanted vaccines (DTwP, DTaP, TT, DT, Td, TT, hepatitis B, combination vaccines, hepatitis A, HPV, PCV 7) and other vaccines including IPV, PPV 23, Hib, inactivated influenza vaccines, meningococcal vaccines, rotavirus vaccines, typhoid vaccines and other brands of varicella vaccines except Varivax TM should be stored at 2 to 8°C, must never be frozen and if accidentally frozen should be discarded. The "Shake Test" can be used to determine if a vaccine vial has been suspected to be frozen at any time. The vial should be shaken so that the sediments, if any, are completely mixed. A frozen control vial should be used to compare with the test vial. During the 15 minutes test time a non-viable test vial will show sediments settling as fast as the control frozen vial. Vaccine vial found in frozen state should be directly discarded and need not undergo shake test. Diluents should never be frozen. They can be stored at 2 to 25°C and can be kept in the door compartments.

Reconstituted lyophilized vaccines (BCG, measles, MMR, Hib, rabies, rotavirus) whether single dose/ multi dose must be stored at

2 to 8°C, protected from light and used within 4 to 6 hours. Multi-dose vials of inactivated liquid vaccines once opened may be used till the expiry date on the container. OPV can be subjected to 10 cycles of freeze-thaw provided that the thawed material is kept refrigerated and the total cumulative duration of the thaw is not more than 24 hours. OPV would lose viability if kept at 22 to 25°C for more than a day. Opened vials of OPV, however, may be used in subsequent sessions at a given health facility if it has been preserved at 2 to 8°C. OPV vials used in the field setting or an outreach facility or during a pulse immunization session must be discarded at the end of the day. Vaccine vials should not be taken out to the field more than 3 times, after that these are best discarded irrespective of whether these have been opened or not.

Vaccines should be transported only in cold boxes or vaccine carriers—vacuum flasks should never be used for this purpose. During shipment and transportation, temperature and time sensitive monitor marks are used to check the cold chain. Transport is the most vulnerable time for the cold injury to vaccines.

Box 7: The WHO policy on multi-dose opened vial

WHO multi-dose opened vial policy

Opened vials of DPT, TT, DT, hepatitis B and OPV vaccines:

- May be used in subsequent immunization sessions for a maximum of one month, provided that each of the following conditions has been met:

  - Expiry date has not passed;

  - Vaccines are stored under appropriate cold chain conditions;

  - The vaccine vial septum has not been submerged in water;

  - Aseptic technique used to withdraw all doses;

Opened vials of measles, BCG & yellow fever vaccines:

- Reconstituted vials of measles, BCG and yellow fever vaccines must be discarded at the end of each immunization session or at the end of six hours, whichever comes first.

Box 8: The recommended time limits for different vaccines

Time limits for using vaccines after reconstitution

- Varicella: 30 min (and protect from light)

- MMRV: 30 min (and protect from light)

- Yellow fever: 1 hour

- Measles/MMR: 4 to 6 hours

- Meningococcal polysaccharide vaccine single dose vial: 30 min

- DTaP/Hib combination: 30 min

However, WHO is actively considering that certain heat stable vaccines like DTwP, DTaP, TT, DT, Td, TT, hepatitis B to be removed from the cold chain because of the following reasons:

- To reach more children beyond the existing cold chain in hard-to-reach rural populations.

- To enable on-time birth doses where home births are common and hepatitis B is endemic.

- To reduce/eliminate the risk of freezing.

References

1. Vaccine Storage Equipment, Vaccine Storage and Handling Toolkit; National Center for Immunization and Respiratory Diseases, CDC available online from http://www.cdc.gov/ vaccines/recs/storage/toolkit/storage-handling-toolkit.pdf.

2. Immunization Handbook for Medical Officers. Ministry of Health and Family Welfare, Government of India, 2008, available online http://nihfw.org/pdf/NCHRC-Publications/ ImmuniHandbook.pdf.

3. Immunization Handbook for Health workers, 2011, Ministry of Health and Family Welfare, Government of India, 2011, available online http://www.searo.who.int /india/topics/ routine_immunization/ Immunization_Handbook_for_Health_Workers_English_2011.pdf.

4. Handbook for Vaccine & Cold Chain Handlers, Ministry of Health and Family Welfare, Govt. of India & UNICEF, 2010, available online http:// www.unicef.org/india/Cold_chain_book_Final_(Corrected19-04-10).pdf.

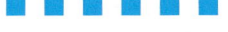

ADVERSE EVENTS FOLLOWING IMMUNIZATION

Reviewed by
Anuradha Bose, Vipin M. Vashishtha

Although vaccines are proven to be extremely safe, there is a potential risk of an adverse reaction, as with any other drug or medication. The Adverse Event Following Immunization (AEFI) is defined as "a medical incident that takes place after immunization, causes concern and is believed to be caused by the immunization".[1] Any untoward medical occurrence which follows immunization and which does not necessarily have a causal relationship with the use of the vaccine is clubbed under AEFI. The adverse event may be any unfavorable or unintended sign, an abnormal laboratory finding, a symptom or a disease.

This risk of AEFI with vaccination is always weighed against the risk of not immunizing a child. It is only when the benefit outweighs the risk, that a vaccine is considered safe. However, even at a relatively low rate, because of the high absolute number of beneficiaries, there is risk of a few serious adverse events in the vaccinated children.[2] These events may be recognized during clinical trials or during post-marketing surveillance (e.g. intussusceptions following human rhesus rotavirus vaccine. Tolerance to vaccine associated adverse events is generally lower as these are administered to healthy children unlike other pharmaceutical products used in morbid populations. Vaccine associated adverse events are more likely to be noticed and communicated and can often significantly impact immunization programs as noticed with MMR and pertussis vaccines.

Importance of AEFI

The vaccines are foreign for human bodies, given to healthy infants and children. In the natural process of developing immunity, a vaccine may cause fever, erythema, local pain, etc. Besides, there is a slight risk of foreign body reaction to the components in the vaccines. These factors are likely to cause some concerns in the caregivers/parents. Whatever the cause, an AEFI may upset people to the extent that they may refuse further vaccination for their children. This may lead to the children much more likely to get a vaccine preventable disease, become seriously ill, disabled, and risk death. AEFI surveillance, therefore, helps to preserve public confidence in the immunization program.[2] Though, the majorities of AEFIs are mild, settle without treatment, and have no long-term consequences; very rarely, serious adverse reaction can occur. The vaccination programs work in a 'paradox' meaning thereby that the focus of attention changes with the implementation of immunization program—when the vaccination coverage increases and disease burden reduces drastically, more cases of AEFI attract the attention of the people than the disease in the community.[3] Figure 1 depicts how AEFI impacts an ongoing immunization program.

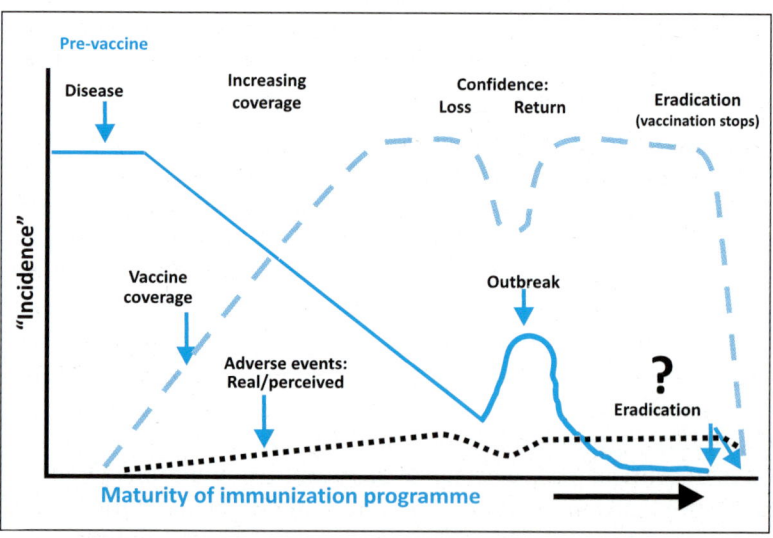

Figure 1. Impact of AEFI on immunization programs
(Adapted from: Chen RT et al, Vaccine 1994; 12: 542–50)

Classification of AEFI

For the programmatic purpose, the AEFIs are classified in five broad categories.[4,5] Table 1 provides brief description of each reaction.

Table 1: Different types of AEFIs
(Source: Adapted from "Immunization Safety Surveillance: Guidelines for managers of immunization programmes on reporting and investigating adverse events following immunization. Manila: World Health Organization, 1999.")

Vaccine reaction	Event caused by the vaccine, e.g., VAPP following OPV; or precipitated by the vaccine when given correctly, e.g. febrile seizure following vaccination in a predisposed child.
Programme error	Event caused by an error in vaccine preparation, handling, or administration, e.g. deaths following measles vaccination due to toxic shock syndrome resulting from improper reconstitution and storage of measles vaccine is the most recent example.
Injection reaction	Event from anxiety about, or pain from, the injection itself rather than the vaccine. Examples include syncope due to pain of vaccination, injection site abscesses, sciatic nerve damage due to gluteal injection.
Coincidental	Event that happens after immunization but not caused by the vaccine—a chance association. Example is the association between immunization and Sudden Infant Death Syndrome (SIDS or cot death), as the incidence of SIDS peaks around the age when infant immunizations are delivered.
Unknown	The cause of the event cannot be determined.

The AEFI reactions can broadly be classified as 'serious AEFIs' (death, disability, cluster and hospitalization) which need to be reported immediately and investigated as per the laid down procedures. The other, i.e. 'minor/non-serious AEFIs' are reported through monthly reporting systems in UIP in Government of India.[2] A serious AEFI is defined as that which is i) fatal or life threatening or ii) results in persistent or significant disability, incapacity or iii) results in or prolongs hospitalization or iv) leads to congenital anomalies/ birth defects. Important adverse reactions that are not immediately life-threatening or do not result in death or hospitalization but may jeopardize the patient should also be considered as serious.

Adverse reactions

An adverse reaction is an undesirable side effect that occurs after a vaccination. Vaccine adverse reactions are classified as a) local, b) systemic, or c) allergic.[6]

a) Local reactions: Most parenteral vaccines induce some degree of local reactions including pain, erythema and induration. Local reactions are more with whole cell pertussis vaccines and aluminium adjuvanted (DTPw, DTaP, DT, Td, Tdap, TT, hepatitis B, hepatitis A, inactivated combination vaccines, HPV and PCV) vaccines. Most studies show the frequency of local reactions to increase with subsequent doses and frequently administered doses (TT). Local reactions may be partly ameliorated by ice application and paracetamol.

b) Systemic reactions: Fever is the most common systemic reaction. Fever is more common with whole cell pertussis vaccines and aluminium adjuvanted vaccines. However, unlike local reactions, the incidence of fever and other systemic reactions usually declines with increasing age and increasing number of doses. Prophylactic administration of paracetamol at the time of administration of vaccine has been found to blunt immune responses of some vaccines, however, it may be used judiciously especially in children predisposed to febrile seizures. Fever due to vaccination does not usually last for more than 48 hours and any fever persisting beyond this time should be evaluated for other causes.

c) Allergic: Severe allergy or anaphylaxis or anaphylaxis like reactions including generalized urticaria or hives, wheezing, swelling of the mouth and throat, difficulty breathing, hypotension, and shock occur rarely at a frequency of 1 per 10,00,000 vaccinees. These reactions are rarely due to the vaccine antigen; they are usually due to other vaccine constituents including residual animal protein (e.g. egg), stabilizers or preservatives (e.g thiomersol). As a precautionary measure, the vaccine should be questioned for any immediate type of hypersensitivity to any of the vaccine constituents. Patients with history of serious allergy to any of the vaccine constituents should not receive the vaccine (exception—children with egg allergy can safely receive measles and MMR vaccines). Since occurrence of anaphylaxis cannot be predicted in most vaccines, all vaccines should be observed for 15 minutes.

Management of anaphylaxis

Although anaphylactic reactions are rare after vaccination, their immediate onset and life-threatening nature require that all personnel and facilities providing vaccinations have procedures in place for anaphylaxis management. All vaccination providers should be familiar with the office emergency plan and be currently certified in cardiopulmonary resuscitation. Anaphylaxis usually begins within minutes of vaccine administration.[6] Rapid recognition and initiation of treatment are required to prevent possible progression to cardiovascular collapse. If flushing, facial edema, urticaria, itching, swelling of the mouth or throat, wheezing, dyspnea, or other signs or symptoms of anaphylaxis occur, the patient should be placed in a recumbent position with the legs elevated if possible.[6] Administration of epinephrine is the management of choice. Additional drugs also might be indicated (Table 2). Maintenance of the airway and oxygen administration might be necessary. After the patient is stabilized, arrangements should be made for immediate transfer to an emergency facility for additional evaluation and treatment.

Table 2: Emergency management of anaphylaxis

1	Administer epinephrine (1:1000 solution) 0.01 ml/kg/dose (max 0.5 ml) intramuscular in anterolateral thigh
2	Set up IV access
3	Lay patient flat and elevate legs if tolerated. Give high flow oxygen and airway/ventilation if needed
4	If hypotensive, set up additional wide bore access and give IV normal saline 20 ml/kg under pressure over 1–2 minutes
5	IM adrenaline may be repeated after 3–5 minutes if required
6	Oral antihistaminics may be given to ameliorate skin symptoms but IV antihistaminics are not recommended. Oral or injectable corticosteroids equivalent to prednisone 1–2 mg/kg may be given but benefit is yet unproven

How to report AEFI from private sector?

The majority of children in India receive immunization through public health facilities. However, it is estimated that approximately 10–20% of total immunization is provided through private sector and by pediatricians.[7] Moreover, the vaccines not part of the UIP in India are provided by the private sector only. There is an evolving AEFI surveillance system in India for UIP vaccines from government sector; however, the reporting from private sector is limited so far. It is important that AEFI from this sector are also reported and investigated, as per the laid down national guidelines, which are applicable to private sector also. Additionally, the AEFI reporting from private sector will provide vital information on the safety of new and underutilized vaccines in India. Once a serious AEFI happens in the private sector at a clinic of pediatricians, in the rural area, she/he should immediately inform medical officer in-charge of nearest primary health center or other health facility. In the urban area, either she/he can inform medical officer-in-charge of nearest urban health center or to the 'District Immunization Officer' (DIO). By all channels, the information should reach DIO as soon as possible.[2]

The private practitioners (including pediatricians) should use the 'First Information Report' (FIR) form for reporting serious AEFI cases to the district officials. Once an AEFI is reported from private sector, the DIO and district AEFI committee members would then investigate the reported AEFI case. The pediatricians should help the investigation team in collection of all the related information.[2]

Online AEFI Reporting Platform for Private Practitioners: IAP, through its IAP Advisory Committee on Vaccines and Immunization Practices (ACVIP) has resolved to collaborate with the National AEFI program by suggesting the following measures:

- Integrate IAP disease surveillance project (IDSURV) with AEFI reporting for a web based and integrated voice recording (IVR) reporting. (www.idsurv.org)

- The IDSURV program will automatically send information to the concerned DIO/state immunization officer.

This 'public–private partnership' (PPP) has been enthusiastically received by Ministry of Health, Government of India for prompt implementation. However, if this system has to be effective, there should be an assurance from the Government that the investigation will focus on system failures rather than on individual punitive action.

Causality assessment of adverse events

Causality is the relationship between two events (the cause and the effect), where the second event is a consequence of the first. The assessment of causality in an AEFI can occur at the population level or at the individual level. The process is available for use in a WHO Manual on assessment of causality. The process should be systematic, and needs to be meticulous and detailed. There are 2 critical questions in the revised WHO causality algorithm: 1) Is there evidence in literature that this vaccine(s) may cause the reported event even if administered correctly? 2) Did the event occur within an appropriate time window after vaccine administration?

Following investigation, causality may be classified as:

i)   Definitely

ii) Probably

iii) Possibly

iv) Unlikely to be related to the vaccine.

However, it must be stated that causality assessment is still an evolving science and despite taking all the measures, and adopting all the available scientific methods, sometimes it is not possible to incontrovertibly prove the causal association of an event with a vaccine. Much more advancement in this arena is needed.

To conclude, AEFIs should be recognized, and reported. Systems should be strengthened so that programmatic errors are minimized. All persons involved with immunization should be aware of AEFIs, the action to be taken in an emergency and the pathway for reporting. Investigation and redressal should focus on identifying areas for rectification, rather than on punitive action.

References

1. World Health Organization. Surveillance of Adverse Events Following Immunization, Field guide for managers of immunization programs. Geneva: World Health Organization; 1997.

2. Chitkara AJ, Thacker N, Vashishtha VM, Bansal CP, Gupta SG. Adverse event following immunization (AEFI) surveillance in India, position paper of Indian Academy of Pediatrics, 2013. Indian Pediatr 2013; 50: 739–741.

3. Chen RT, Rastogi SC, Mullen JR, Hayes SW, Cochi SL, Donlon JA, et al. The vaccine adverse event reporting system (VAERS). Vaccine. 1994; 12: 542–550.

4. Government of India. Adverse Events Following Immunization: Surveillance and Response Operational Guidelines. New Delhi: Ministry of Health and Family Welfare, Government of India; 2010.

5. Government of India. Adverse Events Following Immunization: Surveillance and Response Standard Operating Procedures. New Delhi: Ministry of Health and Family Welfare, Government of India; 2010.

6. General Recommendations on Immunization, Recommendations of the Advisory Committee on Immunization Practices (ACIP), MMWR; Recommendations and Reports / Vol. 60 / No. 2 January 28, 2011.

7. Government of India. Multi Year Strategic Plan (MYP) for UIP of India 2005–10. New Delhi: Ministry of Health and Family Welfare, Government of India; 2010.

■ ■ ■ ■ ■ ■

SCHEDULING OF VACCINES

Reviewed by
Panna Choudhury

Main objectives of scheduling of vaccines are to achieve maximum effectiveness using recommended vaccines for a country while minimizing the number of health care system interactions. Epidemiological, immunological and programmatic aspects are taken into account while scheduling vaccines. In past two decades, many new vaccines have been developed, vaccination schedule is undergoing rapid changes and has become more complex.[1] Traditionally, public sector in developing countries is slow to incorporate newer vaccines as compared to private sector after the vaccine is licensed for use. Cost effectiveness, safety and effectiveness for a given region are important issues for introduction of newer vaccines. As such vaccination schedule in public sector has lesser number of vaccines as compared to those developed by private sector. It often becomes a matter of debate what is the best schedule, but the knowledge of principles that go behind making each schedule will help pediatricians to build an informed opinion.

Rationale for Immunization

Immunized individual gets protection from disease after exposure or infection with organism against which vaccine has been given. When many children in a community are immunized, even unimmunized people get protection from disease due to reduction in transmission of infection, which is known as herd immunity. Thus disease control or elimination requires the induction of protective immunity in a sufficient proportion of population that would restrict the spread of disease and even eradication as happened with smallpox.

Ideal immunization schedule

An ideal immunization schedule is dictated by various considerations foremost being appropriate immunologic response to vaccines and epidemiologic consideration of the vaccine preventable diseases. An optimal and not necessarily best immunological response may be considered appropriate for effective protection at the earliest in a situation where risk of contracting infection at an early age is high. Immunization schedule at individual level and community level often varies considerably as safety and cost effectiveness are taken into consideration. For public sector programs usually it is cost first, efficacy next followed by safety. However, at individual level it is safety first, efficacy next followed by cost. An ideal immunization schedule depends on the following considerations.[2]

Immunological: Minimum age at which vaccine elicit immune response, number of doses required, spacing of doses (interval between primary series and boosters if multiple doses are required).

Epidemiological: Susceptibility for infection and disease. Disease severity and mortality.

Programmatic: Opportunity to deliver with other scheduled interventions.

Minimum age at which the first dose of vaccine should be given

The minimum age at which a vaccine should be given is dependent on factors like disease epidemiology, immunological responsiveness, maternal antibodies:

A. **Disease epidemiology:** Protective immune response must be achieved prior to the most vulnerable age. Most vulnerable age may depend on the disease burden in a country, earlier when the burden is high and vice versa.

B. **Immunological responsiveness:** There is limitation of antibody responses in early life due to the limited and delayed induction of germinal centers in which antigen specific B cells proliferate and differentiate. Therefore, later the age better is the immunological response.

C. **Maternal antibodies:** Maternal antibodies may exert their inhibitory influence on immune responses up to 1 year of age.

D. Booster doses: Immunological principle—after initial immunization, a booster dose is intended to increase immunity against that antigen back to protective levels.

Principles of Antibody Vaccine interactions

Inactivated antigens are generally not affected by circulating antibody, so they can be administered before, after, or at the same time as the antibody. Simultaneous administration of antibody (in the form of immune globulin) and vaccine is recommended for postexposure prophylaxis of certain diseases, such as hepatitis B, rabies, and tetanus.

Live vaccines must replicate in order to cause an immune response. Antibody against injected live vaccine antigen may interfere with replication. If a live injectable vaccine (measles-mumps-rubella [MMR], varicella, or combination measles-mumps-rubella-varicella [MMRV]) must be given around the time that antibody is given, the two must be separated by enough time so that the antibody does not interfere with viral replication. If the live vaccine is given first, it is necessary to wait at least 2 weeks (i.e., an incubation period) before giving the antibody. If the antibody is given before a dose of MMR or varicella vaccine, it is necessary to wait until the antibody has waned (degraded) before giving the vaccine to reduce the chance of interference by the antibody. The necessary interval between an antibody-containing product and MMR or varicella-containing vaccine (except zoster vaccine) depends on the concentration of antibody in the product, but is always 3 months or longer.

Combination vaccines

As more effective vaccines are being developed, the question of the number of needle pricks to which the young infants are subjected to becomes important. More vaccines may also lead to more visits to physicians. Combination vaccines represent one solution to the issue of increased number of injections during a single visit. Among the traditional vaccines DPT combination was a standard for a long time, so was MMR. Logical additions to DPT were Hib, injectable polio, hepatitis B. The preservation of efficacy will need to be continually seen by trials and monitored by surveillance as more such combinations are on the horizon.

Factors that affect the inclusion of a new vaccine in the national immunization program

1. Disease (burden, severity, mortality, national security, risk of importation, competing priorities)

2. Recipient (age, cohort size, politics)

3. Vaccine (local production, availability, cost, efficacy, safety, other vaccines)

In countries still having a high burden of natural disease, disease prevention and controlling the morbidity and mortality is the most important objective, therefore, vaccine with highest effectiveness is chosen for inclusion in the national program, whereas in a country with a low burden of natural disease, the main concerns are low or no side effects of a new vaccine which will decide acceptance of the vaccine. Therefore, a vaccine with a high safety level can only be included in the immunization schedule.

Catch up immunization

Missed immunization does not require restarting of the entire series or addition of doses to the series for any vaccine in the recommended schedule. Two or more inactivated vaccines can be given simultaneously or at any interval between doses without affecting the immune response. An inactive vaccine can similarly be given simultaneously or at any interval with a live vaccine. However, 2 live (intranasal/injectable) vaccines should either be given simultaneously or at least 4 weeks apart. If a dose of DTP, IPV, Hib, pneumococcal conjugate, hepatitis A, hepatitis B, HPV, MMR, or varicella vaccine is missed, subsequent immunization should be given at the next visit as if the usual interval had elapsed. For rota vaccine same principle can be followed, though upper age limit of last dose should be maintained. Minimal interval recommendation should be followed for administration of all doses.

Adolescent immunization

Tdap and HPV are vaccines prescribed for adolescent immunization in India by IAP.[3] Meningococcal conjugate vaccine is recommended for adolescents in the U.S.

WHO recommendations

The World Health Organization monitors vaccination schedules across the world, noting what vaccines are included in each country's program, the coverage rates achieved and various auditing measures (Table 1).[4] WHO gives broad guidelines to help different countries prepare their vaccination schedules according to their epidemiological needs and cost effectiveness. Summary of WHO position papers on Recommendations for Routine Immunization are regularly updated.[5] WHO further subclassifies the vaccines as: (a) Recommendations for all individuals (BCG, hepatitis B, DPT, polio, Hib, PCV, rotavirus, measles, rubella, HPV); (b) Recommendations for individuals residing in certain regions (JE, yellow fever, tick borne encephalitis); (c) Recommendations for individuals in some high-risk populations (typhoid, cholera, meningococcal, hepatitis A, rabies); (d) Recommendations for individuals receiving vaccinations from immunization programs with certain characteristics (mumps, influenza).

Table 1: Vaccination schedule under UIP in India, 2013

Vaccine	When to give	Dose	Route	Site
For pregnant women				
TT-1	Early in pregnancy	0.5 ml	Intra-muscular	Upper arm
TT-2	4 weeks after TT-1*	0.5 ml	Intra-muscular	Upper arm
TT-Booster	If received 2 TT doses in a pregnancy within the last 3 years	0.5 ml	Intra-muscular	Upper arm
For infants				
BCG	At birth or as early as possible till one year of age	0.1 ml (0.05 ml until month of age)	Intra-dermal	Left upper arm
Hepatitis B birth dose	At birth or as early as possible within 24 hours	0.5 ml	Intra-muscular	Antero-lateral side of mid-thigh

Table 1: Vaccination schedule under UIP in India, 2013 *(Contd.)*

Vaccine	When to give	Dose	Route	Site
For infants				
OPV zero dose	At birth or as early as possible within the first 15 days	2 drops	Oral	Oral
OPV 1,2 & 3	At 6 weeks, 10 weeks and 14 weeks	2 drops	Oral	Oral
DPT 1,2 & 3		0.5 ml	Intra-muscular	Antero-lateral side of mid-thigh
Hepatitis B 1,2 & 3		0.5 ml	Intra-muscular	Antero-lateral side of mid-thigh
Hib 1, 2 & 3		0.5 ml	Intra-muscular	Antero-lateral side of mid-thigh
Measles 1st dose	9 completed months–12 months (give up to 5 years if not received at 9–12 months age)	0.5 ml	Sub-cutaneous	Right upper arm
JE 1st dose**	9 completed months	0.5 ml	Sub-cutaneous	Left upper arm
For children and adolescents				
DPT booster	16–24 months	0.5 ml	Intra-muscular	Antero-lateral side of mid-thigh
OPV booster	16–24 months	2 drops	Oral	Oral
Measles 2nd dose	16–24 Months	0.5 ml	Sub-cutaneous	Right upper arm
Rubella***	16–24 months adolescent girls	0.5 ml	Sub-cutaneous	Right upper arm
JE 2nd dose	16–24 months with DPT/OPV booster	0.5 ml	Sub-cutaneous	Left Upper arm
DPT booster 2	5–7 years	0.5 ml	Intra-muscular	Upper arm
TT	10 years and 16 years	0.5 ml	Intra-muscular	Upper arm
Vitamin A****				

* Give TT-2 or booster doses before 36 weeks of pregnancy. However, give these even if more than 36 weeks have passed. Give TT to a woman in labor, if she has not previously received TT.

** JE vaccine (SA 14-14-2) is given in select endemic districts, after the campaign is over in that district.

*** Rubella vaccine will be given as part of measles 2nd dose

**** The 2nd to 9th doses of vitamin A can be administered to children 1–5 years old during biannual rounds, in collaboration with ICDS.

Table 1 summarizes National Immunization Schedule under UIP in India, whereas IAP Immunization Schedule 2013 is included as Appendix 2.

References

1. "History of Vaccine Schedule," Children's Hospital of Philadelphia, last modified June 2010, http:/ / www.chop.edu /service /vaccine-education-center/vaccine-schedule/ history-of-vaccine-schedule.html.

2. Choudhury P. Scheduling of Vaccine. In: IAP Text Book of Vaccines, Eds,Vashishtha VM, Agarwal R, Sukumaran T, Indian Academy of Pediatrics, Jaypee Brothers, New Delhi, 2013.

3. Indian Academy of Pediatrics Committee on Immunization (IAPCOI). Consensus recommendation on Immunization and IAP Immunization Timetable 2012. Indian Pediatr. 2012; 49:560.

4. WHO vaccine-preventable diseases: Monitoring system. 2013 global summary. Available from http://apps.who.int/immunization_monitoring/ globalsummary/schedules. (Accessed on Nov 26, 2013)

5. World Health Organisation (Internet). Updated 1st August 2013. Available from: http://www.who.int/immunization/policy/Immunization_routine_ table1.pdf. (Accessed on Nov 26, 2013)

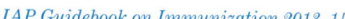

LICENSING PROCEDURE AND INCLUSION OF A VACCINE IN THE NATIONAL IMMUNIZATION PROGRAM (NIP) OF A COUNTRY

2.8

Reviewed by
VG Ramchandran & Panna Choudhury

National Regulatory Authority (NRA) and Licensing Procedure

The National Regulatory Authority (NRA) of a country is a statutory body that performs the task of not only providing license to a particular vaccine to be used in that country, but also acts as a watchdog on all other issues related to performance of that vaccine in the country where it is licensed. NRA supervises the vaccine lot release and performs laboratory inspections along with supervision of post-marketing surveillance for AEFI. NRA also sanctions the vaccine trials, determines the adequacy of the trials by the vaccine companies, supervises the proper conduct of vaccine trials including ethical and humanitarian aspects and has the power to discontinue even an ongoing trial if some irregularities are noted. It is also the duty of NRA to redress all the issues pertaining to safety, efficacy, and effectiveness of a vaccine after licensing.[1]

The vaccines licensing authority in India, i.e. the NRA is Drugs Controller General of India (DCGI) which is approved by WHO. The FDA (Food and Drug Administration) is the government agency responsible for regulating food, dietary supplements, drugs, cosmetics, medical devices, biologics and blood products in the United States.[2] NRA /DCGI are the equivalent agency in India that performs almost all these tasks.

For licensing of a new vaccine, the vaccine manufacturer should conduct the phase I, II, and III trials and must submit their results to NRA for its approval. There are both central and state licensing authorities. Good Clinical Practice (GCP) and ethical guidelines (by ICMR) for approval exist. Licensing of products in India is by the Central Licensing Approval Authority (CLAA). The Drug

Technology Advisory Board (DTAB) approves introduction of vaccines into the immunization services, while all vaccine approval and clinical trials is by the CLAA. The state licensing authority inspects and grants licensing for retail.[3]

Imported products are considered on a case-to-case basis; if trials meet the requirements of the NRA, there is no insistence on clinical trials in the country for registration. The advisory committee that review the information follow published guidelines, directed by a responsible person. External clinical experts may be asked for advice on a case-to-case basis.

After licensing, the vaccine manufacturer should undertake a large post-marketing surveillance (phase IV) to further ensure the safety of their products. Any complaint regarding the safety, efficacy, etc of the licensed vaccine should be directed to NRA. Once the vaccine is licensed in the country, it can be used both by the private as well as the public sector.[3] Figure 1 displays various steps undertaken in vaccine approval and development in India.

Introduction of a new vaccine in the NIP

The issue of introduction of a new vaccine in the National Immunization Program (NIP) is a bit complex. There are several factors that determine introduction of a new vaccine in NIP for mass/public use that include disease burden, cost-effectiveness of a vaccination program, suitability of vaccine products available in the world market, safety and efficacy of the vaccine, programmatic issues, etc. Although inclusion of a new vaccine in national schedule adds to the cost of vaccine and logistics to the health budget of a country, it also results in savings by reduction of the disease burden. Still, the decision to include a new vaccine in national schedule is not straightforward and there are numerous issues in prioritizing investments of a NIP. These issues need to be tackled systematically, providing best possible immunization schedule as per the needs and resources of the country.[4]

The Ministry of Health & Family Welfare (MOHFW)/ Government of India (GOI) has an advisory committee to give recommendations to it on inclusion of any new vaccine in the NIP, i.e. National Technical Advisory Group on Immunization (NTAGI), where IAP too has its representation through its national president who is an important member of this committee.

Issues in decision making

Issues involved in decision are not only policy issues (whether introduction of the new vaccine is in sync with immunization policy of the country), but also technical or programmatic (whether implementation of the decision is technically feasible). Table 1 lists various issues involved in the decision making.

Table 1: Issues involved in introduction of a new vaccine in National Immunization Program

Policy issues
• Assessment of public health priority
➢ Assessment of disease burden in the country
➢ Other preventive measures available (including other vaccine, if any)
• Assessment of candidate vaccine
➢ Efficacy, quality and safety
➢ Economic / financial issues
Technical / programmatic issues
• Vaccine presentation
• Programmatic strength (logistic issues)
• Supply availability

Assessment of public health priority

Prioritization of various public health measures within limited resources is the most challenging task for any country. Public health importance of a disease varies from country to country. Hence, assessment of the burden of the disease in question vis-à-vis other diseases is the first important step in decision making. Introduction of vaccine against the disease with highest disease burden will naturally have greatest impact on infant/childhood mortality and morbidity on national basis. This is one of the most important evidence to convince the policy makers to introduce the candidate vaccine.

The disease burden is assessed not only in terms of incidence and prevalence, but also in terms of annual hospitalizations, disability rate and mortality rate of the disease in question. Ideally, either data from surveillance systems of the country or well designed, multi-centric studies or meta-analyses of studies from the country should form the basis of such assessment. However, in the absence of local studies, data from countries with similar social and demographic characteristics can be used. If the data available is incomplete, mathematical models can be used (with due caution) in assessment of disease burden.

For assessment of disease burden, data on causative organism rather than clinical syndrome is needed. For example, in India, diarrhea and pneumonia remain the leading causes of non-neonatal mortality accounting for 20% and 19% of all under 5 deaths respectively. However, only a proportion of these are preventable by vaccines (Rotavirus, *Haemophilus influenzae* type b and pneumococcus).

Since policy decision for introduction of a vaccine in national immunization schedule has socio-political implication, mass acceptability of a vaccine is very important in a democratic country. The more important and visible the disease is, and safer and more effective is the vaccine perceived to be, the better is the acceptance and uptake of the new vaccine. Any misconception or opposition to the vaccine should be cleared using various channels of communication. This helps in arriving at a decision faster.

When deciding about the priority of a particular vaccine, it is also important to consider other vaccines which are likely to be available in the near future. Similarly, vaccine introduction could be postponed if it is likely that another vaccine would become available in the near future against another disease that presents a greater burden.

Assessment of other interventions available

The proposed vaccine should be compared with other preventive measures (including any existing vaccine) available in terms of effectiveness, safety and feasibility before making a decision on introduction of the vaccine in national immunization schedule.

Assessment of efficacy, quality and safety of the vaccine

The vaccine needs to be efficacious in preventing the disease in immunized individuals. However, it must be noted that the data on efficacy should also be preferably taken from countries with similar disease epidemiology to one considering the use of a hitherto alien vaccine. This is because the efficacy of a vaccine can vary with nutritional status, genetic 'makeup' of the vaccine, co-infections and other factors (Figure 1).

The vaccine being considered for introduction should meet international standards of quality and safety. The data on safety should be obtained not only from clinical trials but also from

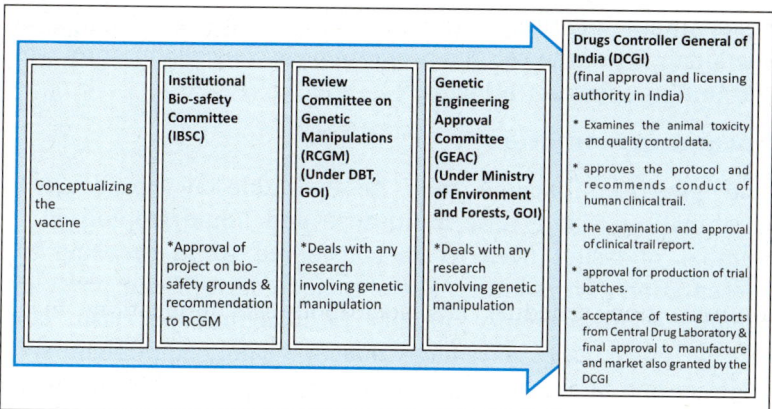

Figure 1: Vaccine approval and development path in India

post-marketing surveillance from other countries with similar profile.[5] Such data, if available, is very useful as it can throw light on rarer adverse events associated with the vaccine. The effect of introduction of a "new" vaccine on the efficacy and safety of other vaccines given at the same time also needs to be explored. It is also important to note that the risk: benefit ratio of a vaccine can vary from country to country depending upon disease burden.

Economic/financial issues

The vaccines other than EPI vaccines are "expensive", when cost is compared on dose-to-dose basis. Hence, cost-effectiveness analysis is essential before any decision on the vaccine introduction is taken by a developing country.[6] The total cost (cost of vaccine and logistics) is compared to the potential savings as a result of reduction in the number requiring treatment of the disease. The cost-effectiveness is also compared with that of another vaccine or another public health program under consideration.

Various methods and tools adopted by the WHO for cost-effectiveness analysis can be used for this purpose. Due care is taken to assess financial sustainability (over medium to long term) of the immunization program after introduction of the new vaccine. If any financial shortfall is expected, appropriate sources of funding also need to be explored before finalizing introduction of the vaccine. If a donor agency is supporting introduction of a new vaccine into the NIP of a country, it is imperative for the national government of that country to look into the long-term sustainability of the vaccine program once the collaboration with the funding agency terminates.[7]

Vaccine presentation

The proposed vaccine may be available as monovalent/ combination, single dose/multi-dose and liquid/lyophilized. A number of issues need to be considered while choosing the presentation /formulation. These include current and proposed immunization schedule, number of injections per visit, cold storage space, vaccine wastage, injection safety equipment, staff training and supervision, recording and reporting mechanisms, and program costs, possibility of bulk imports from producer company/country and bottling at user country utilizing existing facilities in the situations of user country with a proviso for premature termination of contracted bulk-supply if another preparation, perceived to be a better one by the user country becomes available with minimal or no financial riders. If the preferred presentation is unavailable, the country can either postpone introduction or start with another option and switch to preferred option later.

Vaccine supply, availability and quality

This is a crucial issue for developing countries with large populations. The newer vaccines are often manufactured by a limited number of manufacturers and it takes some time to augment production following introduction of vaccine in national immunization program. In addition to current supply situation, future trends need to be assessed carefully before decision-making. A country may decide on phased introduction depending on supply availability. The introduction of conjugated pneumococcal vaccine has been delayed in most countries because of logistic and procurement issues.

Assessment of required doses would obviously depend on target population, estimated coverage and wastage. For vaccine doses requirement in next few years, we need to estimate the increase in target population as well as vaccine coverage. Not only quantity, but the quality of vaccine to be procured also needs to be assessed. Many developing countries prefer to use vaccines procured through UNICEF. These vaccines are already prequalified by the

WHO through a standardized procedure and packaging and transporting conditions are identified for proper cold chain maintenance. In case the country decides to procure its own vaccines, a number of issues are to be looked into. A technical committee should review the technical issues including efficacy and data of the brand concerned as well as the packaging and transportation conditions required. Further, post-marketing surveillance is critical to ensure vaccine quality after licensing. An elaborate protocol must be formulated for strict compliance later on.

Programmatic strength

The NIP of the country must be functioning well with existing vaccines before finalizing introduction of the new vaccine.[8] Otherwise, vaccine addition would further worsen the failing system and will have long-term repercussions. Careful assessment of requirement of additional cold chain capacity, safe injection supplies and disposal, adequate staff, staff training and supervision, advocacy and awareness programs (IEC activities) is essential before finalizing introduction of the new vaccine. Any shortfall in this regard (financial or otherwise) must be addressed beforehand for smooth introduction of the vaccine.

In the Indian context, the feasibility of insisting the producer company to apportion a certain percent of profit generated by the sale of their product as a corpus and vest it with a responsible and credited trustee for providing insurance cover or other financial needs that may arise as a result of mass vaccine-use, post-licensure, may be explored.

References

1. Central Drugs Standard Control Organization. Guidance for Industry on Submission of Clinical Trial Application for Evaluating Safety and Efficacy. Available from http://cdsco.nic.in/CDSCO-GuidanceForIndustry.pdf. (Accessed on Dec 15, 2013)

2. FDA. Vaccines, Blood and Biologics. Available from http://www.fda.gov/ BiologicsBloodVaccines/default.htm. (Accessed on Dec 15, 2013)

3. Yewale V, Vashishtha V. Reply: Newer vaccines-Indian Scenario. Indian Pediatrics, 2009; 46: 1025–1026.

4. World Health Organization. Vaccine introduction guidelines—adding a vaccine to a national immunization program: Decision and implementation,

2005. Available at: http://whqlibdoc.who.int/hq/2005/WHO_IVB_05.18.pdf.

5. Chen RT, Hibbs B. Vaccine safety: Current and future challenges. Pediatr Ann 1998; 27: 445–455.

6. Kumar P, Vashishtha VM. The issues related to introduction of a new vaccine in National Immunization Program of a developing country. J Pediatric Sciences. 2010;5:e44

7. WHO. Economics of immunization: A guide to the literature and other resources, Geneva, 2004. Available at: http: // whqlibdoc.who.int/hq/2004/WHO_V&B_04.02.pdf. (Accessed on Dec 15, 2013)

8. Tapia-Conyer R, Betancourt-Cravioto M, Saucedo-Martínez R, Motta-Murguía L, Gallardo-Rincón H. Strengthening vaccination policies in Latin America: an evidence-based approach. Vaccine 2013; 3: 3826–3833.

■ ■ ■ ■ ■ ■

Licensed Vaccines

BACILLUS CALMETTE GUERIN (BCG) VACCINE

3.1

Reviewed by
A.K. Patwari

Background

Globally, about 1 million cases of pediatric tuberculosis are estimated to occur every year accounting for 10–15% of all tuberculosis (TB).[1] The exact burden of childhood TB in India is unknown due to diagnostic difficulties but it is estimated to be 10% of the total adult incidence.[2] The proportion of pediatric TB cases registered under RNTCP has shown an increasing trend, from 5.6% in 2005 to 7% in 2011.[3] Prevention of childhood tuberculosis is thus an important priority. However, in comparison to other EPI vaccines, efficacy of BCG vaccine is limited. Several new vaccines against tuberculosis are in development phase, and many are designed to boost pre-existing immunity induced by BCG[4] and some candidates aim to ultimately replace BCG as the priming vaccine.[5]

Vaccine

BCG vaccine is derived from the bovine tuberculosis strain and was first developed in 1921. It was the result of painstaking efforts by the French microbiologist, Albert Calmette, and the veterinary surgeon, Camille Guerin, who performed 231 repeated subcultures over 13 years. It continues to be the only effective vaccine against tuberculosis. The two common strains in use are Copenhagen (Danish 1331) and Pasteur, of which the former was produced in India at the BCG Laboratories, Guindy, Tamil Nadu till recently. BCG induces cell-mediated immunity, but the protective efficacy is a matter of debate and is very difficult to quantify. It has an efficacy of 75–86 % for prevention of miliary and meningeal form of the disease. Protective efficacy for pulmonary tuberculosis is 50%.[6]

The vaccine contains 0.1–0.4 million live viable bacilli per dose. It is supplied as a lyophilized (freeze-dried) preparation in vacuum sealed, multi-dose, dark colored ampoules or 2 ml vials with normal saline as diluent. The vaccine is light sensitive and deteriorates on exposure to ultra violet rays. In lyophilized form, it can be stored at 2 to 80°C for up to 12 months without losing its potency. The long necked, BCG ampoule, should be cut carefully by gradual filing at the junction of its neck and body, as sudden gush of air in the vacuum sealed ampoule may lead to spillage of the contents. Diluent should be used for reconstitution. Sterile normal saline may be used if diluent is not available. As the vaccine contains no preservative, bacterial contamination and consequent toxic shock syndrome may occur if kept for long after reconstitution. The reconstituted vaccine should be stored at 2 to 8°C, protected from light and discarded within 4–6 hours of reconstitution.

The recommended dose is 0.1 ml or 0.05 ml as suggested by the manufacturer of the vaccine. Dosage does not depend on the age and weight of the baby. Injection of BCG should be strictly intradermal, using a tuberculin syringe and a 26G / 27G needle. The convex aspect of the left shoulder at level of deltoid insertion is preferred for easy visualization of the BCG scar and for optimum lymphatic drainage. Other sites such as thigh should be avoided. The selected site may be swabbed clean using sterile saline and local antiseptics should be avoided. A wheal of 5 mm at the injection site indicates successful intradermal administration of the vaccine. Subcutaneous administration of BCG is associated with an increased incidence of BCG adenitis. The injected site usually shows no visible change for several days. Subsequently, a papule develops after 2–3 weeks, which increases to a size of 4–8 mm by the end of 5–6 weeks. This papule often heals with ulceration and results in a scar after 6–12 weeks. The ulcer at vaccination site may persist for a few weeks before formation of the final scar. No treatment is required for this condition.

Secondary infection at the vaccination site may require antimicrobials. Ipsilateral axillary/cervical lymphadenopathy may develop a few weeks/months after BCG vaccination. Antitubercular therapy is of no benefit in such situations and should not be administered. The nodes regress spontaneously after a few months. It should also be noted that if fine needle aspiration cytology of the nodes is carried out, stain for acid-fast bacilli may be positive. These are bovine vaccine bacilli and should not be misconstrued as being suggestive of tuberculous disease. In some children, the nodes may even liquefy and result in an abscess. Surgical removal of the nodes or repeated needle aspiration is the treatment of choice; again antitubercular therapy is not recommended. Disseminated BCG infection is extremely unusual but may occur in children with cellular immunodeficiency. BCG should be avoided in the immunocompromised, especially those with cellular immunodeficiency; it may, however, be given at birth to children born to HIV positive mothers.

BCG may be given with other vaccines on the same day or at any interval with the exception of measles/ measles mumps rubella (MMR) vaccine where a gap of 4 weeks between the two vaccines is recommended.

Recommendations for use

Individual use

The recommended age of administration is at birth (for institutional deliveries) or at 6 weeks with other vaccines. Catch up vaccination with BCG is recommended till the age of 5 years. Routine tuberculin testing prior to catch up vaccination is not necessary. BCG may be repeated once in children less than 5 years of age in the absence of a reaction/ scar presuming that BCG has not been taken up (even though most patients with absent reactions/ scars have shown in vitro evidence of cell-mediated immunity against tuberculosis). Here again, tuberculin testing prior to administration of the second dose of BCG is not necessary.

Public health perspectives

IAP ACVIP believes that despite the poor efficacy of the current BCG vaccine against pulmonary TB, it is safe, has relatively high protective efficacy against miliary and meningeal TB, does not interfere with the efficacy of other vaccines given simultaneously, and is inexpensive. Considering a very high disease burden of TB in India, the committee recommends continuation of BCG vaccine in the national immunization program of India (UIP). However, the development of new, improved TB vaccine should remain a national priority.

The failure of BCG to affect disease incidence, the growing HIV/AIDS pandemic and the appearance of multi-drug resistant *Mycobacterium tuberculosis* threaten to overwhelm current TB control strategies in many endemic areas.[7] However, until an improved vaccine is available, efforts to control the spread of TB must rely on optimal use of the tools currently available: Early diagnosis, directly observed therapy, appropriate preventive treatment and public health and infection control measures.

BCG VACCINE

Routine vaccination:

- Should be given at birth or at first contact

Catch up vaccination:

- May be given up to 5 years

References

1. World Health Organization. Guidance for National Tuberculosis Programmes on the Management of Tuberculosis in Children, WHO, Geneva, 2006.

2. Nelson LJ, Wells CD. Global epidemiology of childhood tuberculosis. Internat J Tubercul Lung Dis. 2004; 8: 636–647.

3. Central TB Division. Tuberculosis India 2012. Annual Report of the Revised National Tuberculosis Control Programme, Directorate of General Health Services, Ministry of Health and Family Welfare, Government of India, 2012.

4. Hoft DF, Blazevic A, Abate G, et al. A New Recombinant BCG Vaccine Safely Induces Significantly Enhanced TB-specific Immunity in Human Volunteers. J Infect Dis. 2008; 198(10): 1491–1501.

5. Hanekom WA, Hazel M, Dockrell HM, et al. Immunological Outcomes of New Tuberculosis Vaccine Trials: WHO Panel Recommendations PLoS Medicine July 2008, 5: 1033–1036.

6. Rodrigues LC, Diwan VK, Wheeler JG. Protective Effect of BCG against Tuberculous Meningitis and Miliary Tuberculosis: A Meta-Analysis. Int J Epidemiol 1993; 22 (6): 1154–1158.

7. BCG Vaccine, WHO position paper, Weekly epidemiological record 2004; 79: 25–40. Available from: http://www.who.int /wer/2004 /en/wer7904.pdf.

In contrast to OPV, IPV produces excellent humoral immunity as well as local pharyngeal immunity. In a study from Vellore, monkeys given 3 doses of IPV resisted infection after oral inoculation with wild poliovirus for up to 12 months. This can be explained by the fact that though IPV induces only low levels of IgA antibodies, it generates strong humoral immunity (IgG) and it has been postulated that the spill over of IgG antibodies has inhibitory influence on local infection. So ultimately the degree of mucosal immunity more closely correlates with the titre of homologous humoral antibodies.[8] Mucosal immunity is good when vaccine efficacy is higher as in case of IPV, bOPV or mOPV than tOPV.

Herd effect with polio vaccines

The phenomenon of immunized individuals affecting the epidemiology of infection (and consequently disease) in the unimmunized segment of population is referred to as herd effect. Higher the vaccine efficacy and coverage, greater the herd effect. In industrialized countries, two factors contribute to a high herd effect: 1. There is an excellent gut immunity due to a high OPV immunogenicity and 2. contact immunization of the non-immunized children due to spread of the vaccine virus from the vaccines ('contact immunity'). Both these attributes are weak in developing countries. The herd effect seen in the industrialized countries is not visible in India and is evident by the following facts: 1. Repeated doses of OPV have to be given to the same group of children, with virtually 100% coverage, before wild virus transmission could be stopped, 2. The median age of polio in India was not shifted to the right and remained stationary at 12–18 months from prior to introducing immunization till just before the elimination. On the contrary, IPV with its high immunogenicity and efficacy induces high levels of antibodies which spill over to the gut and thus prevent transmission potential of immunised individuals besides protecting them. Thus contrary to the conventional teaching, IPV exhibits a demonstrable herd effect.[6]

Recommendations for use[9]

Individual use

In the light of remarkable achievement in the field of polio eradication in India over the last few years, the committee has now decided to adopt a sequential IPV- OPV schedule.[9] This will pave the way to ultimate adoption of all-IPV schedule in future considering the inevitable cessation of OPV from immunization schedules owing to its safety issues (VAPP and cVDPVs). This policy is in accordance with the recent decision taken by GPEI where phased removal of Sabin viruses, beginning with highest risk (type 2) would be undertaken. This will result in elimination of VDPV type 2 in 'parallel' with eradication of last wild polioviruses by switching from tOPV to bOPV for routine EPI and campaigns. This switch will result in much early introduction of IPV than anticipated, at least in high risk areas for VDPVs, to provide type 2 protection.

There is considerable evidence to show that sequential schedules that provide IPV first, followed by OPV, can prevent VAPP while maintaining the critical benefits conferred by OPV (i.e., high levels of gut immunity). Data from several studies show that sequential schedules considerably decrease the risk of VAPP. There is moderate level of scientific evidence that sequential immunization schedules starting with two or more doses of IPV and followed by two or more doses of OPV(at an interval of 4–8 weeks) induce protective immunological responses to all three poliovirus serotypes in more than 90% of vaccines. However, the committee has retained the birth dose of OPV as recommended earlier. Providing the first OPV dose at a time when the infant is still protected by maternally-derived antibodies may, at least theoretically, also prevent VAPP. Though OPV at birth is not immunogenic, it enhances serocoversion of subsequent polio vaccines, both OPV and IPV considerably. A birth dose of OPV is considered necessary in countries where the risk of poliovirus transmission is high.

The primary schedule

The committee recommends birth dose of OPV, three primary doses of IPV at 6, 10 and 14 weeks, followed by two doses of OPV at 6 and 9 months, another dose (booster) of IPV at 15–18 months and OPV at 5 years. Alternatively, two doses of IPV can be used for primary series at 8 and 16 weeks, though this schedule is immunologically superior to EPI schedule and the number of IPV doses is reduced, but will be more cumbersome due to extra visits and incompatibility with combination formulations. Further, the child would be susceptible to WPV infection for the first two months of life considering the epidemiology of WPV in India till quite recently. Since IPV administered to infants in EPI schedule (i.e. 6 weeks, 10 weeks and 14 weeks) results in suboptimal seroconversion, hence, a supplementary dose of IPV is recommended at 15–18 months. IPV should be given intramuscularly (preferably) or subcutaneously and may be offered as a component of fixed combinations of vaccines. However, the committee recommends that if IPV is unaffordable or unavailable, the primary series must be completed with three doses of OPV given at 6, 10, and 14 weeks. No child should be left without adequate protection against wild poliovirus (i.e. three doses of either vaccine). All OPV doses (mono-, bi- or trivalent) offered through supplemental immunization activities (SIAs), should also be provided.

Why sequential schedule?

The committee believes that the polio vaccines contained in the schedule should have some strategic purpose. In the previous 'combined' schedule, both OPV and IPV were administered simultaneously with the objective of maximizing immune responses in an individual. It was the need of the hour since wild poliovirus circulation was unhampered despite intensive SIAs at that time. However, since the achievement of elimination of wild poliovirus since 2011, the focus has now shifted to safety issues, VAPP for individual protection, and VDPV for public health needs. The provision of IPV before OPV will take care of VAPP in an individual. Birth dose of OPV does not lead to VAPP.

The reasons behind not proposing 'all IPV' schedule are:

- Committee believes OPV is still needed as long as the risk of wild poliovirus importation from neighbouring countries exists;
- OPV provides critical benefit of superior gut immunity in comparison of IPV,
- Since IAP is committed to support GPEI activities conducted in the country, and SIAs employing OPVs are still going on, it would be neither appropriate nor feasible to avoid complete contact with OPV.

Catch-up schedule

IPV may be offered as 'catch up vaccination' for children less than 5 years of age who have completed primary immunization with OPV. IPV can be given as three doses; two doses at two months interval followed by a third dose after 6 months of last dose. This schedule will ensure a long lasting protection against poliovirus disease.

Recommendations for travellers

The committee has now issued the following recommendations for travelers to polio-endemic countries or areas:[9]

- For those who have previously received at least 3 doses of OPV or IPV should be offered another dose of polio vaccine as a once—only dose before departure.

- Non-immunized individuals should complete a primary schedule of polio vaccine, using either IPV or OPV. Primary series includes at least three doses of either vaccine.

- For people who travel frequently to polio-endemic areas but who stay only for brief periods, a one-time only additional dose of a polio vaccine after the primary series should be sufficient to prevent disease.

Public health perspectives

IAP is signatory to Scientific declaration on polio eradication and fully support Global Polio Eradication and End Game Strategic Plan developed by GPEI and launched in April 2013.[10]

The Polio Eradication and Endgame Strategic Plan 2013–2018[10] was developed by GPEI in 2013 to capitalize on this new opportunity to end all polio disease. It accounts for the parallel pursuit of wild poliovirus eradication and cVDPV elimination, while planning for the backbone of the polio eradication effort to be used for delivering other health services to the world's most vulnerable children.

The four main objectives of the Plan are

1. Poliovirus detection and interruption.

2. Routine immunization strengthening and OPV withdrawal.

3. Containment and certification.

4. Legacy planning.

A proposed timeline of various events is summarized in Figure 1. More details on Polio Eradication and End Game Plan can be found on http://www.polioeradication.org/Resourcelibrary/ Strategyandwork/Strategicplan.aspx

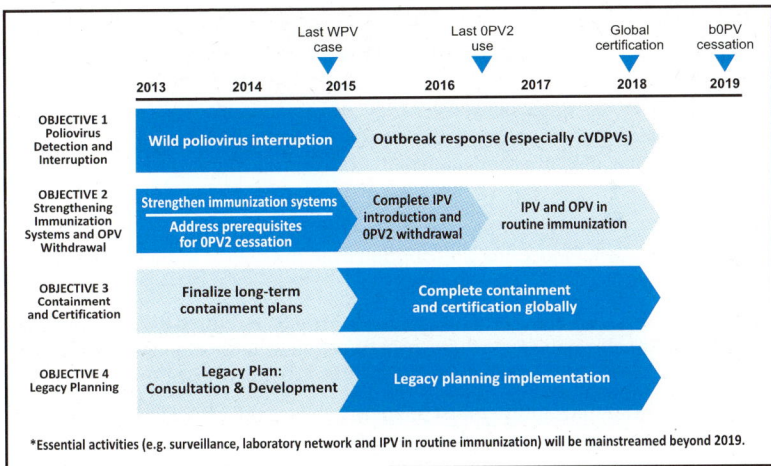

Figure 1: A proposed timeline and component of Polio Eradication & Endgame Strategic Plan 2013–2018.

POLIOVIRUS VACCINES

Routine vaccination

- Recommended schedule: Birth dose of OPV, three primary doses of IPV at 6, 10 and 14 weeks, followed by two doses of OPV at 6 and 9 months, another dose (booster) of IPV at 15–18 months, and OPV at 5 years.
- Birth dose of OPV usually does not lead to VAPP.
- OPV in place of IPV, if IPV is unfeasible, minimum 3 doses.
- Additional doses of OPV on all SIAs.
- IPV: Minimum age — 6 weeks.
- IPV: 2 instead of 3 doses can also be used if primary series started at 8 weeks and the interval between the doses is kept 8 weeks.
- No child should leave your facility without polio immunization (IPV or OPV), if indicated by the schedule!!

Catch-up vaccination

- IPV catch-up schedule: 2 doses at 2 months apart followed by a booster after 6 months of previous dose.

References

1. www.polioeradication.org. (Accessed on 24-11-2013)

2. John TJ, Vashishtha VM. Eradicating poliomyelitis: India's journey from hyperendemic to polio-free status. Indian J Med Res. 2013; 137: 881–894.

3. Sutter RW, Kew OM, Cochi SL. Poliovirus vaccine live. Chapter 26; in Vaccines 5th edition 2008, pp 643–664. Eds SA Plotkin, Orenstein WR and Offit PA, Philadelphia, Saunders, Elsevier.

4. Grassly NC, Fraser C, Wenger J, Deshpande JM, Sutter RW, Heymann DL, et al. New strategies for the elimination of polio from India. Science 2006; 314: 1150–1153.

5. Kohler KA, Banerjee K, Gary Hlady W, Andrus JK, Sutter RW.Vaccine-associated paralytic poliomyelitis in India during 1999: Decreased risk despite massive use of oral polio vaccine, Bull World Health Organ. 2002; 80(3): 210–216.

6. John TJ. Understanding the scientific basis of preventing polio by immunization. Pioneering contribution from India. Proc Indian Natn Sci Acad B 2003; 69 No. 4, pp 393–422.

7. Grassly NC, Jafari H, Bahl S, Durrani S, Wenger J, Sutter RW, Aylward RB. Asymptomatic Wild-Type Poliovirus Infection in India among Children with Previous Oral Poliovirus Vaccination. J Infect Dis 2010; 201:000–000

8. John TJ. Immunization against polioviruses in developing countries. Reviews in Medical Virology 1993;Vol 3: 149–160.

9. Indian Academy of Pediatrics Committee on Immunization (IAPCOI). Consensus recommendations on immunization and IAP immunization timetable 2012. Indian Pediatr2012; 49: 549–564.

10. Polio Eradication & Endgame Strategic Plan 2013-2018. Available from: http://www.polioeradication.org/Portals/0/Document/Resources/StrategyWork/PEESP_EN_US.pdf. (Accessed on 24-11-2013)

HEPATITIS B (Hep B) VACCINE

Reviewed by
Ajay Kalra, S.G. Kasi

Background

Hepatitis B Virus (HBV) is the major cause of chronic liver disease and hepatocellular carcinoma. In India, 2–4% of individuals are chronic carriers of HBV that place us in intermediate endemicity.[1] Infection with HBV may occur perinatally (vertical transmission), during early childhood (the so-called horizontal spread), through sexual contact or nosocomially. Chronic HBV infection in India is acquired in childhood, presumably before 5 years of age, through horizontal transmission. It should be noted that, in our country, horizontal route (e.g. child to child) and the vertical route (i.e. mother to child) are the major routes of transmission of hepatitis B. According to a recent study, the Seropositivity of hepatitis B was found to be 2.9% amongst pregnant women in India.[2] The risk of infection in a child born to a hepatitis B positive mother ranges from 10 to 85% depending on the mother's HBeAg status. Younger the age of acquisition of HBV infection, higher the chances of becoming a chronic carrier. It is believed that as many as 90% of those who are infected at birth go on to become chronic carriers and up to 25% of chronic carriers will die of chronic liver disease as adults. HBV genotypes A and D are prevalent in India, which are similar to the HBV genotypes in the West.[1] Infection with HBV is one of the most important causes of chronic hepatitis, cirrhosis of liver and hepatocellular carcinoma. These outcomes are all preventable by early childhood immunization. It is for this reason that the World Health Organization has recommended universal hepatitis B vaccination.[3]

Vaccines

The plasma-derived hepatitis B vaccine is no longer available. The currently available vaccine containing the surface antigen of hepatitis B is produced by recombinant technology in yeast and adjuvanted with aluminium salts and preserved with thimerosal (thimerosal-free vaccines are also available). Hepatitis B vaccine is available as single and multi-dose vials and should be stored at 2 to 8°C. The vaccine should not be frozen; frozen vaccine should be discarded.[3]

Immunogenicity, efficacy and effectiveness: The protective efficacy of hepatitis B vaccination is related to the induction of anti-HBs antibodies, but also involves the induction of memory T-cells. An anti-HBs concentration of 10 mIU/ml measured 1–3 months after administration of the last dose of the primary vaccination series is considered a reliable correlate of protection against infection.[5] The primary 3-dose vaccine series induces protective antibody concentrations in > 95% of healthy infants, children and young adults.[3]

Dosage & administration: The dose in children and adolescents (aged less than 18 years) is 0.5 ml/ 10 µg and in those 18 years and older is 1 ml/ 20 µg. It should be injected intramuscularly in the deltoid/anterolateral thigh. Gluteal injections should be avoided due to low immunogenicity. The vaccine is extremely safe and well tolerated.

Immunization schedules: The classical schedule is 0, 1 and 6 months. The vaccine is highly immunogenic and seroconversion rates are greater than 90% after a three dose schedule. Seroconversion rates are lower in the elderly, the immuno-compromised and those with chronic renal failure. Four doses at 0, 1, 2 and 12 months of double dose may be given in these patients.[4] Routine testing for anti-HBsAg levels 1 month after completion of the immunization schedule is recommended in children born to HBsAg positive mothers, health care workers and those with co-morbidities. Antibody titers greater than 10 mIU/ml signify a response and are considered protective.[5] Non-responders should be tested for hepatitis B carrier status. If found to be negative, the same three dose schedule should be repeated. Almost all respond to a 3 dose revaccination schedule.

Although the 0-1-6 schedule is the preferred schedule, hepatitis B vaccine schedules are very flexible and there are multiple options for adding the vaccine to existing national immunization schedules without requiring additional visits for immunization. These include:

(i) Birth, 6 and 14 weeks

(ii) 6, 10 and 14 weeks

(iii) Birth, 6 weeks, 6 months

(iv) Birth, 6 weeks, 10 weeks, 14 weeks

As of now, from the data available, none of the above schedules needs a booster. However, data are limited regarding long-term protection for schedules with shorter intervals. Schedules with a birth dose are necessary in all areas of high and moderate endemicity to prevent perinatal transmission.

Duration of protection: The standard three-dose hepatitis B vaccine series consists of two priming doses administered 1 month apart and a third dose administered 6 months after the first dose. This schedule results in very high antibody concentrations. Increasing the interval between the first and second dose of hepatitis B vaccine has a little effect on immunogenicity or final antibody concentration, whereas longer intervals between the last two doses result in higher final antibody concentrations. The higher the peak anti-HBs concentrations following immunization, the longer it usually takes for antibody levels to decline to ≤ 10 mIU/ml.[3] Several studies have documented the long-term protective efficacy of this schedule in preventing HBsAg-carrier status or clinical HBV-disease even when the anti-HBs concentrations decline to ≤ 10 mIU/ml over time. Even an absent anamnestic response following booster vaccination may not necessarily signify susceptibility to HBV in such individuals. Furthermore, observational studies have shown the effectiveness of a primary series of hepatitis B vaccine in preventing infection up to 22 years postvaccination of infants.[3] However, hepatitis B vaccine is a T-cell dependent vaccine and the titers at the end of immunization schedule may not be important so far as it is well above the protective level. An anamnestic response would occur, with the titers going up, should there occur contact with the virus again in future.

Need of boosters: Routine boosters are not needed in healthy children and adults. Studies have shown that individuals who had responded to the vaccination series and had levels of 10 mIU/ml after vaccination are protected against hepatitis B disease for life even if the levels drop to below protective levels or are undetectable later. This is due to immune memory. In the immunocompromised and those with co-morbidities such as chronic renal disease, levels should be checked periodically and booster vaccination given whenever levels drop to below protective levels.

Hepatitis B Immunoglobulin (HBIG)

HBIG provides passive immunity and is indicated along with hepatitis B vaccine in management of perinatal/ occupational/ sexual exposures to hepatitis B in susceptible individuals. The dose of HBIG in adults is 0.06 ml/kg and in neonates/ infants 0.5 ml. HBIG should be stored at 2 to 8°C and should not be frozen. HBIG provides temporary protection lasting 3–6 months. HBIG should never be given intravenously. HBIG is also used alone following exposure to hepatitis B in patients who are non-responders to hepatitis B vaccination (genetic reasons/ immunocompromised status). In this situation two doses of HBIG 1 month apart are indicated. A few intravenous preparations of HBIG (like Hepatect CP) are also available in the market; however, they are not adequately evaluated for their efficacy.

Recommendations for use

Individual use

The committee has now revised its recommendations for hepatitis B vaccination for routine use in office practice and recommended the following schedule: The first dose of a three-dose schedule should be administered at birth, second dose at 6 weeks, and third dose at 6 months (i.e. 0–6 week–6 month). This schedule also conforms to the latest ACIP recommendations, wherein the final (third or fourth) dose in the hepatitis B vaccine series should be administered no earlier than age 24 weeks and at least 16 weeks after the first dose.[6] This schedule will replace the existing schedule of 0–6 week–14 week. However, the hepatitis B vaccine may be given through other schedules as described above, considering the programmatic implications and logistic issues.

The committee stresses the significance and need of a birth dose. The birth dose can reduce perinatal transmission by 18–40%.

Delay in the administration of the first dose beyond the 7th day of life has been shown to be associated with higher rates of HBsAg acquisition in later childhood. The WHO position paper of 2009 clearly states that "since perinatal or early postnatal transmission is an important cause of chronic infections globally, the first dose of hepatitis B vaccine should be given as soon as possible (< 24 hours) after birth even in low-endemicity countries".[3]

Catch up vaccination

Hepatitis B vaccine as a 0-1-6 schedule should be offered to all children/adolescents who have not been previously vaccinated with hepatitis B vaccine. This is to address problems related to horizontal mode of transmission of the virus. Prevaccination screening with anti-HBsAg antibody is not cost effective and is not recommended. Catch up vaccination is particularly important for contacts of HBsAg positive patient. Prevaccination screening for HBsAg should be done in these contacts. All available brands of hepatitis B vaccine are equally safe and effective and any may be used. Interchange of brands is permitted but not routinely recommended. Combination vaccines containing hepatitis B are discussed separately.

Management of an infant born to hepatitis B positive mother

Pregnant women should be counseled and encouraged to opt for HBsAg screening. If the mother is known to be HBsAg negative, hepatitis B vaccine can be given in the 0–6 weeks–6 months schedule. If the mother's HBsAg status is not known, it is important that hepatitis B vaccination should begin within a few hours of birth so that perinatal transmission can be prevented.

If the mother is HBsAg positive (and especially HBeAg positive), the baby should be given hepatitis B Immunoglobulin (HBIG) along with hepatitis B vaccine within 12 hours of birth, using two separate syringes and separate sites for injection. The dose of HBIG is 0.5 ml intramuscular. HBIG may be given up to 7 days of birth but the efficacy of HBIG after 48 hours is not known. Two more doses of hepatitis B vaccine at 1 month/6 weeks and 6 months are needed. If HBIG is not available (or is unaffordable), hepatitis B vaccine may be given at 0, 1 and 2 months with an additional dose between 9 and 12 months. The efficacy of prophylaxis with both HBIG and hepatitis B vaccine is 85–95% and that with hepatitis B vaccine alone (1st dose at birth) is 70–75%. All infants born to HBsAg positive mothers should be tested for HBsAg and anti-HBsAg antibodies at the age of 9–15 months to identify carriers/non-responders.[7]

Immunization of preterm infants

Preterm infants and low birth weight infants with birth weight less than 2000 grams have a decreased response to hepatitis B vaccines administered before the age of one month. However, by the chronological age of one month, preterm babies irrespective of their initial birth weight and gestational age are likely to respond as adequately as full term infants.[3,7]

Recommendations for preterm infants

- Greater than 2000 grams: As for full term infants.

- Less than 2000 grams:

    ➢ Mother HBsAg Negative: Dose 1 at 30 days of age, dose 2 and 3 as per schedule adopted for full term infants.

    ➢ Mother HBsAg positive: Hepatitis B vaccine + HBIG (within 12 hours of birth), continue vaccine series with 3 more doses beginning at 4–6 weeks of age as per schedule for full term infants. Immunize with 4 doses, do not count birth dose as part of vaccine series.[7] Check anti-HBs and HBsAg one month after completion of vaccine series.

Hepatitis B vaccination should be routinely offered to persons in high-risk settings that includes health care workers, public safety workers, trainees in blood or blood-contaminated body fluid healthcare fields in schools of medicine, dentistry, nursing, laboratory technology, and other allied health professions.

Adults with risk factors for HBV infection can begin and should be administered on a 0, 1, and 6 month schedule. An accelerated schedule may be required as dose 1 of the series at any visit, dose 2 at least 4 weeks after dose 1 and dose 3 at least 8 weeks after dose 2 and at least 16 weeks after dose 1.

Post-exposure Prophylaxis (PEP) to Prevent Hepatitis B Virus Infection in Exposed Healthcare Personnel(HCP)

Healthcare Personnel (HCP) are defined as persons (including non-medical employees, students, medical personnels, public-safety workers, or volunteers) whose occupational activities involve contact with patients or with blood or other body fluids from patients in a healthcare, laboratory, or public-safety setting.[8] Hepatitis B vaccine should be offered to all HCP who have a reasonable expectation of being exposed to blood and body fluids on the job. It is preferable that medical students and trainees be offered the vaccine, as exposure is more common during the training period.

All HCP, including trainees, who have direct patient contact or who draw, test or handle blood specimens should have post-vaccination testing for antibody to hepatitis B surface antigen (anti-HBS). Post-vaccination testing should be done 1–2 months after the last dose of vaccine. For immunocompetent HCP, periodic testing or periodic boosting is not needed.

An exposure that might place HCP at risk for HBV infection includes percutaneous injuries (e.g., a needle stick or cut with a sharp object) or contact of mucous membrane or non-intact skin with blood, tissue, or other body fluids that are potentially infectious.[8]

In addition, HBV has been demonstrated to survive in dried blood at room temperature on environmental surfaces for at least 1 week. The potential for HBV transmission through contact with environmental surfaces is well established. The risk of HBV infection in the exposed HCP is primarily related to the degree of contact with blood in the work place and also to the hepatitis B e antigen (HBeAg) status of the source person.

Following a percutaneous or mucosal exposure to blood, 3 factors need to be considered when deciding the nature of PEP. These include

1. HBsAg status of the source
2. Vaccination status of the exposed HCP
3. Vaccination response status of the HCP

The PEP recommendations are given in Table 1.

Table 1: Recommendations for postexposure prophylaxis after percutaneous or mucosal exposure to HBV in HCP
(Adapted from "Updated U.S. PHS Guidelines for the Management of Occupational Exposures to HBV, HCV, and HIV and Recommendations for Postexposure Prophylaxis," MMWR, 6/29/01, Vol. 50 (RR-11)

Vaccination and antibody response status of exposed persons[1]	Treatment		
	Source is HBsAg positive	Source is HBsAg negative	Source is unknown on not tested
Unvaccinated	HBIG[2] x I and begin a hepatitis B vaccine series	Begin a hepatitis B vaccine series	If the source is suspected to be high risk, refer to the column "Source is HBsAg positive." If not, begin a hepatitis B vaccine series.
Fully vaccinated and known responder[3]	No treatment	No treatment	No treatment
Vaccinated with 3 doses and known nonresponder[3]	HBIG[2] x I and begin a hepatitis B revaccination series[4]	No treatment	If the source is suspected to be high risk, refer to the column "Source is HBsAg positive." If not, begin a hepatitis B revaccination series.
Vaccinated with 6 doses and known nonresponder[3]	HBIG[2,5] x 2	No treatment	Treat based on known or suspected risk of source
Fully vaccinated with 3 doses but antibody titer unknown	Test for anti-HBs.[6] If adequate,[3] no treatment. If inadequate, HBIG[2] x I and hepatitis B vaccine booster.	No treatment	If the source is suspected to be high risk, refer to the column "Source is HBsAg positive." If not, test for anti-HBs.[6] If adequate,[3] no treatment, If inadequate, give vaccine booster and check anti-HBs in 1–2 months

1. Persons known to have had HBV infection in the past or who are chronically infected do not require HBIG or vaccine.
2. Hepatitis B immune globulin (0.06 mL/kg) administered IM.
3. Adequate response is anti-HBs of at least 10 mIU/mL after vaccination.
4. Revaccination = additional 3-dose series of hepatitis B vaccine administered after the primary series.
5. First dose as soon as possible after exposure and the second dose 1 month later.
6. Testing should be done as soon as possible after exposure.

Public health perspectives

Hepatitis B vaccination is great public health significance. Though the Government of India initiated hepatitis B vaccination since 2002, but still its utilization through UIP is suboptimal. The IAP ACVIP believes that all infants should receive their first dose of hepatitis B vaccine as soon as possible after birth, preferably within 24 hours. In countries where there is high disease endemicity and where HBV is mainly spread from mother to infant at birth or from child to child during early childhood, providing the first dose at birth is particularly important, but even in countries where there is intermediate endemicity or low endemicity an important proportion of chronic infections are acquired through early transmission.[3] Delivery of hepatitis B vaccine within 24 hours of birth should be a performance indicator for all immunization programmes, and reporting and monitoring systems should be strengthened to improve the quality of data on the birth dose.

HEPATITIS B (HEP B) VACCINE

Routine vaccination

- Recommended schedule: The first dose of a three-dose schedule should be administered at birth, second dose at 6 weeks, and third dose at 6 months (i.e. 0–6 weeks–6 months).

- Minimum age: Birth

- Administer monovalent hepatitis B vaccine to all newborns within 48 hours of birth.

- Monovalent hepatitis B vaccine should be used for doses administered before age 6 weeks.

- Administration of a total of 4 doses of hepatitis B vaccine is permissible when a combination vaccine containing hepatitis B is administered after the birth dose.

- Infants who did not receive a birth dose should receive 3 doses of a hepatitis B containing vaccine starting as soon as feasible.

- The ideal minimum interval between dose 1 and dose 2 is 4 weeks, and between dose 2 and 3 is 8 weeks. Ideally, the final (3rd or 4th) dose in the hepatitis B vaccine series should be administered no earlier than age 24 weeks and at least 16 weeks after the first dose, whichever is later.

- Hepatitis B vaccine may also be given in any of the following schedules: Birth, 1 and 6 months, birth, 6 and 14 weeks; 6, 10 and 14 weeks; birth, 6, 10 and 14 weeks, etc. All schedules are protective.

Catch-up vaccination

- Administer the 3-dose series to those not previously vaccinated.
- In catch-up vaccination, use 0, 1, and 6 months schedule.

References

1.   Acharya SK, et al. Viral hepatitis in India. Natl Med J India 2006; 19:203–217.

2.   Mehta KD, et al. Seropositivity of hepatitis B, hepatitis C, syphilis, and HIV in antenatal women in India. J Infect Dev Ctries 2013; 7:832–837.

3.   Hepatitis B vaccines. WHO Position Paper. Wkly Epidemiol Rec 2009; 84: 405–420.

4.   Damme PV, Ward J, Shouval D, et al. Hepatitis B vaccines. In:Plotkin SA, Orenstein WA, Offit PA (Eds). Vaccines, 6th edition, Philadelphia: Saunders Elsevier; 2012. pp. 205–234.

5.   Jack AD et al. What level of hepatitis B antibody is protective? Journal of Infectious Diseases, 1999,179:489–492.

6.   Consensus Recommendations on Immunization and IAP Immunization Timetable 2012 Indian Academy of Pediatrics Committee On Immunization (IAPCOI)Indian Pediatrics Volume 49 July16, 2012, pg 549–564.

7.   MMWR. A Comprehensive Immunization Strategy to Eliminate Transmission of Hepatitis B Virus Infection in the United States. Recommendations of the Advisory Committee on Immunization Practices (ACIP). December 23, 2005 / Vol. 54 / No. RR-16. Available from: http://www.cdc.gov / mmwr / PDF / rr / rr5416.pdf

8.   CDC. Immunization of Health-Care Personnel; Recommendations of the Advisory Committee on Immunization Practices, MMWR, 2011; 60(7):1–48, Available from: www.cdc.gov/mmwr/pdf/rr/rr6007.pdf

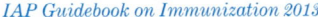

DIPHTHERIA, TETANUS AND PERTUSSIS VACCINES

Reviewed by
Vipin M. Vashishtha, A.J. Chitkara

Background

The morbidity and mortality due to diphtheria, tetanus and pertussis has reduced significantly in India since introduction of the whole cell vaccines in EPI. However, coverage with 3 doses of the whole cell vaccine DTwP vaccine is still low (71.5%) and only 41.4% children in the age group of 18–23 months had received first DTwP booster.[1] The need of completing the schedule and boosters should be stressed upon by the pediatrician.

Epidemiology

Diphtheria: The use of DTP vaccines has had significant impact at the burden of diphtheria. However, the disease is still persisting in a few states and published reports of the disease do exist in Indian literature indicating outbreaks, secular trends and a shifting epidemiology over the years.[2–4] The reported incidence for diphtheria has been 4233 and 2525 cases in the years 2011 and 2012, respectively[5] but underreporting is high likely. The corresponding figures for the year 1980, 1990, and 2000 were 39231, 8425, and 5125, respectively (Figure 1).[5] Diphtheria, however, remains endemic in countries in Africa, Latin America, Asia, the Middle East, and parts of Europe, where childhood immunization with diphtheria toxoid-containing vaccines is suboptimal.

Pertussis: In India, the incidence of pertussis declined sharply after launch of UIP. Prior to UIP, India reported 200,932 cases and 106 deaths in the year 1970 with a mortality rate of <0.001%. During the year 1987, the reported incidence was about 163,000 cases which came down to 40, 508 in 2010 and 39, 091 in 2011 reflecting a decline of about 75% (Figure 1).[6] Amongst different states, AP, MP, Jharkhand, WB, and Bihar reported the maximum cases in 2010. In 2010 only 6 and in 2011 a total of 11 deaths were reported.[6] However, a large number of cases go unreported, and many non-pertussis cases are reported and clubbed under the head of 'whooping cough' cases. The actual number may be high considering the low coverage with primary and booster doses of DTP vaccine in the country. The data on pertussis disease and infection in adolescents and adults is sorely lacking. Further, there is no data on Bordetella pertussis infection rates in the community that may be responsible for appearance of typical pertussis disease in infants and children.[7]

Tetanus: The incidence of tetanus in India has also declined sharply from 45,948 cases in 1980 and 23,356 cases in 1990 to only 2,404 cases in 2012.[5] But the worrying part is persistence of neonatal tetanus, and as many as 588 cases were reported in 2012 (Figure 1).[5]

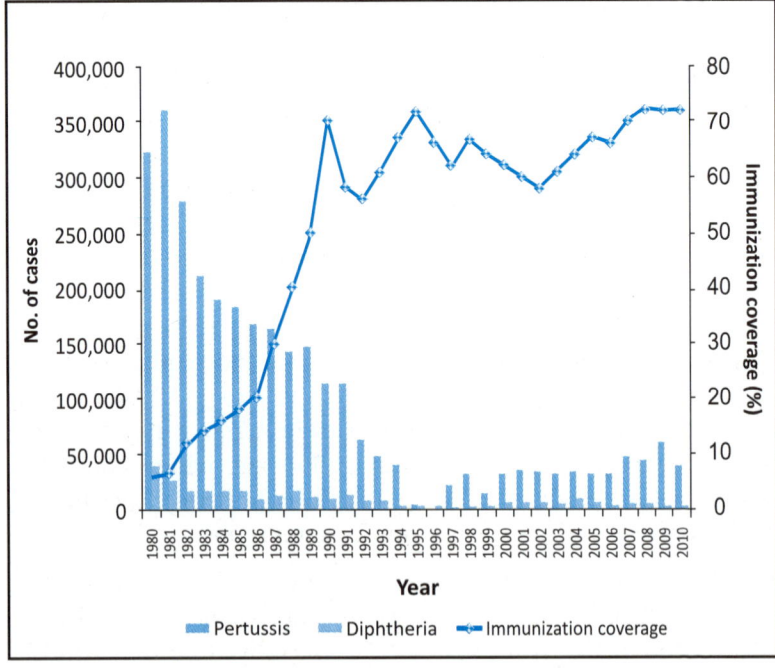

Figure 1: Trends in the reported cases of diphtheria and pertussis from 1980–2010

DTP VACCINES

I. DTwP Vaccines

Popularly known as triple antigen, DTwP is composed of tetanus and diphtheria toxoids as well as killed whole cell pertussis bacilli adsorbed on insoluble aluminium salts which act as adjuvants. The content of diphtheria toxoid varies from 20 to 30 Lf and that of tetanus toxoid varies from 5 to 25 Lf per dose. The vaccines need to be stored at 2 to 8°C. These vaccines should never be frozen, and if frozen accidentally, should be discarded. The dose is 0.5 ml intramuscularly and the preferred site is the anterolateral aspect of the thigh. The immunogenicity (protective titer for diphtheria > 0.1 IU/ml and for tetanus > 0.01 IU/ml) and effectiveness against diphtheria/ tetanus of three doses of the vaccine exceeds 95%. Disease may occur in vaccinated individuals but is milder.

Efficacy

The efficacy of different whole cell pertussis (wP) products vary substantially not only in different studies in different parts of the world but also varies with the case definition of the disease employed.[7] For higher efficacy trials, the efficacy estimates vary from 83% to 98% and 36% to 48% in lower efficacy trials. The pooled efficacy of wP vaccine against pertussis in children was 78% according to a systematic review in 2003.[8] The efficacy of wP alone ranged from 61% to 89%, and the efficacy of combination DTwP vaccines ranged from 46% to 92%.[8] There is no known immune correlate of protection for pertussis vaccines. Immunity against all three components wanes over the next 6–12 years and thus regular boosting is needed.

Adverse effects

Most adverse effects are due to the pertussis component. Minor adverse effects like pain, swelling and redness at the local site, fever, fussiness, anorexia and vomiting are reported in almost half the vaccinees after any of the 3 primary doses. Serious adverse effects have been reported with DTwP vaccines but are rare. The frequency of these side effects/ 1000 doses is 0.2–4.4 for fever more than 40.5°C, 4–8.8 for persistent crying, 0.06–0.8 for hypotonic hyporesponsive episodes (HHE), 0.16–0.39 for seizures and 0.007 for encephalopathy.

The frequency of systemic reactions reduces and that of local reactions increases with increasing number of doses. Children with history of a reaction following vaccination are more likely to experience a reaction following future doses. Catastrophic side effects such as sudden infant death syndrome (SIDS), autism, chronic neurologic damage, infantile spasms, learning disorders and Reye's syndrome were attributed to use of the wP vaccines in the past. It has now been proved beyond doubt that the wP vaccine is not causally associated with any of these adverse events. Absolute contraindications to any pertussis vaccination (including DTwP vaccine) are history of anaphylaxis or development of encephalopathy within 7 days following previous DTwP vaccination. In case of anaphylaxis, further immunization with any diphtheria/ tetanus/ pertussis vaccine is contraindicated as it is uncertain which component caused the event. For patients with history of encephalopathy following vaccination, any pertussis vaccine is contraindicated and only diphtheria and tetanus vaccines may be used. Events such as persistent inconsolable crying of more than 3 hours duration/ hyperpyrexia (fever > 40.5°C)/ HHE within 48 hours of DTwP administration and seizures with or without fever within 72 hours of administration of DTwP are considered as precautions but not contraindications to future doses of DTwP because these events generally do not recur with the next dose and they have not been proven to cause permanent sequelae. Progressive/evolving neurological illnesses is a relative contraindication to first dose of DTwP immunization. However, DTwP can be safely given to children with stable neurologic disorders.

Recommendations for use

The standard schedule is three primary doses at 6, 10 and 14 weeks and two boosters at 15–18 months and 5 years. Early completion of primary immunization is desirable as there is no maternal antibody for protection against pertussis. The schedule for catch up vaccination is three doses at 0, 1 and 6 months. The 2nd childhood booster is not required if the last dose has been given beyond the age of 4 years. DTwP is not recommended in children aged 7 years and older due to increased risk of side effects. It is essential to immunize even those recovering from diphtheria, tetanus and pertussis as natural disease does not offer complete protection.

II. DTaP Vaccines

Background

The introduction of the whole cell vaccines paid rich dividends in terms of decline in disease morbidity and mortality. Once disease rates declined, concerns about frequent local side-effects, as well as public anxiety about the safety of wP vaccines, led to the development of aP vaccines in Japan in 1981. These were licensed in the US in 1996 and have now replaced the whole cell vaccines in many developed countries.

Vaccine

All aP vaccines are associated with significantly lesser side-effects, and thus the replacement of the wP vaccines was mainly driven by the safety-profile of these vaccines. The other important advantage of the aP vaccines is the reproducible production process with its use of purified antigens and the removal of LPS and other parts of the bacterial cell wall during the purification of soluble antigenic material. These vaccines contain ≥ 1 of the separately purified antigens pertussis toxin (PT), filamentous hemagglutinin (FHA), pertactin (PRN), and fimbrial hemagglutinins 1, 2 & 3 (FIM type 2 and type 3). Vaccines differ from one another not only in the number and quantity of antigen components, but also with regard to the bacterial clone used for primary antigen production, methods of purification and detoxification, incorporated adjuvants, and the use of preservatives, such as thiomersal.[9] Nearly two dozens aP vaccines were designed, many were evaluated in immunogenicity and reactogenicity trials, and the efficacy and safety of a number were evaluated in field trials.

Efficacy and preference of a particular aP vaccine product

The efficacy and duration of protection with DTaP vaccines against diphtheria/ tetanus and pertussis is similar to that afforded by the whole cell vaccines. There is considerable controversy on the relative efficacy of different aP vaccines with varying number of components. Several randomized pertussis vaccine efficacy studies were conducted in Europe and Africa to compare the safety and efficacy of the aP and the wP vaccines for the prevention of laboratory-confirmed pertussis disease in infants.[7] All DTaP vaccines show better efficacy against severe disease than mild disease. The efficacies in these trials varied from 54% to 89%.[7] However, a few countries like Japan, Denmark, Sweden, etc have shown consistent control of pertussis disease with aP vaccines in their national immunization program.

There is as yet no consensus about the antigenic composition of an ideal aP vaccine. The exact contribution of the different aP antigens to protection is not clear. Current generation of aP available from different manufacturers should be considered as different and unique products because of the presence of one or more different components in different concentrations, and with different degree of adsorption to different adjuvants. Further, these individual antigens may be derived from different strains of *B. pertussis* and have been purified by different methods.[10] This is the reason why direct comparison of protective efficacy of different aP vaccines in human is not possible.

Different researches have studied the impact of number of components in an aP vaccine on relative protective efficacy of different aP products. In a recent retrospective study in US following a huge outbreak of pertussis in California, the researchers found that 5-component aP vaccine had an estimated efficacy of 88.7% (95% CI, 79.4–93.8%).[11] According to a systematic review involving 49 RCTs, aP vaccines containing 3 or more components had much higher absolute efficacy (80–84%) than those containing only 1- and 2-components (67–70%).[12] A Cochrane review by Zhang et al after studying 6 aP vaccine efficacy trials and 52 safety trials concluded that the efficacy of multi-component (≥3) aP vaccines varied from 84% to 85% in preventing 'typical whooping cough' and from 71% to 78% in preventing mild disease. In contrast, the efficacy of one- and two-component vaccines varied from 59% to 75% against 'typical whooping cough' and from 13% to 54% against mild disease.[13] Though a few countries have demonstrated high levels of effectiveness of mono- and bi- component aP products in preventing pertussis by employing them in their immunization programs,[9] the available evidence overwhelmingly favors multi-component (≥ 3) aP vaccines over mono- or bi- component aP vaccines.[7]

The effectiveness of vaccination programmes on a national level depends not only on the efficacy of the vaccine but also other factors such as the vaccination schedule and adherence, transportation and storage of the vaccine, and herd immunity in the population. Therefore, successful control of pertussis infections by two-component vaccines in a few countries does not necessarily exclude the potential additional benefits of large-scale vaccination with multi-component vaccines. Furthermore, analysis of the results of the four placebo-controlled trials of two one-component, two two-component, two three-component and one five-component vaccine unequivocally demonstrate the multi-component vaccines to have better protective efficacy against both mild and typical pertussis than one- and two-component vaccines.

Adverse effects

The DTaP vaccines score over the whole cell vaccines in terms of adverse effects. Broadly speaking the incidence of both minor and major adverse effects is reduced by two thirds with the acellular vaccines. The incidence of adverse effects is similar with all currently licensed DTaP vaccines. The absolute contraindications to DTaP vaccines are same as those for whole cell vaccines and include history of anaphylaxis/encephalopathy following past pertussis vaccination. Serious adverse events following previous pertussis vaccination (listed in DTwP section) though less likely as compared to DTwP may still occur with DTaP and are similarly considered as precautions while using the vaccine. After the primary series, the rate and severity of local reactions tend to increase with each successive DTaP dose.

Correlate of protection of wP and aP vaccines

Till date there is no single absolute or surrogate correlate of protection is known for pertussis disease and vaccines. Antibody levels against PT, PRN and FIM can be used as markers of protection, but no established protective antibody levels are known. The mechanism of immunity against *B. pertussis* involves both humoral and cellular immune responses which are not directed against a single protective antigen. In addition to the pertussis toxin, the vaccines usually contain one or more attachment factors, which also may be protective. Immune response to current wP vaccines mimics the response to infection in animal models and differs from the response to aP vaccines. The 'murine intracerebral challenge test' has been considered as a 'gold standard' for wP vaccines and has been used to standardize and assess the potency of wP vaccines.[14] But until now there has been no animal model in which protection correlates with aP vaccines efficacy in children, and these vaccines do not pass the original 'murine intracerebral challenge test'. The respiratory challenge by aerosol or intranasal of immunized mice model has been used to study pertussis pathogenesis and immunity and can correlate with efficacy of aP vaccines, but not yet accepted as a regulatory tool. In animal model, duration of protection is longer after wP vaccines compared to aP vaccines, suggesting a role for cell-mediated immunity for long-term protection (Table 1).

Table 1. Composition of available aP vaccines (in combination) brands in India

Product	Infanrix	Tripacel	Pentaxim*	Adacel**	Boostrix**
Tetanus toxoid	5 Lf	5 Lf	5 Lfv	5 Lf	5 Lf
Diphtheria toxoid	15 Lf	15 Lf	15 Lf	2 Lf	2.5 Lf
Acellular Pertussis:					
Pertussis toxoid (PT)	25 µg	10 µg	25 µg	2.5 µg	8 µg
Filamentous haemagglutinin (FHA)	25 µg	5 µg	25 µg	5 µg	8 µg
Pertactin (PRN)	8 µg	3 µg	---	3 µg	2.5 µg
Fimbriae types 2 and 3 (FIM)	---	5 µg	---	5 µg	----
2 and 3 (FIM)					

* A combination of acellular pertussis, IPV and Hib vaccines.
** Tdap vaccines

Recommendations for use

The vaccines should be stored at 2 to 8°C and the recommended dose is 0.5 ml intramuscularly. DTaP vaccines are not more efficacious than DTwP vaccines, but have fewer adverse effects. It must also be remembered that serious adverse effects are rare phenomena even with the wP vaccines unlike popular belief. The schedule is same as with DTwP vaccines. Like DTwP vaccines, DTaP vaccines must not be used in children 7 years or older because of increased reactogenicity. All licensed DTaP vaccines are of similar efficacy and safety as of currently available data and any one of them may be used. DTaP combination vaccines will be discussed separately.

Recent outbreaks of pertussis and choice of wP versus aP vaccines

Since 2009, large outbreaks of pertussis are regularly reported from many industrialized countries like USA, UK, Australia, employing aP vaccines despite having very high vaccination coverage.[7] A few outbreaks have also been reported from countries using wP vaccines like the one reported recently from Khairpur District of Sindh province of Pakistan.[7] There may be multiple factors responsible for the recent resurgence of pertussis in industrialized countries but the major concern today is the fact that aP vaccines are found to be less potent than wP vaccines.[7] Waning of protective immunity is noted with both wP and aP vaccines, and also after acquisition of immunity after natural infection. Whereas a little is known about the duration of protection following aP vaccination in developing countries, many studies in industrialized world documented faster waning with aP vaccines and showed that protection waned after 4–12 years.[11, 15–18]

Several randomized trials conducted in the 1990s to document efficacy of aP vaccines also compared their efficacy with wP vaccines. At least five trials found that wP vaccines had greater efficacy than aP vaccines.[7] Many later trials have also hinted that the efficacy of the aP vaccine may not be as robust as reported in the initial studies.[19–21] Studies after the recent outbreaks in US, UK and Australia have now concluded that the change from wP to aP vaccines contributed to the increase in pertussis cases.[22–24] Recent data from US and Australia have suggested reduced durability of vaccine-induced immunity after the aP vaccination in comparison of wP vaccines.[11,18] World over, the experts have now convinced that aP vaccines may be less effective than previously believed when contrasted with wP vaccines.[19,22,23] These findings suggest that priming with wP is more effective at sustained prevention of pertussis disease than aP vaccines. The current evidence is tilted heavily in favor of wP vaccines as far as effectiveness of the pertussis vaccines is concerned.[7] However, the industrialized world would not take the risk of reverting to wP vaccines considering the low acceptance of these vaccines by the public in the past. A few middle income group countries sitting on the fence and on the verge of shifting to acellular products would like to wait further till a better alternative is available.[7] Table 2 summarizes a few key differences in different attributes related to wP and aP vaccines.

Table 2. Comparative evaluation of whole-cell pertussis (wP) and acellular pertussis (aP) vaccines in terms of different attributes

Characteristics	wP vaccines	aP vaccines
Mechanism of action	Th-1 bias	Th-2 bias
Correlate of protection	Not known	Not known
Animal model (for potency)	known	Not known
Immunogenicity data (India)	Available	Available
Efficacy (Global)	Robust data	Exaggerated data
Efficacy (India)	No trial	No trial
Effectiveness (Global)	Well established	Not established universally
Effectiveness (India)	Established	No data
Priming	Superior	Inferior
Duration of protection/waning	Longer	Shorter
Herd effect	Documented	No herd effect
Minor adverse effects	1 episode in 2–10 injections	Equal to control
Serious adverse effects	Very rare	Very rare (at par with wP)
Acceptance (Global)	Poor	Good
Acceptance (India)	Good (no documentation of resistance)	Good

III. Tdap Vaccine

Vaccination of adolescents and adults

Pertussis in adolescents and adults is responsible for considerable morbidity in these age groups and also serves as a reservoir for disease transmission to unvaccinated/partially vaccinated young infants.[7] Pertussis is increasingly reported from older children, adolescents and adults. According to one serological study from US, 21% (95% confidence interval [CI], 13–32%) of adults with prolonged cough had pertussis.[25] The pertussis burden is believed to be substantially more than the number of reported cases; approximately 600,000 cases are estimated to occur annually just among adults.[26] There is no data on the incidence of adolescent and adult pertussis in India but is perceived to be significant, especially in those states where childhood immunization coverage is good and reduced natural circulation of pertussis leads to infrequent adolescent boosting.[7]

Objectives and rationale of adolescents and adult pertussis vaccination: There are two main objectives—first, to protect vaccinated persons against pertussis, and second, to reduce the reservoir of pertussis in the population at large and thereby potentially decrease exposure of persons at increased risk for complicated infection (e.g., infants).[7] There is a definite need of protecting very young infants not covered by current vaccination recommendations.

Vaccines

Immunity against pertussis following primary/booster DTwP/DTaP vaccination wanes over the next 6–12 years. Henceforth, several developed countries have instituted routine booster immunization of adolescents and adults with standard quantity tetanus toxoid and reduced quantity diphtheria and acellular pertussis vaccine (Tdap) instead of Td. The standard strength DTwP and DTaP vaccines cannot be used for vaccination of children 7 years and above due to increased reactogenicity.

Table 1 provides details of available Tdap vaccines in India. The vaccine should be stored between 2 and 8°C, must not be frozen. The dose is 0.5 ml IM intramuscularly. Immunogenicity studies have shown that antibody response to a single dose of Tdap booster in previously vaccinated children/adolescents is similar to that following 3 doses of full strength DTwP or DTaP vaccines. Vaccine efficacy against clinical disease exceeds 90%. Commonest side effect with Tdap is pain at the local injection site in about 70% of vaccinees, followed by redness and swelling. Systemic side effects like fever, headache and fatigue are rarely seen. Serious adverse events have not been reported. The contraindications are serious allergic reaction to any component of the vaccine or history of encephalopathy not attributable to an underlying cause within 7 days of administration of a vaccine with pertussis component.

Global experience with Tdap

Several developed countries have instituted routine booster immunization of adolescents and adults with Tdap instead of Td in their national immunization programs.[9] The IAP has also recommended only a single one-time dose of Tdap to adolescents aged 10–12 years of age.[7] The CDC-ACIP recommended routine administration of Tdap booster for adolescents in 2005, the vaccine coverage still remains low, with only 56% of adolescents and 8.2% of adults vaccinated in 2012.[27] There is no data on the coverage of Tdap in adolescents and adults in India since it is being used exclusively in private health sector.

Efficacy and effectiveness of Tdap

Wei et al. evaluated effectiveness of Tdap booster among adolescents in the Virgin Islands in 2007, and found effectiveness of 61.3% (95% CI: -52.5–90.2) and 68.3% (95% CI: -126.4–95.6) against probable and laboratory-confirmed pertussis, respectively.[21] A recent unpublished trial reported that Tdap was modestly effective [vaccine effectiveness: 55.2% (95% CI: 44.1–64.1%, p < 0.001)] at preventing PCR-confirmed pertussis among Kaiser Permanente Northern California (KPNC) adolescents and adults. According to ACIP data presented in February 2013 meeting, the Tdap effectiveness was noticed ranging from 66 % to 78% in field observational studies. The preliminary data suggest effectiveness wanes within 3–4 years among aP vaccine recipients and there was no evidence of herd immunity.[7]

Maternal immunization to prevent infant pertussis

Immunization of adolescents and adults, and postpartum administration of Tdap failed to have appreciable impact on laboratory-confirmed pertussis in very young infants.[7] Several strategies like maternal immunization including pregnant women, cocooning, neonatal immunization, have been proposed to reduce the burden of pertussis in those infants too young to have been immunized. Amongst all these strategies, immunization during pregnancy appears to be most effective strategy to have the most impact on infantile pertussis, especially during the first few weeks after birth. The effective transplacental transmission of maternal pertussis antibodies would protect the infant against pertussis during the first months of life. Though the transplacentally acquired antibodies may be detectable at least up to first few weeks of life (at 6–8 weeks), the age at which the first pertussis-containing vaccine is due, however, the concentration of antibodies required for protection against pertussis in newborns is not known.[7] In 2011, the ACIP recommended a dose of Tdap to all pregnant women after 20 weeks gestation to provide protection for both the mother and her newborn during the infant's earliest weeks of life.[28]

Safety of Tdap during pregnancy: There are limited safety data on Tdap administration in pregnant women; however, existing Tdap safety data from the CDC, US FDA and the pharmaceutical pregnancy registries do not indicate any adverse safety effect.[29] Even 3–6 doses of wP vaccines were administered during single pregnancy in 5 different clinical trials conducted in US and no serious untoward local or systemic reactions were noted.[30]

There are a few concerns regarding maternal immunization, they include ultimate titters achieved with a dose of Tdap during pregnancy, the duration of maternal antibodies, and finally, the interference with proper take of pertussis vaccines during primary immunization due to high concentrations of maternal antibodies.[7] However, a recent study demonstrated that infants whose mothers had received Tdap vaccine during pregnancy had higher pertussis antibody concentrations between birth and the first vaccine dose than the cohort whose mothers did not receive the vaccine. There was some blunting of the response to the infant series; but the children did develop adequate antibodies by the end of the complete series.[31] The results of this study are quite reassuring and add evidence to support the recommendation of vaccinating pregnant mothers to protect their children against pertussis.

Current status of Pertussis vaccination in India

Pertussis continues to be a serious public health problem in India. India is employing only wP vaccines in their national immunization program since the adoption of EPI in 1978. Though aP vaccines are also licensed and available, they are mainly prescribed by the private sector and coverage is still miniscule. Private health sector is responsible for offering vaccination to only 9% of the population in India.[1] Despite the low coverage of DTwP vaccine in India,[1] there is poor documentation of large scale outbreaks of pertussis in the country unlike the recent large scale outbreaks reported in many developed countries. Either many large scale outbreaks are totally ignored and go unreported or wP vaccines are providing adequate protection. There are two scenarios of pertussis epidemiology in a given population based on coverage of pertussis vaccine. Since the overall coverage is not very high, pertussis in major parts of the country continues mainly to be a problem of young children. However, many states having very good immunization rates behave like developed countries with high coverage in pediatric age group with resultant more frequent disease in adolescents and adults.[7] Regarding the safety of wP vaccines, there is still no report of higher rates of serious AEFIs, and public acceptance of the vaccine is still not a serious concern.[7]

IAP RECOMMENDATIONS ON PERTUSSIS VACCINATION

Public health perspectives

Pertussis is a highly prevalent pediatric illness having significant morbidity and mortality in the country. There is an urgent need of an effective surveillance to evaluate both the burden of infection and the impact of immunization. The current status of pertussis immunization, in the form of DTwP vaccination is still sub-optimal in many states.[1]

The IAP ACVIP unambiguously supports the current immunization policy of employing only wP vaccines (in the form of DTwP) in UIP because of its proven efficacy, safety, adequate public acceptance, and absence of documentation of significant waning. There is insufficient marginal benefit to consider changing from wP-containing vaccine to aP-containing vaccine.[7]

Individual use

Since there is scarcity of data on vaccine efficacies of both wP and aP vaccines in India and other developing countries, most of the recommendations of the academy in regard to pertussis vaccination are based on the experience gained and data obtained from the use of these vaccines in industrialized countries. However, the continuous decline in reported pertussis cases in last few decades has demonstrated good effectiveness of wP vaccine (of whatever quality) in India. There is no data on the effectiveness of aP vaccines in India.

IAP has now issued following recommendations on use of pertussis vaccines for office-practice in private health sector:

Primary immunization: The primary infant series should ideally be completed with 3 doses of wP vaccines. Vaccination must start at 6 weeks. Acellular pertussis (aP) vaccines should be avoided for the primary series of infant vaccination until or unless there is a genuine compelling reason to use aP vaccine in a given child.

There is scarcity of data on comparative safety, immunogenicity, and efficacy of individual wP vaccines produced in various countries. Similarly, there is no data on either the efficacy of individual wP product or comparative evaluation of different available wP combinations in the Indian market. A few brands in India have achieved WHO prequalification, but not all the products have uniformly attained it. IAP urges the GoI to undertake studies on the quality of available wP and aP vaccines in Indian market. The national regulatory authority (NRA) must set indigenous national guidelines to manufacture and market different pertussis vaccines in the country.

The recommendation on the exclusive use of wP vaccine in primary immunization series is based on the following reasons:

- There is no data on the efficacy/effectiveness of aP vaccines in India and almost all the recommendations are based on the performance of these vaccines in industrialized countries. However, many of these countries have now reported upsurge and frequent outbreaks of the disease despite using highest quality aP vaccines with a very high coverage (close to 100%) since mid-1990s (Figure 2).

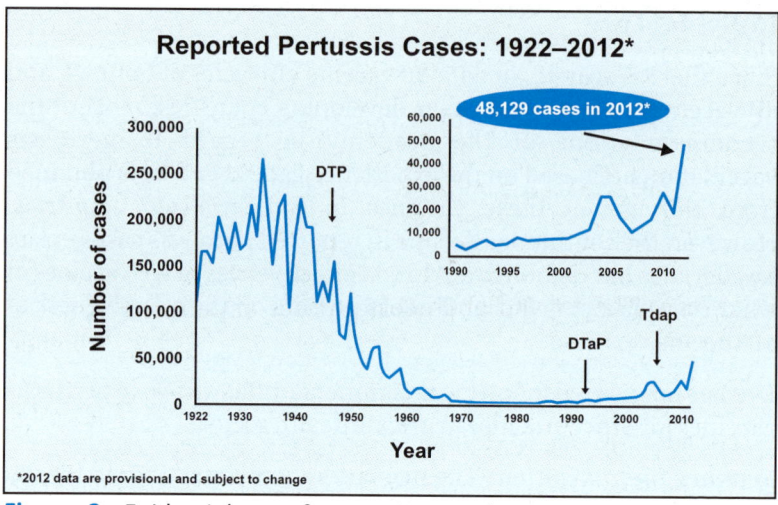

Figure 2. Epidemiology of pertussis in relation to introduction of pertussis vaccines in the USA (*Source: CDC*)

- The aP containing combinations were licensed in India on the basis of immunogenicity studies only. However, in the absence of any known correlate of protection for aP vaccines, mere presence of antibodies cannot be relied as a surrogate for efficacy or protection.

- The studies from USA, Australia and other industrialized countries post-2009 outbreaks have demonstrated superior priming with wP vaccines and more durability of immunity following wP vaccination than aP vaccines.

- There is strong evidence of effectiveness, real life performance of wP vaccines from India where the widespread use of them have markedly reduced the incidence of pertussis after the launch of UIP (Figure 1). We have achieved a good control of pertussis (high effectiveness, not merely the efficacy) with whatever type of wP was available in the country despite with a modest coverage of around 60–70%.

- World over, the widespread use of wP vaccines had almost eliminated pertussis from almost all the countries that had employed them.

The aP vaccine combinations should be avoided for the primary series. However, the aP vaccines may be preferred to wP vaccines in those children with history of severe adverse effects after previous dose/s of wP vaccines or children with neurologic disorders, if resources permit. The parents should be counseled about the probable efficacy related disadvantages of using aP vaccines for the primary series. The schedule is same as with wP (DTwP) vaccines. Like DTwP vaccines, DTaP vaccines must not be used in children 7 years or older because of increased reactogenicity. The contraindications are the same for both the vaccines.

Boosters: The 1st and 2nd booster doses of pertussis vaccines should also be of wP vaccine. However, considering a higher reactogenicity, aP vaccine/combination can be considered for the boosters, if resources permit.

Choice of aP vaccines: Considering the strong evidence in favor of superiority of multi-component (≥ 3) aP vaccines in comparison to one- and two-component aP vaccines from recent systematic reviews and meta-analysis, IAP now recommends that if any aP containing vaccine is used, it must at least have 3 or more components, the more the better.

Administration and schedule: The standard dose of pertussis vaccine is 0.5 ml; this is administered intramuscularly in the anterolateral thigh of children aged <12 months and in the deltoid muscle in older age groups. The standard primary vaccination schedule is three primary doses at 6, 10 and 14 weeks and two boosters at 15–18 months and 5 years. Early completion of primary immunization is desirable as there is no effective maternal antibody for protection against pertussis. The booster should be given ≥ 6 months after the last primary dose. The last dose of the recommended primary series should be completed by the age of 6 months. All infants, including those who are HIV-positive, should be immunized against pertussis.

Schedule for catch up vaccination: Three doses at 0, 1 and 6 months interval should be offered. The 2nd childhood booster is not required if the last dose has been given beyond the age of 4 years. It is essential to immunize even those recovering from pertussis as natural disease does not offer complete protection.

Recommendations for adolescents and adults: Immunity against pertussis following primary/ booster wP/aP vaccination wanes over the next 4–12 years. The academy therefore recommends offering Tdap vaccine instead of Td/TT vaccine to all children/adolescents/adults who can afford to use the vaccine in the schedule discussed below:

- In those children who have received all three primary and the two booster doses of DTwP/DTaP, Tdap should be administered as a single dose at the age of 10–12 years.

- Catch-up vaccination is recommended till the age of 18 years.

- Persons aged 7 through 10 years who are not fully immunized with the childhood DTwP/DTaP vaccine series, should receive Tdap vaccine as the first dose in the catch-up series; if additional doses are needed, Td vaccine should be used. For these children, an adolescent Tdap vaccine is not required.

- A single dose of Tdap may also be used as replacement for Td/TT booster in adults of any age if they have not received Tdap in the past.

- Tdap can now be given regardless of time elapsed since the last vaccine containing tetanus toxoid or diphtheria toxoid.

- There is no data at present to support repeat doses of Tdap.

- IAP recommends decennial Td booster for those who have received one dose of Tdap (5 years for wound management).

Only aP-containing vaccines should be used for vaccination in those aged > 7 years.

Tdap during pregnancy: Maternal immunization, particularly of pregnant women may be an effective approach to protect very young infants and neonates. IAP therefore now suggests immunization of pregnant women with a single dose of Tdap during the third trimester (preferred during 27 through 36 weeks gestation) regardless of number of years from prior Td or Tdap vaccination. Tdap has to be repeated in every pregnancy irrespective of the status of previous immunization (with Tdap). Even if an adolescent girl who had received Tdap one year prior to becoming pregnant will have to take it since there is rapid waning of immunity following pertussis immunization.

Interchangeability of brands: In principle, the same type of wP-containing or aP-containing vaccines should be given throughout the primary course of vaccination. However, if the previous type of vaccine is unknown or unavailable, any wP vaccine or aP vaccine may be used for subsequent doses.

IV. Tetanus Toxoid (TT)

Background

Antibodies to tetanus decline over time and hence regular boosting is needed to ensure adequate levels of antibodies during any apparent/inapparent exposure to tetanus bacilli/ toxin.

Vaccine/Toxoid

TT containing 5 Lf of toxoid is one of the most heat stable and commonly used vaccines. The vaccine should be stored between 2 and 8°C and the dose is 0.5 ml intramuscularly[32]. Administration of boosters more frequently than indicated leads to increased frequency and severity of local and systemic reactions as the preformed antitoxin binds with the toxoid and leads to immune complex-mediated reactions (Swollen limbs & Arthus type 2 reactions).

Recommendations for use

The role of standalone TT vaccines is diminishing and replacement with Td/Tdap is recommended for more comprehensive protection. In individuals who have completed primary and booster vaccination with DTwP/DTaP, TT boosters every 10 years provide sufficient protection.[33]

TT in pregnancy

WHO has evolved exhaustive guidelines for administration of TT in pregnant women and recommends replacement of TT with Td in a phased manner.[32]

- **Unimmunized:** For pregnant women who have not been previously immunized, two doses of TT at least one month apart should be given during pregnancy so that protective antibodies in adequate titers are transferred to the newborn for prevention of neonatal tetanus. The first dose should be administered at the time of first contact/ as early as possible and the second dose of TT should be administered 1 month later and at least 2 weeks before delivery. A single dose of TT would suffice for subsequent pregnancies that occur in the next 5 years; thereafter, 2 doses of TT would again be necessary.

- **Fully immunized:** Five childhood doses (3 primary doses plus two boosters) and one adolescent booster Tdap: No further doses are necessary in pregnancy.

- **Partially immunized:**

  ➢ Three primary doses: For women who have received 3 primary doses in infancy, two doses during the 1st pregnancy are indicated. The 2nd pregnancy requires 1 more dose and gives lasting protection for the reproductive years.

  ➢ Three primary and one childhood booster: 1 dose each in the first and second pregnancy provide lasting protection.

  ➢ Three primary and two childhood boosters: Only 1 dose in the first pregnancy provides lasting protection.

TT in wound management

All patients presenting with skin wounds/ infections should be evaluated for tetanus prophylaxis. Cleaning of the wound, removal of devitalized tissue, irrigation and drainage is important to prevent anaerobic environment which is conducive to tetanus toxin production. The indications for TT and Tetanus immunoglobulin (TIG) are as below (Table 3). Again replacement of TT with Td/Tdap is recommended.

Evidence suggests that tetanus is highly unlikely in individuals who have received 3 or more doses of the vaccine in the past and who get a booster dose during wound prophylaxis, hence passive protection with TIG is not indicated in these patients irrespective of wound severity unless the patient is immunocompromised. For children who are completely unimmunized, catch-up vaccination should be provided by giving three doses of TT at 0, 1 and 6 months. For partially immunized children, catch-up vaccination entails administration of at least 3 doses of TT including previous doses received. Children with unknown / undocumented history should be treated as unimmunized. It is recommended that the TT booster

Table 3. Tetanus prophylaxis in wound management

	Doses of IT	Clean, minor wounds	All other wounds	Given in past
	TT	TIG*	TT	TIG*
Unknown, < 3 doses, immunodeficient	Yes	Yes	Yes	Yes
≥ 3 doses	No**	No	No***	No

Including, but not limited to, wounds contaminated with dirt, feces, soil, saliva; puncture wounds; avulsions; and wounds resulting from missiles, crushing, burns, and frostbite.

* TIG: Tetanus immunoglobulin (250–500 IU IM)

** Yes, if more than 10 years since last dose

*** Yes, if more than 5 years since last dose

doses administered at the time of wound management and for catch-up vaccination be replaced with DTwP/ DTaP/ Td/ Tdap depending on the age of the child and nature of previous doses received for more comprehensive protection.

V. DT Vaccine

This vaccine comprises diphtheria and tetanus toxoid in similar amounts as in DTwP/DTaP, should be stored at 2 to 8°C and the dose is 0.5 ml intramuscularly. It is recommended in children below 7 years of age where pertussis vaccination is contraindicated. Studies with DTwP in school-aged children have shown no serious adverse events attributable to the vaccine. Additionally, boosting of pertussis immunity is important to protect against childhood pertussis.

VI. Td Vaccine

Background

Studies show that diphtheria antibody levels decline over time resulting in increasing susceptibility of adolescents and adults to diphtheria. For diphtheria, the average duration of protection is about 10 years following a primary series of 3 doses of diphtheria toxoid.[34] Considering the current epidemiology of diphtheria in India (i.e. low-endemic), a booster against diphtheria is desirable, but not mandatory. Boosting at the age of 12 months, at school entry and just before leaving school are all possible options.[34] Good childhood vaccination coverage (at least 70%) provides herd effect by reducing circulation of toxigenic strains and prevents outbreaks in adults despite susceptibility. When childhood vaccination programs break down as happened in the former Soviet Union in the early 1990s, massive outbreaks of diphtheria involving primarily adults have occurred. Thus it is desirable to regularly boost adult immunity against diphtheria in addition to tetanus every 10 years. The DTwP, DTaP and DT vaccines cannot be used in children aged 7 years and above due to increased reactogenicity due to the higher diphtheria toxoid and pertussis components.

Vaccine

Td contains the usual dose of tetanus toxoid and only 2 units of diphtheria toxoid, is stored at 2 to 8°C and is administered intramuscularly in a dose of 0.5 ml.

Recommendations for use

This vaccine is indicated as replacement for DTwP/ DTaP/DT for catch-up vaccination in those aged above 7 yrs (along with Tdap) and as replacement for TT in all situations where TT is given.

Diphtheria and tetanus toxoids and pertussis (DTP) vaccine

Routine vaccination

- Recommended schedule: Three primary doses at 6, 10 and 14 weeks and two boosters at 15–18 months and 5 years.
- Minimum age: 6 weeks
- The first booster (4th dose) may be administered as early as age 12 months, provided at least 6 months have elapsed since the third dose.
- DTaP vaccine/combinations should preferably be avoided for the primary series.
- DTaP may be preferred to DTwP in children with history of severe adverse effects after previous dose/s of DTwP or children with neurologic disorders.
- First and second boosters may also be of DTwP. However, considering a higher reactogenicity, DTaP can be considered for the boosters.
- If any 'acellular pertussis' containing vaccine is used, it must at least have 3 or more components in the product.

IAP Guidebook on Immunization 2013–14

Catch-up vaccination

- Catch-up schedule: The 2nd childhood booster is not required if the last dose has been given beyond the age of 4 years
- Catch up below 7 years: DTwP/DTaP at 0, 1 and 6 months;
- Catch up above 7 years: Tdap, Td, and Td at 0, 1 and 6 months.

Tetanus and diphtheria toxoids and acellular pertussis (Tdap) vaccine

Routine vaccination

- Recommended schedule: One dose of Tdap to all adolescents aged 11 through 12 years.
- Minimum age: 7 years (Adacel® is approved for 11–64 years by ACIP and 4 to 64 year old by FDA, while Boostrix® for 10 years and older by ACIP and 4 years of age and older by FDA in US).
- Tdap during pregnancy: One dose of Tdap vaccine to pregnant mothers/adolescents during each pregnancy (preferred during 27 through 36 weeks gestation) regardless of number of years from prior Td or Tdap vaccination.
- Catch-up vaccination
- Catch up above 7 years: Tdap, Td, Td at 0, 1 and 6 months.
- Persons aged 7 through 10 years who are not fully immunized with the childhood DTwP/DTaP vaccine series, should receive Tdap vaccine as the first dose in the catch-up series; if additional doses are needed, use Td vaccine. For these children, an adolescent Tdap vaccine should not be given.
- Persons aged 11 through 18 years who have not received Tdap vaccine should receive a dose followed by tetanus and diphtheria toxoids (Td) booster doses every 10 years thereafter.
- Tdap vaccine can be administered regardless of the interval since the last tetanus and diphtheria toxoid-containing vaccine.

References

1. UNICEF Coverage Evaluation survey, 2009 National Fact Sheet. Available from: http://www.unicef.org/india/National_Fact_Sheet_CES_2009.pdf

2. Singhal T, Lodha R, Kapil A, Jain Y, Kabra SK. Diphtheria—down but not out. Indian Pediatr 2000; 37: 728–737.

3. Patel UV, Patel BH, Bhavsar BS, Dabhi HM, Doshi SK. A retrospective study of diphtheria cases, Rajkot, Gujarat. Indian J Comm Med 2004; 24: 161–163.

4. Khan N, Shastri J, Aigal U, Doctor B. Resurgence of diphtheria in the vaccination era. Indian J Med Microbiol 2007;25: 434–437.

5. WHO Vaccine-Preventable Diseases: Monitoring System 2013 Global Summary. Available at http://apps.who.int / immunization_monitoring/ globalsummary/countries?countrycriteria%5Bcountry%5D%5B%5D=IND& commit=OK

6. National Health Profile (NHP) of India – 2011, Government of India, Central Bureau of Health Intelligence, DGHS. Ministry of Health and Family Welfare. Available from: http://cbhidghs.nic.in/writereaddata/mainlinkFile/08%20 Health%20Status%20%20Indicators%20%202011.pdf

7. Vashishtha VM, Bansal CP, Gupta SG. Pertussis Vaccines: Position Paper of Indian Academy of Pediatrics (IAP). Indian Pediatr 2013; 50: 1001–1009.

8. Jefferson T, et al. Systematic review of the effects of pertussis vaccines in children. Vaccine, 2003, 21: 2003–2014.

9. Pertussis vaccines: WHO position paper. October 2010. Wkly Epidemiol Rec 2010; 85: 385–400.

10. WHO. Guidelines for the production and control of the acellular pertussis component of monovalent or combined vaccines. WHO Technical Report Series No. 878, 1998. Available from:http://www.who.int/biologicals/ publications /trs/areas/vaccines/acellular_pertussis/ WHO_TRS_878_ A2.pdf

11. Misegades LK, et al. Association of childhood pertussis with receipt of 5 doses of pertussis vaccine by time since last vaccine dose, California, 2010. JAMA 2012; 308: 2126–2132.

12. Jefferson T, et al. Systematic review of the effects of pertussis vaccines in children. Vaccine, 2003, 21: 2003–2014.

13. Zhang L, et al. Acellular vaccines for preventing whooping cough in children. Cochrane Database Syst Rev. 2012; 3: CD001478.

14. Kendrick PL, et al. Mouse protection tests in the study of pertussis vaccine; a comparative series using the intracerebral route for challenge. Am J Public Health Nations Health 1947; 37: 803–810.

15. Mills K.H.G. Immunity to Bordetella pertussis. Microbes Infect. 2001; 3: 655–677.

16. Klein NP, et al. Waning protection after fifth dose of acellular pertussis vaccine in children. N Engl J Med. 2012; 367: 1012–1019.

17. Wendelboe AM, et al. Duration of immunity against pertussis after natural infection or vaccination. Pediatr Infect Dis J. 2005; 24: S58–61.

18. Witt MA, et al. Unexpectedly limited durability of immunity following acellular pertussis vaccination in preadolescents in a North American outbreak. Clin Infect Dis. 2012; 54: 1730–1735.

19. Rendi-Wagner P, et al. Hospital-based active surveillance of childhood pertussis in Austria from 1996 to 2003: estimates of incidence and vaccine effectiveness of whole-cell and acellular vaccine. Vaccine 2006; 24: 5960–5965.

20. Lacombe K, et al. Risk factors for acellular and whole-cell pertussis vaccine failure in Senegalese children. Vaccine 2004; 23: 623–628.

21. Wei SC, et al. Effectiveness of adolescent and adult tetanus, reduced-dose diphtheria, and acellular pertussis vaccine against pertussis. Clin Infect Dis. 2010; 51: 315–321.

22. Witt MA, et al. Reduced Risk of Pertussis Among Persons Ever Vaccinated With Whole Cell Pertussis Vaccine Compared to Recipients of Acellular Pertussis Vaccines in a Large US Cohort. Clin Infect Dis. 2013; 56: 1248–1254.

23. Sheridan SL, et al. Number and order of whole cell pertussis vaccines in infancy and disease protection. JAMA 2012; 308: 454–456.

24. Liko J, et al. Priming with whole-cell versus acellular pertussis vaccine. N Engl J Med. 2013; 368: 581–582.

25. Wright SW, et al. Pertussis infection in adults with persistent cough. JAMA 1995; 273: 1044–1046.

26. CDC. Available from: http://www.cdc.gov /mmwr /preview/mmwrhtml/ rr5517a1.htm

27. Stokley S, et al. Adolescent vaccination-coverage levels in the United States: 2006–2009. Pediatrics 2011; 128: 1078–1086.

28. CDC. MMWR Morb. Mortal. Weekly Rep 2011; 60: 1424–1426.

29. Gall SA, et al. Maternal immunization with tetanus-diphtheria-pertussis vaccine: effect on maternal and neonatal serum antibody levels. Am J Obstet Gynecol 2011; 204: 334.e 1–5.

30. CDC. Prevention of pertussis, tetanus and diphtheria among pregnant and postpartum women and their infants. Morbidity and Mortality Weekly Report. Recommendations and Reports, 2008; 57: 1–51.

31. Hardy-Fairbanks AJ, et al. Immune Responses in Infants Whose Mothers Received Tdap Vaccine During Pregnancy. Pediatr Infect Dis J. 2013 Jun 24.

32. Tetanus vaccines: WHO position paper. Weekly Epidemiological Rec. 2006; 81: 196–207.

33. CDC. Available from: http://www.cdc.gov / mmwr /preview /mmwrhtml / mm6001a4.htm

34. Diphtheria vaccine: WHO position paper. Weekly Epidemiol Rec 2006; 81: 24–32.

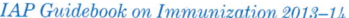

HAEMOPHILUS INFLUENZAE TYPE B (Hib) CONJUGATE VACCINES

3.5

Reviewed by
A.K. Patwari

Background

Capsulated *Haemophilus influenzae* has six serotypes of which type b is most important. *Haemophilus influenzae* type b (Hib) is an important invasive pathogen causing diseases such as meningitis, bacteremia, pneumonia, cellulitis, osteomyelitis, septic arthritis and epiglottitis. Most of invasive Hib disease occurs in children in the first two years of life before natural protective immunity is acquired by the age of 3–4 years. Non-capsulated Hib disease causing bronchitis, otitis media, sinusitis and pneumonia is not amenable to prevention at present and can occur at all ages. Data from the Invasive Bacterial Infections Surveillance (IBIS) group from six referral hospitals in India show that Hib is a common cause of pneumonia and meningitis in India.[1]

Global burden of Hib disease

In spite of the availability of an effective vaccine against Hib for more than a decade, Hib continues to be a leading cause of mortality and morbidity worldwide, especially in developing countries. Globally, in 2010, there were estimated 120 million episodes of pneumonia in children younger than 5 years and of these 14 million progressed to severe episodes. 1·3 million episodes of pneumonia led to death and 81% of deaths occurred in the first 2 years of life.[2]

Global estimates of burden of disease caused by *Haemophilus influenzae* type b in children younger than 5 years suggest that Hib caused about 8.13 million serious illnesses worldwide in 2000 (uncertainty range 7.33–13.2 million) and estimated that Hib caused 371,000 deaths (2,47,000–5,27,000) in children aged 1–59 months.[3] In prospective, microbiology-based studies in childhood pneumonia, the second most common organism isolated in most studies is *H. influenzae* type b (10–30%).[4] In unvaccinated populations, Hib is the dominant cause of non-epidemic bacterial meningitis during the first year of life. Even with prompt and adequate antibiotic treatment, 3–20% of patients with Hib meningitis die. Where medical resources are limited, fatality rates for Hib meningitis may be much higher, and severe neurological sequelae are frequently observed in survivors (in up to 30–40%).[5]

Hib Burden in India

The burden of Hib disease is underestimated in India as cultures are often not sent, the organism is difficult to culture especially when antibiotics have been administered and a large proportion of pneumonia may be non-bacteremic. During 1993–1997, a prospective surveillance was conducted in 5798 patients aged 1 month to 50 years who had diseases likely to be caused by *H. influenzae*. Out of a total of 125 *H. influenza* infections detected, 97% of which were caused by Hib, 108 (86%) isolates were from children aged < 5 years. The clinical spectrum of these children included meningitis (70%), pneumonia (18%) and septicemia (5%). The case-fatality rate was 11% overall and 20% in infants with Hib meningitis.[1]

In 1995, Bahl et al[6] conducted a hospital based study on 110 children < 5 years on severe and very severe pneumonia, and it was found that 19% cases were due to Hib. Another hospital-based study conducted in Delhi by Patwari et al,[7] in 1996, found 15% of 132 children < 12 years suffered from pneumonia due to Hib.

In a later cohort study of 17,951 children aged 0–18 months enrolled from July 2005 to December 2006, the cohort population presented with 227, 231 and 131 events of suspected pneumonia and 164, 72 and 89 events of suspected meningitis at study hospitals at Chandigarh, Kolkata and Vellore, respectively. Amongst hospitalized patients 8–30% children had purulent meningitis and Hib was detected in 20–29 % of cases by culture or Latex Agglutination Test (LAT). Case fatality of pneumonia ranged from 0.77 to 2.35% and that of meningitis ranged from 2.68 to 4.71 % at these study centers.[8]

The WHO estimates for the year 2008 show that 1.828 million children under 5 years die annually in India alone of which 20.3% mortality is due to pneumonia. These statistics coupled with the evidence of large number of Hib pneumonia brought out in the above studies highlights the urgency to take effective measures against Hib disease in India.

Vaccines

All Hib vaccines are conjugated vaccines where the Hib capsular polysaccharide (polyribosylribitol phosphate or PRP) is conjugated with a protein carrier so as to provide protection in the early years of life when it is most needed. Currently available vaccines include HbOC (carrier CRM197 mutant *C. diphtheriae* toxin protein), PRP - OMP (carrier *N. meningitidis* protein outer membrane protein complex) and PRP- T (carrier tetanus toxoid). PRP- D has been withdrawn due to relatively poor efficacy. HbOC and PRP-T vaccines show only a marginal increase in antibody levels after the first dose with a marked increase after the second and even better response after the third dose. On the other hand, PRP-OMP shows an increase in antibody level after the first dose itself with only marginal increases after the second and third doses. The onset of protection with PRP-OMP is thus faster. Additionally, while 3 doses of HbOC and PRP-T are recommended for primary vaccination, only 2 doses of PRP-OMP are recommended for this purpose. Only HbOC and PRP-T are currently available in India. The vaccines should be stored at 2 to 8°C and the recommended dose is 0.5 ml intramuscularly.

Serologic correlate of protection and efficacy

Efficacy trials have demonstrated 90–100% efficacy against culture proven invasive Hib disease for 1 year after vaccination. A trial in Gambian infants has shown 21% protection against episodes of severe pneumonia. The serologic correlate of protection at the time of exposure has been fixed at 0.15 µg/ ml and that for long-term protection as 1 µg/mL. Indirect protection to the unimmunized susceptible children as a result of diminished Hib transmission (~ 50% of children exhibited anti-PRP titers ≥ 5.0 µg/mL; a level that impedes Hib upper respiratory carriage) has also been observed while conducting serological assessment of the Hib immunization program in Mali.[9]

Effectiveness

Developed countries where the vaccine was introduced for universal immunization have witnessed virtual elimination of Hib disease with no serotype replacement. The vaccine has also been shown to impart herd protection by reducing nasopharyngeal carriage. A notable exception in the Hib success story was an increased incidence of Hib disease in vaccinated children between the years 1999–2003 in the UK occurring after a remarkable initial decline in Hib disease in the early 1990's. Most of the cases of invasive Hib disease occurred in the late second year of life. The major factor responsible for this phenomenon was omission of the second year booster.

Waning of immunity and need of boosters

Vaccine induced immunity wanes over time and reduced carriage of the organism in the environment compounds the problem by lack of natural boosting. It is also recognized now that immunological memory is insufficient for protection against Hib disease. Hence a booster dose is mandatory for sustained protection. Primary immunization with either pentavalent vaccine is reported to induce an excellent immunity lasting till the second year of life. A booster dose with DTwP-Hib vaccine effectuated a good anamnestic response to all vaccine components, being especially strong for Hib in children previously vaccinated with pentavalent vaccine.[10]

Safety

Side effects are mild and usually local. The committee reviewed the post-marketing surveillance data on the safety of Hib and Hib containing combination vaccines in India and found a total of 98 (46 serious and 49 non-serious) AEFI episodes for 53.51 million doses (overall frequency 1.83/million doses, and for serious AEFI 0.85/million) from October 2004 through December 2011, suggesting that there was no safety concern of Hib vaccines as reported frequently in lay media. The committee strongly supports the Government of India's efforts to introduce this vaccine in all the states in the country.[11]

Recommendations for use

Public health perspective

The IAP ACVIP recommends offering the Hib vaccine to all children. Hib conjugate vaccines were recommended by IAP in early 2000's, introduced in private sector without much debate on safety issues, except for questions pertaining to its high cost.[12] In April 2008, the Hib and Pneumococcal subcommittee of National Technical Advisory Group on Immunization (NTAGI) in India reviewed the existing Indian, regional and global data on Hib disease epidemiology, vaccine safety and efficacy and cost effectiveness. It concluded that the disease burden of Hib is sufficiently high in India to warrant prevention by vaccination, the vaccine is safe and efficacious. It strongly recommended its immediate introduction in India's Universal Immunization Program (UIP). Observations from a mathematical model developed to compare scenarios with and without Hib vaccination in order to estimate the cost-effectiveness of Hib vaccine in Haryana state suggests that Hib vaccine introduction is a cost-effective strategy in India.[13]

The Government of India's (GOI) decision to introduce Hib vaccine in EPI in a phased manner was challenged in the court of laws in a PIL (public interest litigation) on the grounds that India does not have significant Hib disease burden to warrant use of Hib vaccine in the EPI. However, after hearing the NTAGI's stand on the issue, the GOI introduced pentavalent vaccine, which includes Hib, in Tamil Nadu and Kerala to begin with. Post-introduction evaluation of pentavalent vaccine (DPT+hepatitis B+Hib) in these 2 states has documented the process of new vaccine introduction and successful streamlining in the immunization program in a short time. So far 7 more states have already introduced pentavalent vaccine in their immunization programs.

Hib containing pentavalent vaccine safety issues

Since 2008, Hib vaccine has increasingly been introduced in form of combination pentavalent vaccine into Asian countries immunization programs. A report on Vaccine Safety concerns in Sri Lanka, Bhutan, India and Vietnam describes events following reported AEFIs due to pentavalent vaccine in these countries that include suspension of the vaccine, review of serious AEFIs by independent national and international experts, and then re-introduction of pentavalent vaccine in Sri Lanka and Bhutan. In Vietnam clinical, epidemiological and vaccine quality issues are currently being reviewed. In Sri Lanka and Bhutan none of the fatal cases could be classified as having a consistent causal association with immunization. In Sri Lanka after re-introduction, 6 of 19 infant deaths were found at autopsy to have severe congenital heart disease. Following this finding, in Sri Lanka, children with known severe congenital heart disease are now vaccinated under close medical supervision, and no additional deaths among these children have since been reported in temporal association with PV vaccine administration.[14] In India pentavalent vaccine (Pentavac by M/s Serum Institute of India) was introduced in Kerala and Tamil Nadu in 2011 and later extended to the states of Goa, Pondicherry, Karnataka, Haryana, Jammu and Kashmir, Gujarat and Delhi during the second half of 2012 to the 1st quarter of 2013. To date, 83 AEFI cases, some of which were associated with fatality, have been reported after vaccine introduction from Kerela, Tamil Nadu and Jammu and Kashmir. However, a special causality sub-committee formed by the National AEFI Committee examined these instances and concluded that the infant deaths reported from these states were not causally related to pentavalent vaccine. The NTAGI in 2013 recommends scale-up of the pentavalent vaccine to the remaining states of India with simultaneous strengthening of the AEFI and expansion of sentinel surveillance systems. The Academy also endorses the continued use of pentavalent vaccine in the UIP. The IAP members are using these vaccines in their clinical practice for more than a decade. IAP had conducted a scientific study amongst around 1000 pediatricians and found that more than 80% of them are using this Hib-containing pentavalent vaccine in their clinical practice for more than last 5–15 years. Majority of them had never encountered any serious AEFI, including death.[15]

Individual use

IAP ACVIP recommends use of Hib vaccine for all children below the age of 5 years.

Schedule and doses

The vaccination schedule for Hib consists of three doses when initiated below 6 months, 2 doses between 6 months and 12 months and 1 dose between 12 months and 15 months, with a booster at 16–18 months. For children aged more than 15 months a single dose may suffice. The interval between two doses should be at least 4 weeks. As Hib disease is essentially confined to infants and young children, catch-up vaccination is not recommended for healthy children above 5 years. However, the vaccine should be administered to all individuals with functional/ anatomic hyposplenia irrespective of age. Hib vaccines are now used mostly as combination vaccines with DTwP/ DTaP/Hep B/ IPV.

Catch-up vaccination

When infants and children under 5 years of age have missed scheduled vaccine doses or start of Hib vaccination has been delayed, a catch-up schedule should be commenced. Table 1 is designed to assist in planning a catch-up program .

Table 1. Recommended catch-up schedule when start of Hib vaccination has been delayed

Vaccine	Trade Name	Age now			
		3–6 months	7–11 months	12–14 months	15–59 months
PRP-OMP [(1), (2)]	PedvaxH IB	2 doses, 1–2 months apart and booster at 12 months	2 doses, 1–2 months apart and booster at least 2 months later, at 12–15 months	1 dose, and booster at least 2 months after previous dose [(4)]	Single dose [(3) (4)]
Hib (PRP-OMP) -hepB	Comvax				
HbOC [(3)]	HibTITER	3 doses, months apart, and booster at 12 months	2 doses, 2 months apart, and booster at 12 months and at least 2 months after previous dose	1 dose, and booster at 18 months	Single dose [(3) (4)]
PRP-T [(3)]	Hiberix ActHIB				

(1) Extremely preterm babies (<28 weeks or <1500 grams) who commence catch-up Hib vaccination with PRP-OMP between 3 months and 11 months of age require a 3-dose primary series (not 2 doses). The third dose should be given 1–2 months after the second dose of PRP-OMP. The booster dose should be given at 12 months as usual.

(2) Where possible, use the same brand of Hib vaccine throughout the primary course.

(3) When a booster is given after the age of 15 months, any of the 3 available conjugate Hib vaccines can be used.

(4) Depending on the combination used, further doses of hepatitis B or IPV are required.

HAEMOPHILUS INFLUENZAE TYPE B (HIB) CONJUGATE VACCINE

Routine vaccination:

- Minimum age: 6 weeks

- Primary series includes Hib conjugate vaccine at ages 6, 10, 14 weeks with a booster at age 12 through 18 months.

Catch-up vaccination:

- Catch-up is recommended till 5 years of age.

- 6–12 months; 2 primary doses 4 weeks apart and 1 booster;

- 12–15 months: 1 primary dose and 1 booster;

- Above 15 months: Single dose.

- If the first dose was administered at age 7 through 11 months, administer the second dose at least 4 weeks later and a final dose at age 12–18 months at least 8 weeks after the second dose.

References

1. Invasive Bacterial Infections Surveillance (IBIS) Group of the International Clinical Epidemiology Network. Are Haemophilus influenzae infections a significant problem in India? A prospective study and review. Clin Infect Dis 2002, 34:949–957.

2. Walker CL, Rudan I, Liu L, Nair H, et al. Global burden of childhood pneumonia and diarrhea. Lancet 2013, 381:1405–1416.

3. Watt JP, Wolfson LJ, O'Brien KL, Henkle E, et al and Hib and Pneumococcal Global Burden of Disease Study Team. Burden of disease caused by Haemophilus influenzae type b in children younger than 5 years: Global estimates. Lancet 2009, 374:903–911.

4. Rudan I, Boschi-Pinto C, Biloglav Z, Mulholland K, Campbell H. Epidemiology and etiology of childhood pneumonia. Bull World Health Organ 2008, 86:408–416.

5. WHO Position Paper on *Haemophilus influenzae* type b conjugate vaccines. Wkly Epidemiol Rec 2006, 81: 445–452.

6. Bahl R, Mishra S, Sharma D, Singhal A, Kumari S.A bacteriological study in hospitalized children with pneumonia. Ann Trop Paediatr 1995 Jun; 15(2): 173–177.

7. Patwari AK, Bisht S, Srinivasan A, Deb M, Chattopadhya D. Aetiology of pneumonia in hospitalized children. J Trop Pediatr 1996, 42:15–20.

8. Gupta M, Kumar R, Deb AK, Bhattacharya SK, et al: Hib study working group. Multi-center surveillance for pneumonia & meningitis among children (<2 year) for Hib vaccine probe trial preparation in India. Indian J Med Res 2010, 131: 649–658.

9. Hutter J, Pasetti MF, Sanogo D, Tapia MD, Sow SO, Levine MM. Naturally acquired and conjugate vaccine-induced antibody to *Haemophilus influenzae* type b (Hib) polysaccharide in Malian children: Serological assessment of the Hib immunization program in Mali. Am J Trop Med Hyg 2012, 86: 1026–1031.

10. Sharma H, Yadav S, Lalwani S, Kapre S, et al. Antibody persistence of two pentavalent DTwP-HB-Hib vaccines to the age of 15–18 months, and response to the booster dose of quadrivalent DTwP-Hib vaccine. Vaccine 2013, 31: 444–447.

11. Consensus recommendations on Immunization and IAP Immunization Timetable 2012. Indian Pediatr 2012, 49: 549–564.

12. Vashishtha VM. Introduction of Hib containing pentavalent vaccine in national immunization program of India: The concerns and the reality! Indian Pediatr 2009; 46: 781–782.

13. Gupta M, Prinja S, Kumar R, Kaur M. Cost-effectiveness of *Haemophilus influenzae* type b (Hib) vaccine introduction in the universal immunization schedule in Haryana State, India. Health Policy Plan 2013, 28: 51–61.

14. WHO, Global Advisory Committee on Vaccine Safety, report of meeting held 12-13 June 2013 http://www.who.int/vaccine_safety/committee/ reports/ Jun_2013/en/ (Accessed on December 10, 2013)

15. Vashishtha VM, Dogra V, Choudhury P, Thacker N, Gupta SG, Gupta SK. *Haemophilus influenzae* type b disease and vaccination in India: Knowledge, attitude and practices of pediatricians. WHO South-East Asia Journal of Public Health 2013; (In press).

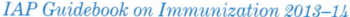

PNEUMOCOCCAL VACCINES

Reviewed by
Vipin M. Vashishtha, Panna Choudhury, & Thomas Cherian

Pneumococcal diseases

Epidemiology: The causative agent *Streptococcus pneumoniae* is a Gram-positive, encapsulated diplococcus and frequently colonizes the human nasopharynx. The polysaccharide capsule is an essential virulence factor and the > 90 distinct pneumococcal serotypes are defined on the basis of differences in the composition of this capsule of which a handful are responsible for most cases of invasive pneumococcal disease (IPD). In general, immunity following infection is serotype-specific, but cross-protection between related serotypes can occur. A definitive diagnosis of pneumococcal infection can be made by isolating the bacterium from blood or other normally sterile body sites, but the etiological diagnosis is problematic in cases of non-bacteraemic pneumococcal pneumonia.

Serotypes distribution: The distribution of serotypes that cause disease varies by age, disease syndrome, disease severity, geographic region, and over time. Prior to introduction of pneumococcal conjugate vaccines, 6–11 serotypes accounted for ≥ 70% of all IPD occurring in children worldwide. While a wide variety of serotypes cause non-invasive diseases such as otitis media and sinusitis, serotypes 1, 5, 6A, 6B, 14, 19F, and 23F are common causes of IPD globally in children < 5 years of age. Serotypes 1, 5, and 14 together account for 28%–43% of IPD across regions and for about 30% of IPD in 20 of the world's poorest countries; serotypes 23F and 19F are responsible for 9%–18% of cases globally. Serotype 18C is common in regions with a large proportion of high-income countries (i.e., Europe, North America, and Oceania). Some serotypes such as 6B, 9V, 14, 19A, 19F, and 23F are more likely than others to be associated with drug resistance.[1]

Spectrum of diseases: Pneumococcal infections include serious diseases such as meningitis, bacteremia, and pneumonia, as well as milder but more common illnesses, such as sinusitis and otitis media. IPD is commonly defined as morbidity associated with the isolation of pneumococci from a normally sterile body site, such as the blood stream, or those secondary to blood stream spread, e.g. meningitis or septic arthritis; it does not include sites such as the middle ear which are infected by contiguous spread from the nasopharynx.[2]

Most illnesses are sporadic. Outbreaks of pneumococcal disease are uncommon, but may occur in closed populations. Children under the age of 2 years are at greatest risk for IPD. On average, about 75% of IPD cases and 83% of pneumococcal meningitis occur in children aged < 2 years, but these incidences vary considerably, as does the distribution of cases in age strata below 2 years. For pneumonia, between 8.7% and 52.4% of cases occur in infants aged <6 months.[2] Case fatality rates (CFR) can be high for IPD, ranging up to 20% for septicaemia and 50% for meningitis in developing countries.[2]

Transmission: *S. pneumoniae*, is transmitted mainly through respiratory droplets. Infants and young children are thought to be the main reservoir of this agent with cross-sectional point prevalence of nasopharyngeal carriage ranging from 27% in developed to 85% in developing countries.

Burden of pneumococcal diseases

Pneumococcal diseases (PDs) occur worldwide, though the incidence of disease and mortality varies by region. Disease occurs in all age groups, with the highest rates of disease in children under 2 years of age and among the elderly. Invasive pneumococcal disease is the easiest to measure and its incidence is often used as a measure of the morbidity of severe PDs.

The greater burden of severe PDs morbidity is from pneumonia. However, the magnitude of morbidity from pneumococcal pneumonia is difficult to ascertain because of the difficulty with its microbiological diagnosis. Culture of lung aspirate has been considered as the best available method for microbiological diagnosis, but wide variations in the proportion of pneumonia caused by pneumococcus using this method, even within the same country.

Global

Disease rates and mortality are higher in developing than in industrialized settings, with the majority of deaths occurring in Africa and Asia. Children with HIV infection are at substantially increased risk of serious pneumococcal disease. Before widespread immunization with 7-valent pneumococcal conjugate vaccine (PCV), the mean annual incidence of IPD in children aged < 2 years was 44.4/100,000 per year in Europe and 167/100,000 in the United States. In comparison, the annual incidence of IPD in children < 2 years in Africa ranged from 60/100,000 to 797/100,000.[2] Because of the difficulties in diagnosing pneumococcal pneumonia and the paucity of data from some parts of the world, mathematical modeling approaches have been used to determine the burden of severe PDs.

India

Burden of PDs: The incidence of invasive pneumococcal disease in India has not been measured in any study. There is no nationally representative study of any PD incidence from the community. Most of the available data on PDs is from hospitals and on meningitis.[4] There is no useful data on the burden of milder pneumococcal illnesses, such as sinusitis and otitis media. According to a two year prospective study at three Bengaluru hospitals in south India, incidence of IPD in the first year of study among less than 2-year old children was found to be 28.28 cases per 100,000 population in which pneumonia contributed 15.91 and acute bacterial meningitis (ABM) 6.82 cases per 100, 000 population. The same study has documented an overall estimated IPD incidence of 17.78 cases per 100,000 1–59 month old with highest burden amongst 6–11 month old population (49.85 cases per 100,000) during the second year of the study.[5]

Pneumonia burden: The pneumonia working group of Child Health Epidemiology Reference Group (CHERG) had estimated an incidence of 0.37 episodes per child year for clinical pneumonia among children < 5 years in India for the year 2004.[6] One Indian study reported the incidence of severe clinical pneumonia ranged from 0.03 to 0.08 per child-year at three study sites.[7] Another Indian study finds that Indian children <5 years of age suffer ~3 episodes of respiratory infection per year, with heavier burden on younger children. Approximately, 1 in 5 episodes is a lower or severe lower respiratory infection.[8] The hospital based Bengaluru study in south India quoted an incidence of 5,032.98 cases per 100,000 population of clinical pneumonia amongst 1–59 month old children, whereas the chest X-ray confirmed incidence was found 1,113.50 cases per 100,000 in the same age group.[5]

There is no systematic review or nationwide study of etiology of childhood pneumonia in India. According to a recent India-specific review, the incidence of pneumonia (ALRI) in India was found to be 290–536 and of severe pneumonia (severe ALRI) was 27–96 per 1000 child-years. Out of these cases, 18–59% of all pneumonia (ALRI) and 53% of all severe pneumonia (severe ALRI) were of bacterial origin. Pneumococci accounted for 5–12% of all severe pneumonia cases across studies; 12–30% of pneumonia cases with a confirmed etiology.[9] Viruses mainly respiratory syncytial virus (RSV), influenza A and B, para-influenza 1, 2 and 3, and-adenovirus are responsible for 22.1% of under five year old children patients with ARI, but only RSV and para-influenza 3 were seen to cause severe ALRI disease.[8] Another systematic review reported that about 12–35% of childhood pneumonias were caused by pneumococci and 10–15% by *H. influenzae* and RSV each.[10]

Meningitis burden: There is also lack of community-based incidence of ABM in India. Only limited data from prospective population-based incidence studies are available not only from India but also from entire Asia. A study from Vellore found an annual incidence of 'possible', 'probable' and 'proven' ABM as 86, 37.4 and 15.9 per 100,000 children per year, respectively. Assuming that the probable and proven cases were truly ABM, the burden of disease was 53/100,000/year in under-five children.[11] According to the recent review on epidemiology of pneumococcal infections in India, pneumococci were responsible for 27–39% of all cases of ABM in children.[9]

Mortality data

Global: WHO estimates that out of estimated 8.8 million global annual deaths amongst children < 5 years of age in the year 2008, 476,000 (95% CL 333,000–529,000) deaths occurred in HIV-uninfected children due to pneumococcal diseases.[2] However, the latest estimates of CHERG found pneumonia was responsible for 1.396 million (UR 1.189–1.642 million, 18.3%) and meningitis 0.180 million (UR 0.136–0.237 million, 2%) deaths of total estimated 7.6 million under-5 deaths globally in 2010.[12]

India: One India-specific estimate for the year 2005 found 136,000 deaths (46,000–253,000) caused by PDs comprising 10% of deaths in Indian children aged 1–59 months.[13] The death rate for pneumococci was 106 per 100,000 (range 36–197), and more than two-thirds of pneumococcal deaths were pneumonia-related. Central and Eastern regions of the country had highest pneumococcal mortality with more than half of all Indian deaths occurring in four states: Bihar, Madhya Pradesh, Rajasthan, and Uttar Pradesh.[13] According to CHERG latest estimates for 2010, pneumonia was responsible for 0.397 million (UR 0.302–0.484 million, 23.6%) of total estimated 1.682 million under-5 deaths in India.[12] Considering that pneumococci constitute around 5–35 % of all pneumonia cases across different studies, the total number of estimated death caused by pneumococcal pneumonia would be ranging from 19, 850 to 138, 950 deaths per year.

Distribution and prevalence of different pneumococcal serotypes in India

The significance of knowing prevalence of distribution of different pneumococcal serotypes in the community is immense since each serotype had a distinct 'personality' and represented a distinct disease.[4] There are many studies highlighting (1, 5, 14–22) distribution and prevalence of different pneumococcal serotypes in the country, including some recent studies done by vaccine manufacturers in India like Pneumonet by M/s Pfizer[5] and alliance for surveillance of invasive pneumococci (ASIP) by M/s GSK.[22] The data on prevalence of different pneumococcal serotypes in the country is sparse and limited to a few hospital-based studies. There are only a few hospital-based studies mostly from South India. The Pneumonet study (2009–11) could do serotyping in only 36 isolates out of 9,950 subjects aging between 28 days and 5 years. Serotypes 6, 14, 18, 5, 19 and 1 were the most frequent serotypes.[5]

Two large studies IBIS and ASIP having 314 and 225 isolates, respectively, are again hospital based. According to IBIS study,[15] the most common serotypes out of total 314 serotypes were 6, 1, 19,

14, 4, 5, 45, 12, and 7 in children under 5 years of age. Serotypes 1 and 5 accounted for 29% of disease.[15] The multi-centric ASIP study[22] is the most recent one and still undergoing, included children from 2 months to 5 years of age. A total of 225 serotypes were isolated from 3572 subjects. Serotypes 14 (16%), 5 (14.6%), 1 (11.1%), 19F (9.7%) and 6B (6.7%) were most frequent serotypes.[22] However, this study also does not have representation from all over the country and major part of central India is not represented. The large studies from Asian and other neighboring countries like PneumoAdip,[17] ANSORP,[18, 19] SAPNA,[20] etc did not have adequate representation of isolates from India. Another hospital-based study from Delhi amongst individuals aged between 2 years and 77 years studied 126 clinical isolates of *Streptococcus pneumonia*. Serotypes 19, 1 and 6 were more frequently isolated. Thirty per cent of the strains were comprised of serotypes 1, 3, 5, 19A and 7F, and 30 new sequence types were encountered in this study.[23] In a recent report from Vellore, out of 244 isolates from IPD patients over a period of January 2007 to June 2011, the most common serotypes in this study were 1, 5, 19 F, 6B, 14, 3, 19A and 6A in that order.[24] This result is similar to the national Indian study from 1999, but with minor differences in order of prevalence, and a decreased prevalence of serogroup 7.[15]

Though a limited number of serotypes cause most IPD worldwide and the serotypes included in existing pneumococcal conjugate vaccines responsible for 49–88% of deaths in developing countries of Africa and Asia where PD morbidity and mortality are the highest,[1] still there is a need of establishing a real-time multi-site comprehensive pneumococcal disease surveillance including both population and hospital-based surveillance arms. The ongoing projects should also include data on zonal distribution and prevalence of different serotypes on annual basis. There is need to incorporate more sophisticated diagnostic tests like immune-chromatography (ICT), latex particle agglutination (LPA), and real-time polymerase chain reaction (PCR) apart from cultures to increase the yields. Since a few serotypes are difficult to grow and under diagnosed by culture (such as serotype 3), the PCR can be used to pick serotypes from culture negative cases as done in a few European countries.[4] The surveillance should not be a one-time project but should be an ongoing initiative to pick natural variations in the sero-epidemiology. The surveillance project should have three important objectives—to collect data on serotype distribution, to guide appropriate pneumococcal conjugate vaccine formulations, to identify trend of antimicrobial resistance amongst different serotypes, and lastly, to assess the impact of vaccine introduction (in national immunization program (NIP) on the serotype distribution and replacement, if any).

Pneumococcal vaccines

Currently two types of vaccines are licensed for use;

(1) Pneumococcal Polysaccharide Vaccine (PPSV)

(2) Pneumococcal Conjugate Vaccines (PCVs).

Pneumococcal polysaccharide vaccine

The unconjugated pneumococcal polysaccharide vaccine is a 23 valent vaccine (PPSV 23) containing 25 µg per dose of the purified polysaccharide of the following 23 serotypes of pneumococcus— 1, 2, 3, 4, 5, 6B, 7F, 8, 9N, 9V, 10A, 11A, 12F, 14, 15B, 17F, 18C, 19F, 19A, 20, 22F, 23F, 33F. These serotypes account for over 80% of serotypes associated with serious diseases in adults. It is a T cell independent vaccine that is poorly immunogenic below the age of 2 years, has low immune memory, does not reduce nasopharyngeal carriage and does not provide herd immunity. The vaccine is administered as a 0.5 ml dose either intramuscularly in the deltoid muscle or subcutaneously. It is stored at 2 to 8°C. It is a safe vaccine with occasional local side effects. Not more than two life time doses are recommended, as repeated doses may cause immunologic hyporesponsiveness.[25]

Immunogenicity: A single dose of PPSV 23 results in the induction of serotype-specific immunoglobulin (Ig) G, IgA, and IgM antibodies; the IgG antibodies predominantly belong to the IgG2 subclass. Though the total antibodies, as measured using the ELISA, are similar between age groups, however, functional antibody responses, are lower in the elderly compared to young adults.

Efficacy and effectiveness: Data on the efficacy and effectiveness of PPV 23 is conflicting.[26,27] A systematic review commissioned by WHO concluded that the evidence was consistent with a protective effect against invasive pneumococcal disease and pneumonia in healthy adults and against invasive pneumococcal disease in the elderly. There was no evidence of efficacy against invasive disease or pneumonia in other high-risk populations with underlying diseases or highly immuno-suppressed individuals in both adults and children.[28] One study in Uganda in HIV-infected adults showed an increased risk of pneumonia among those vaccinated with PPSV23.[29]

Pneumococcal conjugate vaccines

In order to overcome the immunological limitations of PPSV, the individual polysaccharides of a set of pneumococcal serotypes were conjugated to carrier proteins in order to make them immunogenic in infants, confer more long-lasting protection and induce immunological memory.

The serotype composition and the protein carrier(s) for vaccines that were either evaluated in phase 3 clinical trials or are currently undergoing are shown in Figure 1. Three of these vaccines containing 7, 10 or 13 serotypes of pneumococcus, respectively (PCV 7, PCV 10 and PCV 13) were licensed and marketed globally; of these PCV 10 and PCV 13 are currently marketed. A second 7-valent vaccine with the outer membrane protein complex of *Neisseria meningitides* as the protein carrier was evaluated for efficacy against otitis media, but not licensed.[30] A 9-valent vaccine (PCV 9) was evaluated in clinical trials in South Africa and the Gambia,[31, 32] but was reformulated with additional serotypes and marketed as a 13-valent vaccine (PCV 13). Two 11-valent vaccines (PCV 11) formulations with similar serotype composition, but different protein carriers were also evaluated in phase 3 clinical trials. One with diphtheria and tetanus toxoid as the protein carrier was tested in the Philippines, but not further developed or licensed.[33] The other PCV 11 formulation with protein D as the protein carrier, was evaluated for efficacy against acute otitis media, but was further reformulated and licensed as a 10-valent vaccine (PCV 10).[34] An Indian company with active support of Department of Biotechnology (DBT), Government of India is developing 15-valent vaccine containing two additional serotypes, 2 and 12F to existing PCV 13. Merck is also developing 15-valent vaccine with two additional serotypes, 22F and 33F to existing

Formu-lation	Protein carrier	1	2	3	4	5	6A	6B	7F	9V	12F	14	18C	19A	19F	22F	23F	33F
PCV 7	CRM 197				■			■		■		■	■		■		■	
PCV 7	OMP				■			■		■		■	■		■		■	
PCV 9	CRM 197	■			■	■		■		■		■	■		■		■	
PCV 10	Protein D, TT, DT	■			■	■		■	■	■		■	■		■		■	
PCV 11	TT, DT	■		■	■	■		■	■	■		■	■		■		■	
PCV 11	Protein D	■		■	■	■		■	■	■		■	■		■		■	
PCV 13	CRM 197	■		■	■	■	■	■	■	■		■	■	■	■		■	
PCV 15*	CRM 197	■		■	■	■	■	■	■	■		■	■	■	■	■	■	
PCV 15**	CRM 197	■		■	■	■	■	■	■	■		■	■	■	■	■	■	■

Figure 1: Serotype composition of the pneumococcal conjugate vaccine formulations that have been evaluated in phase III clinical efficacy trials or under clinical development.

■ Serotypes in the vaccine   □ Serotypes with cross protection

*Under production in India by the support of DBT

**Under production in US by Merck

PCV 13. Both these formulations are using CRM 197 as a carrier protein.[35]

Vaccine compositions

PCV 13

PCV13 contains polysaccharides of the capsular antigens of *S. pneumoniae* serotypes 1, 5, 7F, 3, 6A and 19A, in addition to the 7 polysaccharides of the capsular antigens of 4, 6B, 9V, 14, 18C, 19F and 23F present in the PCV7, individually conjugated to a nontoxic diphtheria cross-reactive material (CRM) carrier protein (CRM197). A 0.5-mL PCV13 dose contains approximately 2.2 µg of polysaccharide from each of 12 serotypes and approximately 4.4 µg of polysaccharide from serotype 6B; the total concentration of CRM197 is approximately 34 µg. The vaccine contains 0.02% polysorbate 80 (P80), 0.125 mg of aluminium as aluminium phosphate (AlPO4) adjuvant, 5 mL of succinate buffer, and no thimerosal preservative. Except for the addition of six serotypes, P80, and succinate buffer, the formulation of PCV13 same as that of PCV7.

PCV 10

PCV10 covers 3 additional serotypes besides PCV7, i.e. 1, 5, and 7F. Three different carrier proteins are used in this formulation (Table 1). It contains aluminium phosphate as an adjuvant.

Table 1: Antigen concentration of different serotypes and carrier proteins used in the development of PCV10.

Serotypes	1, 5, 6B, 7F, 9V, 14, 23F	4	18C	19F
Antigen concentration	1 mcg	3 mcg	3 mcg	3 mcg
Carrier proteins	Non-typeable *H. influenzae* (NTHi) Protein D		Tetanus toxiod	Diphtheria toxoid

The choice of non-typeable *Haemophilus influenzae* protein D as main carrier protein in PCV 10 was driven in part to avoid carrier-mediated suppression and possible bystander interference with co-administered vaccines. PCV10 is a preservative-free vaccine and adsorbed on aluminium phosphate.

Vaccine immunogenicity and efficacy

Serological correlates of protection: Any new pneumococcal conjugate vaccine has to meet the following criteria laid down by the WHO:[2]

*   IgG (for all common serotyoes collectively and not individually) of equal to or more than 0.35 mcg/ml measured by the WHO reference assay (or an alternative);
*   The serotype-specific IgG geometric concentration ratios.

Immunogenicity: Comparisons of OPA antibody titres of serotypes that are common to the new vaccine and the licensed comparator should focus on serotype-specific GMT ratios rather than the previously used threshold functional titer ≥1:8.

Both the vaccines have comparable immunogenicity in terms of the proportion of subjects achieving serotype specific IgG antibody levels ≥ 0.35 µg/ml in the dosage schedules indicated by the manufacturer. The immunogenicity of the vaccines has also been tested using different schedules.

Efficacy: The efficacy of PCV has been evaluated in different populations in both industrialized and developing countries in different parts of the world and against a number of different clinical outcomes.

i. IPD: IPD was the primary outcome for the pivotal clinical trials of PCV. This outcome is very specific and represents the more serious forms of disease caused by the pneumococcus. While the trials used different formulations of the vaccine administered in infants in either a 6, 10 and 14 weeks schedule or a 2, 4 and 6 month schedule, the efficacy estimates were fairly consistent. In a systematic review and meta-analysis from seven studies, a pooled vaccine efficacy of 80% (95% confidence interval (CI) 58% to 90%, P < 0.0001) was observed against vaccine type invasive disease and 58%(95% CI 29% to 75%, P = 0.001) against total invasive disease (irrespective of serotype).[36]

ii. Pneumonia: Since pneumococcal pneumonia is difficult to diagnose, most trials opted to measure efficacy against pneumonia from any cause that was associated with alveolar consolidation, using a standardized WHO definition and process for interpreting radiographs.[37] The results of 5 trials that used the standardized process are summarized in Table 2.[31–33, 38, 39] Given the diversity in vaccine formulations and vaccination schedules used and in the populations in which the vaccines were tested, the results were remarkably

Table 2: Efficacy of PCV against all-cause radiological pneumonia (defined using WHO criteria)

Study site	Vaccine	Vaccine efficacy (%) (95% CL)	Reference
Northern California, USA	PCV-7	25.5 (6.5, 40.7)	37
Soweto, South Africa (HIV neg.)	PCV-9	25 (4, 41)	30
The Gambia	PCV-9	37 (27, 45)	31
Philippines	PCV-11	23 (−1, 41)	32
Latin America	PCV-10	23 (9, 36)	38

consistent. The pooled estimate of vaccine efficacy against radiologically defined pneumonia was found to be 27%(95% CI 15% to 36%, P < 0.0001).[35] Though most of the reduction is in cases of pneumonia that met the WHO definition for radiologically defined pneumonia, reduction in cases of pneumonia that did not meet this definition have also been observed in clinical efficacy trials.[40] Thus, the full impact of PCV on pneumonia extends beyond the impact on radiologically defined pneumonia. Studies in South Africa have also shown reductions in hospitalization with virus-associated lower respiratory infection, suggesting that co-infection with pneumococcus contributes to severity of disease, resulting in hospitalization; receipt of PCV reduces the risk of severe disease associated with respiratory viruses that requires hospitalization.[41]

iii. Otitis media: The PCVs were efficacious in preventing acute otitis media (AOM) caused by the serotypes of pneumococcus present in the vaccine, with very similar point estimates of efficacy, ranging from 56 to 57.6%. In two of these trials of two different formulations of PCV 7, increases in AOM due to other serotypes of pneumococcus and other organisms increased, such that the overall impact on otitis media was not significant.[30, 42] However, the PCV 7-CRM197 was observed to protect against recurrent or more severe forms of AOM, including otitis requiring tympanostomy tube placement.[43–45] In the third trial with PCV 10, the protection against vaccine-type pneumococcal otitis was not completely offset by increases in otitis by other serotypes of pneumococcus or other bacteria; vaccine efficacy against all otitis media of 33.6% (95% CL 21, 44%) was observed.[34] In this trial, significant protection was also observed against AOM caused by 'Non-typeable *Haemophilus influenzae*' (NTHi) with observed efficacy of 35% (95% CL 1.8, 57.4%); this protection was attributed to the immune response to protein D of NTHi, which was the protein carrier in this formulation of the vaccine.[34]

Vaccine effectiveness

Many countries in which PCVs were introduced as part of routine immunization have shown reduction in vaccine type invasive disease, not only in the targeted children, but also in older populations as a result of the indirect effects of the vaccine through reduction in nasopharyngeal carriage and transmission of the organism.[46-49] Most of the available data on the effectiveness of PCV are with PCV 7. But available data using the newer PCV 10 and 13 formulations also show similar effectiveness, including against the additional serotypes included in these formulations.[50-52] Impact of PCV was seen in developing countries also like Kenya where the vaccine was introduced in 2011 and impressive reductions have been observed in the rates of invasive pneumococcal disease. Several studies have also documented significant reductions in pneumonia hospitalization following the introduction of PCV.[50, 53] Following introduction of PCV13 into the national immunization programs of Argentina, Uruguay, and UK, reductions in hospitalized chest X-ray confirmed pneumonia and empyema cases were noted. Similarly, following PCV-13 introduction in Nicaragua—a low-middle income country, reduction in hospitalization and outpatient visits for pneumonia was found in children 1 year of age However, at least one study failed to document any reduction in radiologically defined pneumonia.[54] One trial using PCV 9, conducted in a high mortality setting in Gambia, reduction in overall mortality of 16% (95% CL 3, 28) was observed.[32]

Duration of protection: In South Africa, results of surveillance showed that 6.3 years after vaccination with PCV9, vaccine efficacy remained significant against IPD (78%; 95% CI, 34–92%). This was consistent with immunogenicity data showing that specific antibody concentrations among HIV-uninfected children remained above the assumed protective levels compared to unvaccinated HIV-uninfected controls during this period.

Effectiveness of incomplete series: In pivotal clinical trials, the effectiveness of 1 dose of PCV13 was estimated as 48%, 2 doses 87% and 2+1 doses 100%. One dose catch up for toddlers showed 83% effectiveness.

Safety

The safety of PCV has been well studied and all formulations are considered to have an excellent safety profile in various studies.[55-57] The main adverse events observed are injection-site reactions, fever, irritability, decreased appetite, and increased and/or decreased sleep that were reported about 10% of the vaccines. Fever with temperature > 39°C was observed in 1/100 to < 1/10 vaccines, vomiting and diarrhea in 1/1000 to < 1/100, and hypersensitivity reactions and nervous system disorders (including convulsions and hypotonic-hyporesponsive episodes) were reported in 1/10 000 to < 1/1000 of the vaccines.[2]

Clinical trials in India

There are no efficacy trials with PCV13 or PCV10 in India. Immunogenicity studies and WHO criteria to license any new PCV were employed to assess the protective efficacy of these formulations. Both the vaccines are now licensed and available in the country. The details about these trials in India and other pivotal trials of both these vaccines are provided in the previous edition of the guidebook.[58]

Serotype replacement

Early observations, which showed that though PCV reduced nasopharyngeal carriage with vaccine serotypes, carriage with non-vaccine serotypes increased, led to concerns about replacement disease due to serotypes not contained in the vaccines. Surveillance in populations in which PCV was first introduced, documented increases in the incidence rates of invasive pneumococcal disease caused by non-vaccine serotypes, though the magnitude of this increase was variable.[45, 46] Because of these observations, the WHO commissioned a systematic review of the data on serotype changes following the introduction of PCV in childhood immunization programmes.[59] The results indicated that while serotype replacement did occur, in all countries there was a net reduction in invasive pneumococcal disease, including pneumococcal meningitis, in children less than 5 years of age. The net benefit in older populations was variable. The predominant serotypes causing replacement disease were those found in the higher valency formulations of PCV. WHO recommends that surveillance for replacement disease should continue, especially in developing countries where the potential for replacement may be different from that in industrialized countries.[2]

PCV 10 versus PCV 13: Coverage of serotypes

According to a few recent Indian studies there is significant difference in the coverage of serotypes contained in both these vaccines and the serotypes responsible for PDs in hospitalized children in India. ASIP study (2011–2012) based on 225 serotypes, estimated the coverage of PCV13 and PCV10 around 73.3% and 64%, respectively.[22] Pneumonet study (2009–2011) based on only 36 pneumococcal serotypes found the coverage of PCV13 and PCV10 to be 91.67% and 63.89%, respectively.[5] Shariff M, et al study (2007–2010) based on 126 serotypes estimated the coverage of PCV 13 and PCV 10 to be 73% and 54%, respectively.[23] ANSORP study (2008–2009) based on 23 isolates estimated the coverage of PCV13 and PCV10 to be 95.7% and 82.6%, respectively.[19] In the Vellore study, the proportion of serotypes that are included in the vaccines PCV7, 10, and 13 for all ages was 29%, 53%, and 64%, respectively, and 54%, 66%, and 71%, respectively, for children <2 years.[24] So, the serotype coverage difference between PCV13 and PCV10 ranges from 9.3% to 27.8% based on these recent studies in India. However, the systematic review commissioned by WHO concluded that the coverage of serotypes included in PCV10 and PCV13 reached ≥ 70% of IPD in every region of the world (range: 70–84% and 74–88%, respectively).[2]

Recommendations for use

I. Pneumococcal polysaccharide vaccine

Individual use

See below the section on recommendations for use of PCV in high-risk children.

Public health perspectives

Many industrialized countries continue to use the vaccine in the elderly and in high-risk populations. In developing countries, with competing priorities, WHO does not recommend the use of this vaccine in high-risk populations with underlying disease, as part of the national immunization program though vaccination to specific high-risk individuals may be administered at the discretion of the attending physician.[28] There is also insufficient evidence to support its use in pregnant women to protect their newborn infants. The only study in a developing country showed no benefit and a suggestion of increased risk among HIV-infected adults[28]. Hence, on the basis of current evidence, IAP ACVIP supports the WHO recommendations and does not recommend broader use of this vaccine alone in high-risk populations with underlying disease.

II. Pneumococcal conjugate vaccines

Individual use

A. Healthy children

Indication: Both PCV10 and PCV13 are licensed for active immunization for the prevention of PDs caused by the respective vaccine serotypes in children from 6 weeks to 5 years of age. In addition, PCV13 is also licensed for the prevention of PD in adults > 50 years of age in India. US (FDA) licensed PCV13 for use in the age group of 6–17 years also, but not as yet in India.

Administration schedule: The vaccines are given by injection into the anterolateral aspect of the thigh in infants and into the deltoid muscle in older age groups. IAP ACVIP recommends following schedule of PCV 10 and PCV 13 (Table 3).

Table 3. Recommended schedule for use of PCV13/PCV10 among previously unvaccinated infants and children by age at time of first vaccination

Age at first dose	Primary series		Booster dose	
	PCV13	PCV10	PCV13	PCV10
6 weeks–6 months	3 doses	3 doses	1 dose at 12–15 months*	1 dose at 12–15 months*
7–11 months	2 doses	2 doses	1 dose during 2nd year	1 dose during 2nd year
12–23 months	2 doses#	2 doses#	NA	NA
24–59 months	1 dose	2 doses#	NA	NA

Abbreviation: NA = not applicable; *At least 6 months after the third dose; #At least 8 weeks apart

Primary schedule (For both PCV10 and PCV13)

- Three primary doses with an interval of at least 4 weeks between doses, plus a booster at least 6 months after the third dose (3p+1 schedule). The first dose can be given as early as 6 weeks of age; the booster dose is given preferably between 12 and 15 months of age.

- Previously unvaccinated infants aged 7–11 months should receive 2 doses, the second dose at least 4 weeks after the first, followed by a third dose in the second year of life.

- For PCV10, unvaccinated children 12 months to 5 years of age should receive 2 doses, with an interval between the first and second dose of at least 2 months.

- For PCV13, unvaccinated children aged 12–24 months should receive 2 doses at least 2 months interval. Children aged 2–5 years should receive a single dose; adults > 50 years of age should receive a single dose.

- Routine use of PCV 10/13 is not recommended for healthy children aged more than 5 years. Minimum age for administering first dose is 6 weeks. Minimum interval between two doses is 4 weeks for children vaccinated at age <12 months, whereas for those vaccinated at age >12 months, the minimum interval between doses is 2 months (8 weeks).

Interchangeability: When primary immunization is initiated with one of these vaccines, the remaining doses should be administered with the same product. Interchangeability between PCV10 and PCV13 has not yet been documented. However, if it is not possible to complete the series with the same type of vaccine, the other PCV product should be used.

PCV13 is administered intramuscularly as a 0.5 mL dose and is available in latex-free, single-dose, prefilled syringes. PCV13 can be administered at the same time as other routine childhood vaccinations, if administered in a separate syringe at a separate injection site. However, there are reports of higher incidence of febrile seizures when one brand of influenza vaccine, Fluzone was co-administered with PCV13 to children 6–23 months old in US and Australia. Hence, PCV13 should preferably be administered one month before this brand of TIV. The safety and efficacy of concurrent administration of PCV13 and PPV23 has not been studied, and concurrent administration is not recommended.

B. High-risk group of children

Administration of PPSV23 after PCV13/PCV10 among children aged 2–18 years who are at increased risk for pneumococcal disease should be undertaken as per following instructions:

- Children aged ≥ 2 years with underlying medical conditions (Table 4) should receive PPSV23 after completing all recommended doses of PCV13/PCV10. These children should be administered 1 dose of PPSV23 at age ≥2 years and at least 8 weeks after the most recent dose of PCV.

Table 4: Children at high risk for pneumococcal disease, suitability of PCV13 versus PCV10 for Indian children

Risk group	Condition
Immunocompetent children	Chronic heart disease (particularly cyanotic congenital heart disease and cardiac failure)
	Chronic lung disease (including asthma if treated with prolonged high-dose oral corticosteroids)
	Diabetes mellitus
	Cerebrospinal fluid leak
	Cochlear implant
Children with functional or anatomic asplenia	Sickle cell disease and other hemoglobinopathies
	Sickle cell disease and other hemoglobinopathies
	Congenital or acquired asplenia, splenic dysfunction
Children with immunocompromising conditions	HIV infection
	Chronic renal failure and nephrotic syndrome
	Diseases associated with treatment with immunosuppressive drugs or radiation therapy (e.g. malignant neoplasms, leukemias, lymphomas, and Hodgkin disease; or solid organ transplantation)
	Congenital immunodeficiency includes B-(humoral) or T-lymphocyte deficiency; complement deficiencies, particularly C1, C2, C3, and C4 deficiency; and phagocytic disorders (excluding chronic granulomatous disease)

- Children who have received PPSV23 previously also should receive recommended PCV13/PCV10 doses.

- For children aged 24 through 71 months with certain underlying medical conditions, administer 1 dose of PCV13/10 if 3 doses of PCV were received previously or administer 2 doses of PCV13/10 at least 8 weeks apart if fewer than 3 doses of PCV were received previously.

- A single dose of PCV13/10 may be administered to previously unvaccinated children aged 6 through 18 years who have anatomic or functional asplenia (including sickle cell disease), HIV infection or an immunocompromising condition, cochlear implant or cerebrospinal fluid leak.

- Administer PPSV 23 at least 8 weeks after the last dose of PCV to children aged 2 years or older with certain underlying medical conditions like anatomic or functional asplenia (including sickle cell disease), HIV infection, cochlear implant or cerebrospinal fluid leak.

- An additional dose of PPSV (i.e. 2nd dose) should be administered after 5 years to children with anatomic / functional asplenia or an immunocompromising condition. No more than two PPSV23 doses are recommended.

- PPSV should never be used alone for prevention of pneumococcal diseases amongst high-risk individuals.

- When elective splenectomy, immunocompromising therapy, or cochlear implant placement is being planned; PCV13/PCV 10 and/or PPSV23 vaccination should be completed at least 2 weeks before surgery or initiation of therapy.

- The ACVIP now stresses the need of treating prematurity (PT) and very-low birth weight (VLBW) infants as another high-risk category for pneumococcal vaccination. These infants have up to 9-fold higher incidence of IPD in VLBW babies as compared to full size babies.[60] PCV 13/10 must be offered to these babies on a priority basis.[4]

The ACVIP reviewed all the available relevant data on the performance of PCV13 and PCV10. The committee maintains that the direct protection rendered by the serotype included in a vaccine formulation is definitely superior to any cross protection offered by the unrelated serotypes even of the same group in any PCV formulation. However, the committee still not convinced about the clinical efficacy of serotype 3 contained in PCV13 despite multiple studies showing good functional immune responses after the infant series and reasonably effectiveness.[4] There has been no consistent PCV13 impact on serotype 3 IPD burden or carriage reported so far. Similarly, the committee still thinks that despite using a different conjugation method (cyanylation versus reductive amination), PCV10 is yet to demonstrate a better clinical efficacy (cross protection) against serotype 19A than shown by PCV7.[4] The presence of 19A in India is confirmed by almost all the recent studies. On the other hand, the committee is convinced about the adequate cross-protection rendered by serotype 6B to 6A based on performance of PCV7 in many European countries and US in decreasing IPDs caused by 6A, and the recent immunogenicity data of PCV10 on Indian children. The committee thinks that though NTHi, a co-pathogen plays some role in the pathogenesis of mucosal disease with *Streptococcus pneumoniae*, its role in childhood pneumonia is still not proven. After appraising in detail the available relevant data, the committee concludes that since there is still limited data on the prevalence of pneumococcal serotypes from all the regions of the country, particularly on the prevalence of different serotypes in the community including serotypes 3, 6A and 19A, and non-typeable *Haemophilus influenzae* (NTHi), it is difficult to comment on the comparative utility of one product over other in context to India. Further, in the absence of head to head trials, it is difficult to determine if either vaccine has a clear advantage over other. Though based on recent pneumococcal serotype surveillance studies from different parts of the country, PCV 13 definitely has some edge over PCV10.

Public health perspectives

IAP believes that despite absence of a nationally representative data, there is significant burden of PDs, particularly pneumonia in the country. The currently available PCV formulations are safe and efficacious and the additional serotypes in PCV 10 and 13 represent significant progress in efforts to control pneumococcal disease. WHO continues to recommend that these vaccines be prioritized for inclusion in the national programs in countries with high child mortality.[2] Based on the available evidence, the committee considers PCV10 and PCV13 of almost comparable safety and efficacy, particularly for mass use. Nevertheless, the choice of formulation will depend on the prevalence of the vaccine serotypes in the country, vaccine supply and pricing.

However, there are some issues to confront with for introducing PCVs in the NIP of the country. The percentages of isolates that are covered by the available licensed PCVs are lower than they were in the U.S. prior to mass vaccination, some of the herd effects that were observed in the U.S. might not occur to the same extent if mass vaccination with PCV10 or PCV13 was started in India.[47] On the other hand, herd effects were observed in Europe despite a 15–20% lower coverage.[48] Hence, the vaccines need to have good effectiveness at community level against pneumonia. There is an urgent need to carry out community-based surveys to establish exact disease burden of various syndromes caused by pneumococci and to establish an effective surveillance system to monitor prevalence of different serotypes in different epidemiological settings, and also to monitor epidemiological changes following vaccine introduction, especially to monitor the occurrence and magnitude of serotype replacement. Lastly, there is need to carry out deft cost effective analysis before any decision to introduce current PCVs into NIP is contemplated. The committee thinks availability of an efficacious yet an affordable indigenous product based on local prevalence of serotypes shall facilitate this decision. Currently data on pneumococcal disease in older age groups in India is insufficient to make any recommendations for use of PCV as part of a national immunization program.

Cost effectiveness: Cost-effectiveness evaluations of PCV have been conducted in several countries with varying results. The variability in results is related to the assumptions used in the analysis. The inclusion of indirect effects of vaccination had a big impact on the outcome of the analysis. One analysis of the cost-effectiveness of PCV in low-income countries that considered only the direct effects of the vaccine concluded that the vaccines would be highly cost-effective in these high mortality settings.[61]

Choice of schedule: The WHO recommends a minimum of three doses of vaccine, given in either a 3p+0 or a 2p+1 schedule. If a 3 dose primary series is used the first dose may be given as early as 6 weeks of age with a minimum of 4 weeks between doses. If 2p+1 schedule is chosen, the first dose may be given as early as 6 weeks of age, preferably with an 8 week interval between the two primary doses and the booster dose administered between 9 and 15 months. In countries where disease incidence peaks before 32 weeks of age, the 2p+1 schedule may leave some infants unprotected during the peak period of risk, especially in the absence of herd effect.[2] Catch-up immunization of children older than 12 months of age at the time of vaccine introduction may accelerate the impact of vaccination through rapid induction of herd immunity. Older children with high risk of disease, e.g. those with asplenia, should also be targeted for vaccination.

Shortened vaccination schedule for public use consideration

Schedules of PCV are an area of intense debate. One exciting prospect will be to study a shortened vaccination schedule as this will moderately cut down the cost incurred on pneumococcal mass vaccination program. Based on data from immunogenicity studies and on effectiveness data in children who received incomplete courses of PCV, several countries adopted schedules other than those used in the initial clinical efficacy trials.

The most common immunization schedules used are 3 primary doses with 1 booster dose (3p+1), 3 primary doses with no booster (3p+0) and 2 primary doses with 1 booster dose (2p+1). Two systematic reviews have been conducted to evaluate the value of the respective schedules.[62,63] Most of the studies are based on PCV7. The primary doses have been given in a 2, 4, and 6 months schedule or in a 6, 10 and 14 weeks schedule, with the booster doses between 9 and 18 months of age. In general, there is evidence to support to use of all three schedules.

3+1 schedule: The gold standard regimen of 3 + 1 has been defined by the US licensure trials.[64] This schedule is three doses in infancy, generally 2 months apart with a booster in the second year of life.

3 + 0 schedule: It consists of 3 primary doses with no booster. However, a limitation of this shortened schedule for countries with a significant burden of disease caused by serotype 1 is that the extended period of susceptibility to serotype 1 and the invasive nature of that serotype may require prolonged levels of antibody in the second year of life, especially after 18 months of age.[65]

2+1 schedule: In the 2p+1 schedule, the GMT of antibody is higher when the two doses are given with an interval of 2 months between doses, as compared to a one month interval. For certain serotypes (6B and 23F), the antibody levels in the interval between the two primary doses and the booster dose may be lower than when 3 primary doses are given, but following the booster dose the antibody levels may exceed those following a 3p schedule. Thus, while the 2p+1 schedule may leave some infants incompletely protected during the interval between the primary series and the booster dose (i.e. between 6 and 12 months of age), it may confer some advantage in terms of protection against serotypes that cause disease slightly later in life (e.g. serotype 1) and in the duration of protection, in comparison to schedules without a booster dose. However, one should refrain from using 2+1 schedule for individual in office practice and can be used only in NIP.

Variant 2+1 schedule: In this schedule, the booster is brought in line with the WHO scheduled visit of 9 months (hence, a 6-week, 14-week, plus 9-month schedule) because there is no further visit around 12 months in the infant EPI schedules. This could also be described as a prolonged variant of the 3 + 0 schedule, which is the final schedule that has been tested in large efficacy trials in South Africa[31] and the Gambia.[32] This schedule may address the limitation of 3+0 schedule, but the effectiveness of this schedule or other prolonged schedules in protection against serotype 1 remains under investigation.[66]

Pneumococcal conjugate vaccines (PCVs)

Routine vaccination:

- Minimum age: 6 weeks

- Both PCV10 and PCV13 are licensed for children from 6 weeks to 5 years of age (although the exact labeling details may differ by country). Additionally, PCV13 is licensed for the prevention of pneumococcal diseases in adults > 50 years of age.

- Primary schedule (for both PCV10 and PCV13): 3 primary doses at 6, 10, and 14 weeks with a booster at age 12 through 15 months.

Catch-up vaccination:

- Administer 1 dose of PCV13 or PCV10 to all healthy children aged 24 through 59 months who are not completely vaccinated for their age.

- For PCV 13: Catch-up in 6–12 months: 2 doses 4 weeks apart and 1 booster; 12–23 months: 2 doses 8 weeks apart; 24 months and above: Single dose

- For PCV10: Catch up in 6–12 months: 2 doses 4 weeks apart and 1 booster; 12 months to 5 years: 2 doses 8 weeks apart

- Vaccination of persons with high-risk conditions:

  - PCV and pneumococcal polysaccharide vaccine [PPSV] both are used in certain high-risk group of children.

  - For children aged 24 through 71 months with certain underlying medical conditions, administer 1 dose of PCV13 if 3 doses of PCV were received previously, or administer 2 doses of PCV13 at least 8 weeks apart if fewer than 3 doses of PCV were received previously.

  - A single dose of PCV13 may be administered to previously unvaccinated children aged 6 through 18 years who have anatomic or functional asplenia (including sickle cell disease), HIV infection or an immunocompromising condition, cochlear implant or cerebrospinal fluid leak.

  - Administer PPSV23 at least 8 weeks after the last dose of PCV to children aged 2 years or older with certain underlying medical conditions.

Pneumococcal polysaccharide vaccine (PPSV23)

- Minimum age: 2 years

- Not recommended for routine use in healthy individuals. Recommended only for the vaccination of persons with certain high-risk conditions.

- Administer PPSV at least 8 weeks after the last dose of PCV to children aged 2 years or older with certain underlying medical conditions like anatomic or functional asplenia (including sickle cell disease), HIV infection, cochlear implant or cerebrospinal fluid leak.

- An additional dose of PPSV should be administered after 5 years to children with anatomic/functional asplenia or an immunocompromising condition.

- *PPSV should never be used alone for prevention of pneumococcal diseases amongst high-risk individuals.*

- **Children with following medical conditions for which PPSV23 and PCV are indicated in the age group 24 through 71 months:**

  - Immunocompetent children with chronic heart disease (particularly cyanotic congenital heart disease and cardiac failure); chronic lung disease (including asthma if treated with high-dose oral corticosteroid therapy), diabetes mellitus; cerebrospinal fluid leaks; or cochlear implant.

  - Children with anatomic or functional asplenia (including sickle cell disease and other hemoglobinopathies, congenital or acquired asplenia, or splenic dysfunction);

  - Children with immunocompromising conditions: HIV infection, chronic renal failure and nephrotic syndrome, diseases associated with treatment with immunosuppressive drugs or radiation therapy, including malignant neoplasms, leukemias, lymphomas and Hodgkin disease; or solid organ transplantation, congenital immunodeficiency.

References

1. Johnson HL, Deloria-Knoll M, Levine OS, et al. Systematic evaluation of serotypes causing invasive pneumococcal disease among children under five: The pneumococcal global serotype project. PLoS Med 2010; 7.pii:e1000348.

2. World Health Organization. Pneumococcal vaccines: WHO position paper-2012. Wkly Epidemiol Rec 2012; ; 87: 129–144.

3. Estimated Hib and pneumococcal deaths for children under 5 years of age, 2008 Available from: http : / / www . who.int / immunization_monitoring/ burden/Pneumo_hib_estimates/en/index.html

4. Indian Academy of Pediatrics Committee on Immunization (IAPCOI). Consensus recommendations on immunization and IAP immunization timetable 2012. Indian Pediatr 2012; 49: 549–564.

5. Nisarga RG, Balter I, et al. Prospective, active hospital-based epidemiologic surveillance for IPD and pneumonia burden among infants and children in Bangalore south zone, India. Presented at the 8th International Symposium on Pneumococci and Pneumococcal Diseases (ISPPD). Iguaçu Falls, Brazil, 11–15 March 2012. Available at: http://isppd.ekonnect.co/ISPPD_297/ poster_22150/program.aspx

6. Rudan I, Boschi-Pinto C, Biloglav Z, Mulholland K, Campbell H. Epidemiology and etiology of childhood pneumonia. Bull World Health Organ. 2008; 86: 408–416.

7. Gupta M, Kumar R, Deb AK, Bhattacharya SK, Bose A, John J, et al. Multi-center surveillance for pneumonia & meningitis among children (< 2 yr) for Hib vaccine probe trial preparation in India. Indian J Med Res 2010; 131: 649–665.

8. Broor S, Parveen S, Bharaj P, Prasad VS, Srinivasulu KN, Sumanth KM, et al. A prospective three-year cohort study of the epidemiology and virology of acute respiratory infections of children in rural India. PLoS One 2007; 2: e491.

9. Johnson HL, Kahn GD, Anne M. Palaia AM, Levine OS, Santosham M. Comprehensive review characterizing the epidemiology of *Streptococcus pneumoniae* in India. The 8th International Symposium on Pneumococci and Pneumococcal Diseases (ISPPD). Iguaçu Falls, Brazil, 11–15 March 2012, Abstract # A-428-0023-00743.

10. Mathew JL, Patwari AK, Gupta P, Shah D, Gera T, Gogia S, et al. Acute respiratory infection and pneumonia in India: A systematic review of literature for advocacy and action: UNICEF-PHFI series on newborn and child health, India. Indian Pediatr 2011; 48: 191–218.

11. Minz S, Balraj V, Lalitha MK, Murali N, Cherian T, Manoharan G, Kadirvan S, Joseph A, Steinhoff MC. Incidence of *Haemophilus influenzae* type b meningitis in India. Indian J Med Res 2008;128: 57–64.

12. Liu L, Johnson HL, Cousens S, Perin J, Scott S, Lawn JE, et al. Global, regional, and national causes of child mortality: An updated systematic analysis for 2010 with time trends since 2000. Lancet 2012; 379: 2151–2161.

13. Johnson HL, Bassani DG, Perin J, Levine OS, Cherian T, O'Brien KL. Burden of childhood mortality caused by *Streptococcus pneumoniae* in India. The 8th International Symposium on Pneumococci and Pneumococcal Diseases (ISPPD). Iguaçu Falls, Brazil, 11–15 March 2012, Abstract # A-428-0023-00743.

14. John TJ, Pai R, Lalitha MK, Jesudason MV, Brahmadathan KN, Sridharan G, Steinhoff MC. Prevalence of pneumococcal serotypes in invasive diseases in southern India. Indian J Med Res 1996; 104 : 205–207.

15. Invasive Bacterial Infections Surveillance (IBIS) Group, International Clinical Epidemiology Network (INCLEN). Prospective multicentre hospital surveillance of *Streptococcus pneumoniae* disease in India. Lancet 1999; 353: 1216–1221.

16. Kanungo R, Rajalakshmi B. Serotype distribution & antimicrobial resistance in *Streptococcus pneumoniae* causing invasive & other infections in south India. Indian J Med Res 2001; 114: 127–132.

17. Levine OS, Cherian T, Hajjeh R, Knoll MD. Progress and future challenges in coordinated surveillance and detection of pneumococcal and Hib disease in developing countries. Clin Infect Dis 2009 ; 48 Suppl 2: S33–36.

18. Shin J, Baek JY, Kim SH, Song JH, Ko KS. Predominance of ST320 among *Streptococcus pneumoniae* serotype 19A isolates from 10 Asian countries. J Antimicrob Chemother 2011; 66: 1001–1004.

19. Kim SH, Song JH, Chung DR, Thamlikitkul V, Yang Y, Wang H, et al. Changing trend of antimicrobial resistance and serotypes in *Streptococcus pneumoniae* in Asian countries: an ANSORP study. Antimicrob Agents Chemother 2012; 56: 1418–1426.

20. Bravo LC; Asian Strategic Alliance for Pneumococcal Disease Prevention (ASAP) Working Group. Overview of the disease burden of invasive pneumococcal disease in Asia. Vaccine 2009; 2: 7282–7291.

21. Vashishtha VM, Kumar P, Mittal A. Sero-epidemiology of *Streptococcal pneumoniae* in developing countries and issues related to vaccination. J Pediatr Sci 2010; 5: e48.

22. Manoharan A. Surveillance of invasive disease caused by *Streptococcus pneumoniae* or *Hemophilus influenzae* or *Neisseria meningitides* in children (<5 Years) in India. Alliance for Surveillance of Pneumococci (ASIP). Poster Discussion 2: Bacterial Infections 1, 13:30 to 15:30 Hours, May 30, 2013 at the 31st Annual Meeting of the European Society for Paediatric Infectious Diseases; May 28eJune 1, 2013. Milan, Italy.

23. Shariff M, Choudhary J, Zahoor S, Deb M. Characterization of *Streptococcus pneumoniae* isolates from India with special reference to their sequence types. J Infect Dev Ctries 2013; 7: 101–109. Available at: http://www.jidc.org/index. php/journal/article/view/23416655/826.

24. Molander V, Ellison C, Balaji V, Backhaus E, John J, Vargheese R et al. Invasive pneumococcal infections in Vellore, India: clinical characteristics and distribution of serotypes. BMC Infectious Diseases 2013; 13: 532. Available from http://www.biomedcentral.com/1471-2334/13/532. (Accessed on Dec 28, 2013)

25. O'Brien KL, Hochman M, Goldblatt D. Combined schedules of pneumococcal conjugate and polysaccharide vaccines: Is hyporesponsiveness an issue? Lancet Infect Dis 2007; 7: 597–606.

26. Moberley SA, Holden J, Tatham DP, Andrews RM. Vaccines for preventing pneumococcal infection in adults. Cochrane Database Syst Rev 2008; (1): CD000422.

27. Huss A, Scott P, Stuck AE, Trotter C, Egger M. Efficacy of pneumococcal vaccination in adults: A meta-analysis. CMAJ 2009; 180: 48–58.

28. World Health Orgainzation. 23-valent pneumococcal polysaccharide vaccine: WHO position paper. Weekly Epidemiological Record 2008; 83: 373–384.

29. French N, Nakiyingi J, Carpenter LM, Lugada E, Watera C, Moi K, et al. 23-valent pneumococcal polysaccharide vaccine in HIV-1-infected Ugandan adults: double-blind, randomised and placebo controlled trial. Lancet 2000; 355: 2106–2111.

30. Kilpi T, Ahman H, Jokinen J, Lankinen KS, Palmu A, Savolainen H, et al. Protective efficacy of a second pneumococcal conjugate vaccine against pneumococcal acute otitis media in infants and children: randomized, controlled trial of a 7-valent pneumococcal polysaccharide-meningococcal outer membrane protein complex conjugate vaccine in 1666 children. Clin Infect Dis 2003; 37: 1155–1164.

31. Klugman KP, Madhi SA, Huebner RE, Kohberger R, Mbelle N, Pierce N, et al. A trial of a 9-valent pneumococcal conjugate vaccine in children with and those without HIV infection. N Eng J Med 2003; 349: 1341–1348.

32. Cutts FT, Zaman SMA, Enwere G, Jaffar S, Levine OS, Okoko JB, et al. Efficacy of nine-valent pneumococcal conjugate vaccine against pneumonia and invasive pneumococcal disease in the Gambia: Randomised, double-blind, placebo-controlled trial. Lancet 2005; 365: 1139–1146.

33. Lucero MG, Nohynek H, Williams G, Tallo V, Simoes EA, Lupisan S, et al. Efficacy of an 11-valent pneumococcal conjugate vaccine against radiologically confirmed pneumonia among children less than 2 years of age in the Philippines: A randomized, double-blind, placebo-controlled trial Pediatr Infect Dis J 2009; 28: 455–462.

34. Prymula R, Peeters P, Chrobok V, Kriz P, Novakova E, Kaliskova E, et al. Pneumococcal capsular polysaccharides conjugated to protein D for prevention of acute otitis media caused by both *Streptococcus pneumoniae* and non-typable *Haemophilus influenzae*: A randomised double-blind efficacy study. Lancet 2006; 367: 740–748.

35. Skinner JM, Indrawati L, Cannon J, Blue J, Winters M, Macnair J et al. Pre-clinical evaluation of a 15-valent pneumococcal conjugate vaccine (PCV15-CRM197) in an infant-rhesus monkey immunogenicity model. Vaccine 2011; 29: 8870–8876.

36. Lucero MG, Dulalia VE, Nillos LT, Williams G, Parreno RA, Nohynek H, et al. Pneumococcal conjugate vaccines for preventing vaccine-type invasive pneumococcal disease and X-ray defined pneumonia in children less than two years of age. Cochrane Database Syst Rev 2009; (4): CD004977.

37. Cherian T, Mulholland EK, Carlin JB, Ostensen H, Amin R, deCampo M, et al. Standardized interpretation of paediatric chest radiographs for the diagnosis of pneumonia in epidemiological studies. Bulletin of the World Health Organization 2005.

38. Hansen J, Black S, Shinefield H, Cherian T, Benson J, Fireman B, et al. Effectiveness of heptavalent pneumococcal conjugate vaccine in children younger than 5 years of age for prevention of pneumonia: Updated analysis using World Health Organization standardized interpretation of chest radiographs. Pediatr Infect Dis J 2006 Sep; 25(9): 779–781.

39. Tregnaghi MW, Saez-Llorens X, Lopez P, Abate H, Smith E, Posleman A, et al. Evaluating the efficacy of 10-valent pneumococcal non-typeable *Haemophilus influenzae* protein-D conjugated vaccine (PHID-CV) against community acquired pneumonia in Latin America. Proceedings of the European Society of Pediatric Infectious Diseases 2011, The Hague, Netherlands. 2011.

40. Madhi SA, Klugman KP. World Health Organisation definition of "radiologically-confirmed pneumonia" may under-estimate the true public health value of conjugate pneumococcal vaccines. Vaccine 2007 Mar 22; 25(13): 2413–2419.

41. Madhi SA, Klugman KP, The Vaccine Trialist Group. A role for *Streptococcus pneumoniae* in virus-associated pneumonia. Nat Med 2004; 10: 811–813.

42. Eskola J, Kilpi T, Palmu A, Jokinen J, Haapakoski J, Herva E, et al. Efficacy of a pneumococcal conjugate vaccine against acute otitis media.[comment] [summary for patients in Can Fam Physician. 2002 Nov;48:1777-9; PMID: 12506948]. N Eng J Med 2001; 344(6): 403–409.

43. Fletcher MA, Fritzell B. Pneumococcal conjugate vaccines and otitis media: An appraisal of the clinical trials. Int J Otolaryngol 2012; 2012:312935. doi: 10.1155/2012/312935. Epub 2012 Jun 3.

44. Sarasoja I, Jokinen J, Lahdenkari M, Kilpi T, Palmu AA. Long-term effect of pneumococcal conjugate vaccines on tympanostomy tube placements. Pediatr Infect Dis J. 2013; 32: 517–520.

45. Poehling KA, Szilagyi PG, Grijalva CG, Martin SW, LaFleur B, Mitchel E, et al. Reduction of frequent otitis media and pressure-equalizing tube insertions in children after introduction of pneumococcal conjugate vaccine. Pediatrics 2007; 119(4): 707–715.

46. Singleton RJ, Hennessy TW, Bulkow LR, Hammitt LL, Zulz T, Hurlburt DA, et al. Invasive pneumococcal disease caused by nonvaccine serotypes among alaska native children with high levels of 7-valent pneumococcal conjugate vaccine coverage. JAMA 2007; 29: 1784–1792.

47. Pilishvili T, Lexau C, Farley MM, Hadler J, Harrison LH, Bennett NM, et al. Sustained reductions in invasive pneumococcal disease in the era of conjugate vaccine. J Infect Dis 2010; 201: 32–41.

48. Miller E, Andrews NJ, Waight PA, Slack MP, George RC. Herd immunity and serotype replacement 4 years after seven-valent pneumococcal conjugate vaccination in England and Wales: An observational cohort study. Lancet Infect Dis 2011; 11: 760–768.

49. Poehling KA, Talbot TR, Griffin MR, Craig AS, Whitney CG, Zell E, et al. Invasive pneumococcal disease among infants before and after introduction of pneumococcal conjugate vaccine. JAMA 2006; 295: 1668–1674.

50. Grijalva CG, Pelton SI. A second-generation pneumococcal conjugate vaccine for prevention of pneumococcal diseases in children. Curr Opin Pediatr 2011; 2: 98–104.

51. Miller E, Andrews NJ, Waight PA, Slack MP, George RC. Effectiveness of the new serotypes in the 13-valent pneumococcal conjugate vaccine. Vaccine 2011; 29: 9127–9131.

52. Palmu AA, Jokinen J, Borys D, Nieminen H, Ruokokoski E, Siira L, et al. Effectiveness of the ten-valent pneumococcal *Haemophilus influenzae* protein D conjugate vaccine (PHiD-CV10) against invasive pneumococcal disease: A cluster randomised trial Lancet. 2013; 381(9862): 214–222. doi: 10.1016/ S0140-6736(12)61854-6. Epub 2012 Nov 16.

53. Jardine A, Menzies RI, McIntyre PB. Reduction in hospitalizations for pneumonia associated with the introduction of a pneumococcal conjugate vaccination schedule without a booster dose in Australia. Pediatr Infect Dis J 2010; 29: 607–612.

54. O'Grady KF, Carlin JB, Chang AB, Torzillo PJ, Nolan TM, Ruben A, et al. Effectiveness of 7-valent pneumococcal conjugate vaccine against radiologically diagnosed pneumonia in indigenous infants in Australia. Bull World Health Organ 2010; 88: 139–146.

55. Dicko A, Odusanya OO, Diallo AI, Santara G, Bary A, Dolo A, et al. Primary vaccination with the 10-valent pneumococcal non-typeable *Haemophilus influenzae* protein D conjugate vaccine (PHiD-CV) in infants in Mali and Nigeria: A randomized controlled trial. BMC Public Health 2011; 11: 882 doi: 10.1186/1471-2458-11-882.

56. Lalwani S, Chatterjee S, Chhatwal J, Verghese VP, Mehta S, Shafi F, et al. Immunogenicity, safety, and reactogenicity of the 10-valent pneumococcal non-typeable *Hemophilus influenzae* protein D conjugate vaccine (PHiD-CV) when co-administered with the DTPw-HBV/Hib vaccine in Indian infants: A single-blind, randomized, controlled study. Human vaccines & immunotherapeutics 2012, 8: 612–622.

57. Vanderkooi OG, Scheifele DW, Girgenti D, Halperin SA, Patterson SD, Gruber WC, Emini EA, Scott DA, Kellner JD: Safety and immunogenicity of a 13-valent pneumococcal conjugate vaccine in healthy infants and toddlers given with routine pediatric vaccinations in Canada. Pediatr Infect Dis J 2012; 31: 72–77.

58. IAP Guidebook on Immunization 2009–2011. Eds. Yewale V, Choudhury P, Thacker N. 2011. Published by Indian Academy of Pediatrics. 2011; P 94–108.

59. Review of serotype replacement in the setting of PCV7 use and implications for the PCV10/PCV13 Era. Geneva: World Health Organization; 2011.

60. Shinefield H, Black S, Ray P, Fireman B, Schwalbe J, Lewis E. Efficacy, immunogenicity and safety of heptavalent pneumococcal conjugate vaccine in low birth weight and preterm infants. Pediatr Infect Dis J 2002; 21: 182–186.

61. Sinha A, Levine O, Knoll MD, Muhib F, Lieu TA. Cost-effectiveness of pneumococcal conjugate vaccination in the prevention of child mortality: An international economic analysis. Lancet 2007; 369: 389–396.

62. Conklin L, Knoll MD, Loo J, Fleming-Dutra K, Park D, Johnson TS, et al. Landscape analysis of pneumococcal conjugate vaccine dosing schedules: A systematic review Sub-report on the 3-dose schedules A Project of the AVI Technical Assistance Consortium (AVI-TAC) Final Report 1.0. Geneva: World Health Organization; 2011 Oct 17.

63. Scott P, Rutjes AW, Bermetz L, Robert N, Scott S, Lourenco T, et al. Comparing pneumococcal conjugate vaccine schedules based on 3 and 2 primary doses: Systematic review and meta-analysis. Vaccine 2011; 29: 9711–9721.

64. Black S., Shinefield H., Fireman B., et al: Efficacy, safety and immunogenicity of heptavalent pneumococcal conjugate vaccine in children. Northern California Kaiser Permanente Vaccine Study Center Group. Pediatr Infect Dis J 2000; 19: 187–195.

65. Klugman KP, Madhi SA, Adegbola RA, et al: Timing of serotype 1 pneumococcal disease suggests the need for evaluation of a booster dose. Vaccine 2011; 29: 3372–3373.

66. Klugman KP, Black S, Dagan R, Malley R, Whitney CG. Pneumococcal conjugate vaccine and pneumococcal common protein vaccines. In: Plotkin S, Orenstein WA, Offit P, editors. Vaccines. 6th ed. Philadelphia: WB Saunders; 2013. p. 504–541.

■ ■ ■ ■ ■ ■

ROTAVIRUS VACCINES

3.7

Reviewed by
Panna Choudhury

Epidemiology

Rotaviruses are globally the leading cause of severe, dehydrating diarrhea in children aged <5 years. In low-income countries 80% of primary rotavirus infection occur among infants <1 year old, whereas in high-income countries, the first episode may occasionally be delayed until the age of 2–5 years. According to Global Enteric Multicenter Study (GEMS), the four most common pathogens responsible for moderate-to-severe diarrhea amongst children in sub-Saharan Africa and south Asia were Rotavirus, Cryptosporidium, enterotoxigenic *Escherichia coli*, and Shigella.[1]

In most developing countries, rotavirus epidemiology is characterized by one or more periods of relatively intense rotavirus circulation against a background of year-round transmission, whereas in high income countries with temperate climates, distinct winter seasonality is typically observed. WHO estimates that in 2008, approximately 453,000 (420,000–494,000) rotavirus gastroenteritis (RVGE)-associated child deaths occurred worldwide. These fatalities accounted for about 5% of all child deaths and cause-specific mortality rate of 86 deaths per 100,000 population aged < 5 years.[2] More than 80 % due to rotavirus diarrhea occur in low-income countries.[3]

Rotavirus morbidity and mortality in India

Indian Academy of Pediatrics carried out a systematic review (unpublished) of burden of rotavirus diarrhea in under-five Indian children. An analysis of 51 studies from all over India over last four decades dealing with hospitalization with rotavirus diarrhea showed a stool positivity rate of 22.1%. Stool positivity rate for rotavirus is about 39% when studies year 2000 onwards are only included. In community settings, analysis of 16 studies with

IAP Guidebook on Immunization 2013–14 | 205

diarrhea showed stool positivity for rotavirus at 18.6%. Rotavirus was identified as an etiological agent in 16.1% cases of nosocomial diarrhea. Most cases of rotavirus diarrhea were found to occur in the first two years of life. The most commonly affected age group was 7–12 months both in hospital and community settings. Highest number of cases were recorded in winter months.

It is difficult to estimate the impact of rotavirus diarrhea on under five mortality in India. As per the 2007 update of Indian Rotavirus Strain Surveillance Network (IRSSN), the proportion of diarrheal hospitalizations due to rotavirus was 39%.[4] The Million Death Study, a nationally representative sample of 6.3 million people in 1.1 million households within the Sample Registration System, recorded approximately 334, 000 diarrheal deaths in India during 2005, i.e., 1 in 82 Indian children died from diarrhea before the age of 5 years.[5] As per the IRSSN data, rotavirus was estimated to cause approximately 34% (113,000; 99% confidence interval, CI: 86,000–155,000) of all diarrheal deaths in under-5 children. Taken together, there was an estimated mortality rate of 4.14 (99% CI: 3.14–5.68) deaths per 1000 live births during 2005 suggesting that approximately 1 in 242 children will die from rotavirus infection before reaching their fifth birthday.

Healthcare associated rotavirus infections
Rotavirus accounts for 31–87% of health care associated gastroenteritis out of which one third is severe. The incidence is 0.3 to 4.8 per 1000 hospital days.

Seasonality of rotavirus infections
In temperate countries, there is a marked seasonal pattern with peaks encompassing winter and spring months when the ambient temperature and humidity is low. Such a marked seasonality is not seen in the tropical countries but the activity is higher during winter months. When minimal seasonality occurs, rotaviruses circulate at a relatively higher level all year round, resulting in children exposed at an early age and experiencing severe illness. Rotavirus diarrhea accounts for 2,000,000 outpatient visits, 457,000–884,000 hospitalizations, and 122,000–153,000 deaths in under-5 children in India annually. There is huge economic impact of rotavirus diarrhea. It is estimated India spends Rs 2.0–3.4 billion (US$ 41–72 million) annually in medical costs to treat rotavirus diarrhea.[6]

Pathogen

Rotavirus is an icosahedral RNA virus and seven sero groups have been described (A–G); group A rotaviruses cause most human disease. The viral outer capsid is made of VP7 and VP4 proteins. The VP7 protein determines the G serotypes and the VP4 protein the P serotypes. Variability of genes coding for the VP7 and VP4 proteins is the basis of classification into genotypes. All G genotypes correspond with serotypes; there are more P genotypes than serotypes. Each rotavirus strain is designated by its G serotype number followed by P serotype number and then P genotype number in square brackets, e.g. G1P1A[8]. The disease is spread mostly through person-to-person contact rather than poor hygienic or sanitary conditions. Transmission is by fecal-oral spread, close person-to-person contact and by fomites. Rotaviruses are probably also transmitted by other modes such as respiratory droplets. The increasing role of rotavirus in the etiology of severe childhood diarrhea is likely attributable to the fact that this pathogen is often transmitted from person to person and is difficult to control through improvements in hygiene and sanitation, which have had greater impact on the prevention of diarrhea caused by bacterial and parasitic agents over the past two decades. The universal occurrence of rotavirus infections even in settings with high standards of hygiene testifies to the high transmissibility of this virus.

In the systematic review (unpublished) carried out by Indian Academy of Pediatrics, a total of 47 studies could be identified which dealt with serotyping of rotavirus. Overall, G1 was the most common serotype isolated in Indian studies (32%), followed by G2 (24%) and G-untypable (15%). Emergence of G9 and G12 has been noticed in recent years. In P serotyping, P[4] was most prevalent (23%) all over India, followed by P[6] (20%) and P untypable/others (13%). Several studies have reported different G-P combinations, novel serotypes, group B and group C rotavirus. Data from IRSSN showed that the most common types of strains were G2P[4] (25.7% of strains), G1P[8] (22.1%), and G9P[8] (8.5%); G12 strains were seen in combination with types P[4], P[6], and P[8] and together comprised 6.5% of strains.[4]

Protective Immunity

Protection against rotavirus infection is mediated by both humoral and cellular components of the immune system. Following the first infection, the serological response is directed mainly against the specific viral serotype (i.e. a homotypic response), whereas a broader, heterotypic antibody response is elicited following ≥ 1 subsequent rotavirus infections.[7] A study from Mexico showed that children with 1, 2, or 3 previous infections had progressively lower risk of subsequent rotavirus infection (adjusted relative risk, 0.62, 0.40, and 0.34, respectively) or of diarrhea (adjusted relative risk, 0.23, 0.17, and 0.08) than children who had no previous infections. Subsequent infections were significantly less severe than first infections (p = 0.02) and second infections were more likely to be caused by another G type (p = 0.05)[8] However, study from India reported that the risk of severe disease continued after several reinfections. Levels of reinfection were high, with only approximately 30% of all infections identified being primary. Protection against moderate or severe disease increased with the order of infection but was only 79% after three infections. With G1P[8], the most common viral strain, there was no evidence of homotypic protection.[9]

Vaccines

Currently two live oral vaccines are licensed and marketed worldwide, human monovalent live vaccine and human bovine pentavalent live vaccine. A vaccine based on Indian neonatal strains, 116E has undergone Phase III clinical trials and has demonstrated strong efficacy and excellent safety profile.

Human monovalent live vaccine (RV1)

Human monovalent live rotavirus vaccine contains one strain of live attenuated human strain 89-12 [type G1P1A(8)] rotavirus. It is provided as a lyophilized power that is reconstituted before administration. Each 1-ml dose of reconstituted vaccine contains at least 106 median culture infective units of virus. The vaccine contains amino acids, dextran, Dulbecco's modified Eagle medium, sorbitol and sucrose. The diluents contain calcium carbonate, sterile water and xanthan. The vaccine contains no preservatives of thiomersal. The vaccine and the diluents should be stored at 2 to 8°C and must not be frozen. The vaccine should be administered promptly after reconstitution as 1 ml orally.

Human bovine pentavalent live vaccine (RV5)

Human bovine pentavalent live vaccine is a Human bovine reassortant vaccine and consists of five reassortants between the bovine WC23 strain and human G1, G2, G3, G4 and P1A[8] rotavirus strains grown in vero cells and administered orally. Each 2-ml vial of vaccine contains approximately 2×106 infectious units of each of the five reassortant strains. The vaccine viruses are suspended in the buffer solution that contains sucrose, sodium citrate, sodium phosphated monobasic monohydrate, sodium hydroxide, plysorbate 80, and tissue culture media. The vaccine contains no preservatives of thiomersal. The vaccine is available as a liquid virus mixed with buffer and no reconstitution is needed. It should be stored at 2 to 8°C.

Indian neonatal rotavirus live vaccine, 116 E

This vaccine developed by Bharat Biotech of India is a live, naturally attenuated vaccine containing monovalent, bovine-human reassortant strain characterized as G9 P [11], with the VP4 of bovine rotavirus origin, and all other segments of human rotavirus origin. The vaccine strain was isolated from asymptomatic infants, with mild diarrhea by Indian researchers in 1985 at AIIMS, New Delhi. Follow up of these infants indicated that they were protected against severe rotavirus diarrhea for up to 2 years. This strain was sent for vaccine development to the NIH by DBT-India and later transferred to Bharat Biotech International Limited in 2001 for further development. In a phase II study, both low (10^4 ffu) and high (10^5 ffu) dosages of 116E were found safe in infants between 8 and 20 weeks of age with low prevalence of adverse effects. IgA immunogenicity rates for the 105 ffu dosage were 64.7% after 1 dose, and 89.7% after 3 doses. Vaccine virus was shed in ~20% infants.[10]

Rotavirus vaccines' efficacy and effectiveness

Although the composition of the two vaccines (RV1 and RV5) is different, their field effectiveness and, largely, mechanism of action are similar. Both prevent effectively severe rotavirus gastroenteritis (RVGE) but are less efficacious against mild RVGE or rotavirus infection. Field effectiveness of these vaccines in

Europe and the USA against severe RVGE has been above 90% and in Latin America around 80%. Trials in Africa have yielded efficacy rates between 50 and 80%. In Malawi, the effectiveness of RV1 was 49 percent, compared to about 77 percent in South Africa. This study showed that a rotavirus vaccine significantly reduces the episodes of severe rotavirus gastroenteritis in African children during the first year of life. The overall efficacy of the vaccine was lower than that observed in European studies and Latin American studies. The possible reasons include poor nutritional status, co-infections with other enteral pathogens, interference by breastfeeding due to presence of high levels anti-rotavirus neutralizing antibodies in breast milk, and interference by maternal antibody or by co-administration of the oral poliovirus vaccine, which may reduce rotavirus antibody levels.[11]

Based on 11 RCTs of RV1 and 6 RCTs of RV5, a recent Cochrane review showed protection against severe RVGE after 1 and/or 2 years of follow up, ranging from approximately 80–90% with modest waning over the period of observation in regions with very low or low child and adult mortality as compared to approximately 40–60% efficacy over 2 years of follow up in regions with high child and very high adult mortality.[12] However, since the incidence of severe rotavirus disease is significantly higher in high child mortality settings, the numbers of severe disease cases and deaths averted by vaccines in these settings are likely to be higher than in low mortality settings, despite the lower vaccine efficacy.

Observational studies in Mexico and Brazil after the introduction of RV1 reported a reduction in diarrhea related deaths in infants and young children. After RV1 introduction, Mexico saw a 35% (95% CI: 29–39) reduction in the rate of diarrheal deaths predominantly during the usual rotavirus season among children age appropriate for the vaccine.[13] After RV1 introduction in Brazil in 2006, 30% (95% CI: 19–41) and 39% (95% CI: 29–49) decreases in gastroenteritis mortality were noted in 2007 and 2008, respectively, when compared to the mortality rates in 2004–2005.[14] Thus, introduction of the vaccine into countries is likely to have a greater effect than that predicted on the basis of the efficacy trials. RV5 was also reported to reduce the number of cases of severe RVGE by nearly half (48 percent) in infants evaluated in developing countries in Asia (Bangladesh and Vietnam) and by

39 percent in infants evaluated in developing countries in Africa (Ghana, Kenya, and Mali) through nearly two years of follow-up. These were the first studies demonstrating efficacy for any rotavirus vaccine in developing countries in Asia. For the two vaccines that are currently licensed for use in many countries, 22.1% of the strains identified in this study would be covered by RV1 and 47.9% by RV5, if only homotypic immunity is induced by vaccination, although reports from Europe indicate cross-protection across genotypes with use of RV1.

Studies in India

There is no efficacy study of the two rotavirus vaccines, RV1 and RV5, conducted in India. Both of these vaccines were licensed on the basis of immunogenicity studies. The only efficacy study conducted in the country so far was with Indian neonatal rotavirus vaccine, 116E. A randomized, double-blind, placebo-controlled phase III clinical trial (unpublished) amongst 6,799 infants was conducted at three sites in India. The first year efficacy against severe RGE was 56.4% (95% CI: 36–70%) with protection continuing into the second year of life also. The vaccine also showed 20% efficacy against all cause severe diarrhea admission.

In the immunogenicity studies of RV1 and RV5 conducted in India, the seroconversion rate was reported to be comparable with the results obtained from other studies done in the developing countries (i.e. Latin America, South Africa, and Bangladesh). Studies show no interference between rotavirus vaccines and other childhood vaccines including IPV, pneumococcal, Hib, DTaP and hepatitis B. Data is insufficient for pertussis immunity. Immunogenicity studies about simultaneous administration of rotavirus vaccines with OPV are available for RV1 and RV5, which show no reduction in immunogenicity against polio and no significant reduction in immunogenicity against rotavirus.[15, 16]

Safety and risk of acute intussusceptions of rotavirus vaccines

The available new generations of rotavirus vaccines are considered quite safe and the risk of acute intussusception is very small in comparison to previous vaccine. The committee reviewed the emerging data on intussusception related to current rotavirus vaccines following large-scale use of these vaccines in Mexico,

Brazil, Australia and US.[17] Based on post-marketing surveillance data, the current rotavirus vaccines have been associated with an increased risk of intussusceptions (about 1–2/100,000 infants vaccinated) for a short period after administration of the first dose in some populations.[17] This risk is 5–10 times lower than that observed with the previously licensed vaccine (1 case per 10,000 doses). There are no published reports on incidence/rates of acute intussusception following rotavirus vaccination in India. However, the post-marketing surveillance data (unpublished) of Indian manufacturers revealed 13 cases of acute intussusceptions associated (causality not yet proved) with rotavirus vaccines administration since the launch of RV1 in India till December 2011, and two cases following RV5 during a five-month surveillance period (May–September 2011) in India.[17] After reviewing recent data, the committee concludes that there is definite albeit a small risk of acute intussusceptions following use of current generation of rotavirus vaccines. However, the benefits of rotavirus vaccination against severe diarrhea and death from rotavirus infection far exceed the miniscule risk of intussusceptions.

Recommendations for use

Public health perspectives

The ACVIP acknowledges the morbidity and mortality burden of rotavirus and need for a effective rotavirus vaccine. Such a vaccine would be most needed in the national immunization program as the disease consequences are the most serious in the underprivileged. Given the minimal impact that water and sanitation measures have had on the burden of rotavirus in developing areas, there is wide agreement that effective vaccination represents the most promising prevention strategy against the disease. However, the committee is concerned regarding the overall effectiveness/efficacy of the currently available vaccines in high burden countries, including India. Though these vaccines had comparatively higher impact on the overall disease morbidity and mortality in high burden countries than in low burden countries despite poor efficacy in the former, there is need to evaluate efficacy in much larger cohorts and to undertake strategies to further optimize immune responses of the currently available vaccines to provide better protection. The committee thinks that well studied economic evaluation in the form of impeccable cost-effective analysis of these vaccines is mandatory before any decision on inclusion of these vaccines into UIP is taken. The NTAGI has already initiated the consultations on the potential introduction of rotavirus vaccines in UIP and referred the matter to a special Standing Technical Sub-Committee (STSC) to review the evidence on the subject. The availability of an indigenous, cheap rotavirus vaccine shall facilitate a favorable decision. It is expected that Indian neonatal strain rotavirus vaccine, once approved by regulatory authorities will cost as low as Rs. 54 per dose.[18]

Individual use

Administration schedule: Vaccination should be strictly as per schedule discussed below, as there is a potentially higher risk of intussusceptions if vaccines are given to older infants. Vaccination should be avoided if age of the infant is uncertain. There are no restrictions on the infant's consumption of food or liquid, including breast-milk, either before or after vaccination. Vaccines may be administered during minor illnesses.

Though there is limited evidence on safety and efficacy of rotavirus vaccines in preterm infants, vaccination should be considered for these infants if they are clinically stable and at least 6 weeks of age as preterms are susceptible to severe rotavirus gastroenteritis. Vaccination should be avoided in those with history of hypersensitivity to any of the vaccine components or previous vaccine dose. Vaccination should be postponed in infants with acute gastroenteritis as it might compromise efficacy of the vaccine. Immunocompromised infants are susceptible to severe and prolonged rotavirus gastroenteritis but safety and efficacy of either of the two vaccines in such patients is unknown. Risks versus benefits of vaccination should be considered while considering vaccination for infants with chronic gastrointestinal disease, gut malformations, previous intussusceptions and immuno-compromised infants.

Rv1 and RV5 vaccines when started at 8 weeks of age and given at 2 or 3 dose schedule respectively, has been found to be highly effective in preventing rotavirus gastroenteritis.[19] WHO position paper[2] recommends that 1st dose of rotavirus vaccination should be given with 1st dose of DPT vaccination both for RV1 and RV5, which effectively means starting the schedule at 6 weeks in India. It is a well-known fact that first dose of RV1 administered at 6 weeks along with OPV is nonimmunogenic. Several studies from South Africa, Vietnam, and Philippines have indicated that the older the infant when they receive the first dose of vaccine, the better the immune response in terms of seroconversion and GMCs. In a study conducted in South Africa, the seroconversion of first dose of RV1 when administered at 6 weeks along with OPV was found to be only 13%, whereas when the same dose was administered at 10 weeks along with IPV, the seroconversion rose to 43%. In the same study, the anti-rotavirus IgA antibody seroconversion rates were higher for the 10–14 weeks schedule (55–61%) compared to the 6–10 weeks schedule (36–43%).[20] The titers of circulating maternal antibody in the infants and OPV co-administration have a negative impact on the immune response of the first rotavirus vaccine dose (lower seroconversion rates and reduced GMCs).

In Africa trial, the 2-dose and 3-dose schedule of RV1 starting at 6 weeks of age showed that vaccine efficacy against severe rotavirus diarrhea for the first year with 2-dose schedule was 58.7 (95% CI 35.7 –74) while for 3-dose schedule the same was 63.7 (95% CI 42.4 – 77.8).[18] There was no difference on the first year efficacy of both the schedules in Malawi, but a definite gradient favoring 3- dose schedule in South Africa (81.5, 95% CI, 55.1–93.7 for 3-dose versus 72.2, 95% CI, 40.4–88.3 for 2-dose). However, when second year efficacy against severe rotavirus diarrhea was considered, there was significant difference in the efficacy of the two schedules in both the countries (85% for 3-dose versus 32% for 2-dose in South Africa, and 49% versus 18%, respectively in Malawi).[21-23]

Recently a randomized, 3-arm (1:1:1) trial of RV1 was carried out in a peri-urban slum in Karachi, Pakistan. IgA seroconversion rate in the 3-dose arm (6, 10 and 14 weeks), 2-dose 6, 10 weeks arm and 2-dose 10,14 weeks arm were 36.7% (95% CI: 29.8%, 44.2%), 36.1% (95% CI: 29.0%, 43.9%) and 38.5% (95% CI: 31.2%, 46.3%) respectively. Similar low response in all the arms needs to be taken note of in the background of settings of slum; 2-dose 6, 10 weeks arm gave lowest response albeit insignificantly.[24]

However, another 3-arm (1:1:1) similar study from rural Ghana clearly showed superiority of 3-dose schedule for RV1. Among baseline seronegative participants in Groups 1(6,10 weeks), 2(10,14 weeks) and 3(6,10,14 weeks), seroconversion rates were 28.9%, 37.4%, and 43.4% respectively(p=0.014 by Fisher's exact test for the primary comparison of Group 3 versus Group 1). Post-vaccination IgA geometric mean titers (GMT) were 22.1 (95% CI: 17.4, 28.2) for Group 1, 26.5 (95% CI: 20.7., 34.0) for Group 2, and 32.6 (95% CI: 24.7, 43.2) for Group 3 (t-test Group 1 versus Group 3: p=0.038). Amongst 2 dose series, Group 2 had better response than Group 1 though the difference was not statistically significant[25].

Overall, most of the comparative studies with 2 versus 3-dose schedule have employed RV1 in 10, 14 weeks instead of recommended 6, 10 weeks schedule. An immunogenicity study from India has shown that RV1 given in a 2-dose schedule, with 1st dose between 8 and 10 weeks and 2nd dose between 12 and 16 weeks is immunogenic and well tolerated in healthy Indian infants.[15] Pentavalent vaccine given in 3 doses has shown adequate immunogenicity in Indian infants when started at 6 weeks of age.[16] A 3-dose schedule of RV 116E starting at 8 weeks demonstrated a robust immune response.[10] Considering all the abovementioned facts, the IAP ACVIP opined that if RV1 vaccine is to be administered in a 2-dose schedule, the first dose should start at 10 weeks of age instead of 6 weeks in order to achieve better immune response. The second dose can be administered at 14 weeks to fit with existing national immunization schedule. However 3-dose schedule of any rotavirus vaccine can start at 6 weeks of age with minimum interval of 4 weeks between the doses.[26]

Upper limits of immunization: Immunization should not be initiated in infants 15 weeks or older because of insufficient safety data for vaccines use in older children. All the doses of either of the vaccines should be completed within 8 months (32 weeks) of age. Both vaccines should not be frozen. Rotavirus vaccine must not be injected. Programmatic errors have been reported. Large vaccine volume requires full insertion of vial tip into infant's mouth. Contact with infant's mouth contaminates the vial and complicates development of multi-dose vials.

Special situations

Regurgitation of vaccine

Re-administration need not be done to an infant who regurgitates, spits out, or vomits during or after administration of vaccine though the manufacturers of RV1 recommend that the dose may be repeated at the same visit, if the infant spits out or regurgitates the entire vaccine dose. The infant should receive the remaining recommended doses of rotavirus vaccine following the routine schedule (with a 4-week minimum interval between doses).

Interchangeability of Rotavirus Vaccines

Ideally, the rotavirus vaccine series should be completed with the same product. However, vaccination should not be deferred because the product used for previous doses is unavailable. In such cases, the series should be continued with the product that is available. If any dose in the series was RV5, or if the product is unknown for any dose in the series, a total of three doses should be administered.

ROTAVIRUS (RV) VACCINES

Routine vaccination:

- Minimum age: 6 weeks for both RV-1 [Rotarix] and RV-5 [RotaTeq])

- Only two doses of RV-1 are recommended at present.

- RV1 should preferably be employed in 10 and 14 week-schedule, instead of 6 and 10 weeks; the former schedule is found to be far more immunogenic than the later.

- RV5 should be employed in a three-dose 6, 10, and 14 week-schedule. If any dose in series was RV5 or vaccine product is unknown for any dose in the series, a total of 3 doses of RV vaccine should be administered.

Catch-up vaccination:

- The maximum age for the first dose in the series is 14 weeks, 6 days .

- Vaccination should not be initiated for infants aged 15 weeks, 0 days or older.

- The maximum age for the final dose in the series is 8 months, 0 days.

Missed opportunity

It is not necessary to restart the series or add doses because of a prolonged interval between doses with either of the vaccines.

Contraindications

Rotavirus vaccine should not be administered to infants who have a history of a severe allergic reaction (e.g., anaphylaxis) after a previous dose of rotavirus vaccine or to a vaccine component. History of intussusception in the past is also an absolute contraindication for rotavirus vaccines administration. Latex rubber is contained in the RV1 oral applicator, so infants with a severe (anaphylactic) allergy to latex should not receive RV1 vaccine. The RV5 dosing tube is latex-free.

References

1. Kotloff KL, Nataro JP, Blackwelder WC, Nasrin D, Farag TH, Panchalingam S, et al. Burden and aetiology of diarrhoeal disease in infants and young children in developing countries (the Global Enteric Multicenter Study, GEMS): a prospective, case-control study. Lancet 2013; 382: 209–222.
2. Rotavirus vaccine. WHO Position Paper 2013. Weekly epidemiological record. 2013; 88: 49–64.
3. Parashar UD, Gibson CJ, Bresse JS, Glass RI. Rotavirus and severe childhood diarrhoea. Emerg Infect Dis 2006; 12: 304–316.
4. Kang G, Arora R, Chitambar SD, Deshpande J, Gupte MD, Kulkarni M, et al. Multicenter, hospital-based surveillance of rotavirus disease and strains among Indian children aged < 5 years. J Infect Dis. 2009; 200: S147–153.
5. Bassani DG, Kumar R, Awasthi S, Morris SK, Paul VK, Shet A, et al. Million Death Study Collaborators. Causes of neonatal and child mortality in India: A nationally representative mortality survey. Lancet 2010; 376: 1853–1860.
6. Tate JE, Chitambar S, Esposito DH, Sarkar R, Gladstone B, Ramani S, et al. Disease and economic burden of rotavirus diarrhoea in India. Vaccine. 2009; 27: F18–24.
7. Angel J, Franco MA, Greenberg HB. Rotavirus immune responses and correlates of protection. Current Opinion in Virology, 2012, 419–425.
8. Velazquez FR, Matson DO, Calva JJ, Guerrero L, Morrow AL, Carter-Campbell S et al. Rotavirus infection in infants as protection against subsequent infections. New England Journal of Medicine, 1996, 335: 1022–1028.
9. Gladstone BP, Ramani S, Mukhopadhya I, Muliyil J, Sarkar R, Rehman AM, et al. Protective effect of natural rotavirus infection in an Indian birth cohort. N Engl J Med 2011; 365: 337–346.
10. Bhandari N, Sharma P, Taneja S, Kumar T, Rongsen-Chandola T, Appaiahgari MB, et al. A dose-escalation safety and immunogenicity study of live attenuated oral rotavirus vaccine 116E in infants: a randomized, double blind, placebo-controlled trial. J Infect Dis 2009; 200: 421–429.
11. Vesikari T. Rotavirus vaccination: a concise review. Clin Microbiol Infect 2012; 18 (Suppl. 5): 57–63.
12. Soares-Weiser K, Maclehose H, Bergman H, Ben-Aharon I, Nagpal S, Goldberg E, et al. Vaccines for preventing rotavirus diarrhoea: Vaccines in use. Cochrane Database Systematic Review, 2012, 11: CD008521. doi: 10.1002/14651858. CD008521.pub3. Review.

13. Richardson V, Hernandez-Pichardo J, Quintanar-Solares M, Esparza-Aguilar M, Johnson B, Gomez-Altamirano CM, et al. Effect of rotavirus vaccination on death from childhood diarrhea in Mexico. N Engl J Med 2010; 362: 299–305.

14. Lanzieri TM, Linhares AC, Costa I, Kolhe DA, Cunha MH, Ortega-Barria E, et al. Impact of rotavirus vaccination on childhood deaths from diarrhea in Brazil. Int J Infect Dis 2011; 15: e206–210.

15. Narang A, Bose A, Pandit AN, Dutta P, Kang G, Bhattacharya SK, et al. Immunogenicity, reactogenicity and safety of human rotavirus vaccine (RIX4414) in Indian infants. Hum Vaccin 2009; 5: 414–419; PMID: 19276664.

16. Lokeshwar MR, Bhave S, Gupta A, Goyal VK, Walia A. Immunogenicity and safety of the pentavalent human-bovine (WC3) reassortant rotavirus vaccine (PRV) in Indian infants. Hum Vaccin Immunother 2013; 9: 172–176. doi: 10.4161/hv.22341

17. Indian Academy of Pediatrics Committee on Immunization (IAPCOI). Consensus recommendations on immunization and IAP immunization timetable 2012. Indian Pediatr 2012; 49: 549–564.

18. http://www.thehindu.com/sci-tech/health/medicine-and-research/india-unveils-first-indigenous-rotavirus-vaccine/article4714757.ece. (Accessed on 28th Oct 2013)

19. Payne DC, Boom JA, Staat MA, Edwards KM, Szilagyi PG, Klein EJ, et al. Effectiveness of pentavalent and rotavuris vaccines in concurrent use among US children < 5 years of age, 2009–2011. Clin Infect Dis 2013; 57: 13–20.

20. Steele AD, De Vos B, Tumbo J, Reynders J, Scholtz F, Bos P, et al. Co-administration study in South African infants of a live-attenuated oral human rotavirus vaccine (RIX4414) and poliovirus vaccines. Vaccine 2010; n28: 6542–6548.

21. Madhi SA, Cunliffe NA, Steele D, Witte D, Kirsten M, Louw C, et al. Effect of human rotavirus vaccine on severediarrhea in African infants. N Engl J Med 2010; 362: 289–298.

22. Cunliffe NA, Witte D, Ngwira BM, Todd S, Bostock NJ, Turner AM, et al. Efficacy of human rotavirus vaccine against severe gastroenteritis in Malawian children in the first two years of life: a randomized, double-blind, placebo controlled trial. Vaccine 2012; 30 (Suppl 1): A36–43.

23. Madhi SA, Kirsten M, Louw C, Bos P, Aspinall S, Bouckenooghe A, et al. Efficacy and immunogenicity of two or three dose rotavirus-vaccine regimen in South African children over two consecutive rotavirus-seasons: A randomized, double-blind, placebo-controlled trial. Vaccine 2012;30 (Suppl 1): A44–51.

24. Ali SA, Kazi M, Cortese M, Fleming J, Parashar U, Jiang B et al. Impact of Different Dosing Schedules on the Immunogenicity of the Human Rotavirus Vaccine in Children in Pakistan – a Randomized Controlled Trial(Abstract). Proceedings of the Vaccine for Enteric Disease. 2013 Nov 6–8; Bangkok, Thailand.

25. Armah G, Lewis K, Cortess M, Parashar U, Ansah A, Gazley L et al. Immunogenicity of the Human Rotavirus Vaccine Given on Alternative Dosing Schedules in Rural Ghana. Proceedings of the Vaccine for Enteric Disease. 2013 Nov 6-8; Bangkok, Thailand.

26. Vashishtha VM, Kalra A, Bose A, Choudhury P, Yewale VN, Bansal CP et al. Indian Academy of Pediatrics (IAP) Recommended Immunization Schedule for Children Aged 0 through 18 years – India, 2013 and Updates on Immunization. Indian Pediatr 2013; 50: 1095–1108.

■ ■ ■ ■ ■

MEASLES, MUMPS AND RUBELLA VACCINES

Reviewed by
Panna Choudhury, Sashi Vani

MEASLES

Measles elimination contributes significantly in achieving Millennium Development Goal 4 (MDG-4). "One of the three indicators for monitoring progress towards achieving MDG 4 is the "proportion of 1-year-old children immunized against measles".[1]

With the help of measles vaccination, globally number of measles deaths have dropped considerably to the tune of about 74%, between the years of 2000 and 2011.The number of measles deaths during this period have reduced from 542,000 to 158,000 and number of reported new cases have dropped by 58% to 355,000.[2] Reduction in measles-related deaths have contributed to overall decline of 23% of under 5 mortality between 1990 and 2008.[3] However, measles death is still unacceptably high at about 450 deaths everyday or 18 deaths every hour. All 194 WHO member countries have committed to reduce measles deaths by 95% by year 2015.[4]

In developed countries, measles is no longer endemic and the 2005 goal set by the World Health Assembly (WHA) to halve measles deaths worldwide (compared to 1999 levels) was achieved on time.[5] This has been made possible by a multi-pronged strategy including improved routine coverage, provision of second dose through routine immunization or periodic supplementary immunization activities, careful surveillance and appropriate case management.[6] Emphasis is also being given on laboratory backed surveillance, outbreak preparedness, research and development and also on communication to build public confidence and demand for immunization.[7]

In many developing countries, measles continues to be a serious public health problem. India has also recognized importance of elimination of measles and introduced measles vaccination through National Universal Immunization program since the year 1985. The measles deaths have been reduced from 106,000 in 2005 to 65000 in 2010 and 29336 in 2012(8,9). Still India contributes to almost 47% of the Global Measles deaths, reflecting poor performance.[10] In 2012 and 2013 (till 31st May)India reported 74 and 61 measles outbreaks. Most measles cases are reported between 1 to 9 years. With the highest birth cohort in the world, highest number of measles deaths and relatively poor vaccine coverage, India poses a challenge for the Global Measles Eradication goal.

To control measles country needs sustained > 95% vaccination coverage. A recent vaccination coverage survey in India showed overall 71% coverage for measles vaccine (given during 9 to 12 months of age). Accepting 85% vaccine effectiveness for vaccination at 9 months, actual protection was offered to only 60% of annual birth cohorts (71% × 85% = 60%). In other words, 40% remained susceptible to measles.

Amongst different states in India, there is a considerable difference in vaccination coverage. States like Kerala, Goa, Sikkim and Punjab demonstrate almost 90% coverage, whereas states like U.P., Bihar, M.P., Rajasthan report have less than 70% coverage. Least coverage is reported from U.P. and Bihar with large number of measles cases.[11]

Vaccine

A safe, effective and reasonably inexpensive vaccine is available against measles for the past 5 decades. All currently used vaccines are live attenuated vaccines. Most of the currently used live attenuated measles vaccine strains originate from the original Edmonston strain and include Schwarz, Edmonston Zagreb, Moraten and Edmonston-B strains. Indian vaccines are usually formulated from the Edmonston Zagreb strain grown on human diploid cells or purified chick embryo cells. Each dose contains at least 1000 infective units and has no preservative. It is supplied freeze-dried in single dose or multidose vials with distilled water as a diluent. The vaccine may be stored frozen or at 2–8°C (shelf life 2 years). Reconstituted vaccine is destroyed by light and is very heat labile (loses 50% potency at 20°C and 100% at 37°C after

1 hour) and is susceptible to contamination as it does not have any preservative. For these reasons reconstituted vaccine should be protected from light, kept at 2–8°C and used within 4–6 hours of reconstitution. This is particularly applicable to multidose vials. The dose is 0.5 ml subcutaneously or intramuscularly, preferably over the upper arm / anterolateral thigh. Immunogenicity depends on the age of administration due to interference by preexisting maternal antibodies. Seroconversion rates are around 60% at the age of 6 months, 80–85% at the age of 9 months and beyond 95% at the age of 12–15 months. While antibody titers wane over the years measles specific cellular immunity persists and provides lifelong protection. Secondary vaccine failures rarely occur. Immunogenicity is lower in the immunocompromised including HIV. In HIV infected infants superior seroconversion rates are seen at 6 months as compared to 9 months due to progressive immunodeficiency with age. Vaccine efficacy studies from India have reported varying efficacies ranging from 60–80% when given at the age of 9 months. Adverse reactions apart from local pain and tenderness include a mild measles like illness 7–12 days after vaccination in 2–5% of the vaccinees. Thrombocytopenic purpura may occur at a frequency of 1/30,000 vaccinees. Though depression of cell-mediated immunity may occur, it recovers within 4 weeks and is considered harmless even for those with early HIV or latent/ unrecognized tuberculosis. There is no data to support causal relationship between measles vaccine and encephalitis, Guillain Barre Syndrome, subacute sclerosing encephalitis and autism. There is no transmission of the vaccine virus from the vaccinees to the contacts. Measles vaccine has been the cause of several infant deaths in several states of India due to toxic shock syndrome[12] and use of succinylcholine instead of distilled water as the diluents.[13] Measles vaccine vial can get contaminated when the cap is punctured, leading to bacterial growth in the vial as it does not contain preservative. Bacteria like staphylococci excrete several exotoxin and can cause severe shock in recipients. TSS can be prevented by adhering to injection safety and if reconstituted multidose measles vaccine is used within 4–6 hours. Left over doses after this period must be discarded. The vaccine is contraindicated in the severely immunocompromised, in those with history of severe allergic reactions to the constituents and in pregnancy. The vaccine should be administered to those

with HIV infection unless severely immunocompromised as here the benefits outweigh the risks. The vaccine may be given to those with history of egg allergy. The vaccine may be given along with all childhood vaccines with the exception of BCG vaccine.

Recommendations for use

Overwhelming evidence has demonstrated that measles vaccination preferably combined with rubella containing vaccines are among the most cost effective public health tools available currently, provided universal coverage of not less than 95% is achieved. Vaccine immunogenicity and efficacy are best when the vaccine is administered beyond the age of 12 months. However, in India a significant proportion of measles cases occur below the age of 12 months. Hence in order to achieve the best balance between these competing demands of early protection and high seroconversion, completed 9 months of age has been recommended as the appropriate age for measles vaccination in India.

Individual use

Measles vaccine given at 9 months is an epidemiological compulsion and has almost 20% primary vaccine failure due to maternal antibodies. Therefore at least 2 or 3 measles containing vaccines are required for protection and in spite of this 5–8% may remain susceptible. Thus additional doses of measles vaccine preferably as MMR vaccine at the age of 15 months and again between 4.5 years and 5 years give durable and possibly lifelong protection against measles.

In case of an outbreak, the vaccine can be given to infants as young as completed 6 months. Administration of the vaccine within 2 days of exposure protects and or modifies the severity of clinical disease. The vaccine should be given irrespective of prior history of measles as any exanthematous illness is often confused as measles.

Public health perspectives

For reducing measles mortality in the country, National Technical Advisory Group on Immunization (NTAGI), reviewing data on measles epidemiology and case fatality rate, has recommended the second dose of measles in India for all states through state-specific delivery strategies.[14] These are as follows:

- A second dose of measles vaccine should be introduced in the UIP at the time of DPT booster dose (at 16–24 months of age) in states with ≥ 80% evaluated coverage with the first dose of measles vaccine.

- Catch-up measles vaccination campaigns should be implemented for children 9 months to age 10 years in states with < 80% evaluated coverage with the first dose of measles vaccine and that detailed action plans for these SIAs should be finalized immediately in states with low coverage and high measles mortality burden.

In 14 states with MCV1 coverage less than 80% — measles SIA for 9 months to 10 years age group followed 6 months later by MCV2 under routine immunization. In 21 states with MCV1 coverage more than 80%, MCV2 under routine immunization at 16 to 24 months age group. Under MCUP (Measles Catch-up Program) all children in target group are to be vaccinated irrespective of previous doses of vaccine received and irrespective of the previous history of measles disease. This age group covers about 18 to 25% of the population with a target of 135 million children. Expected coverage is more than 90%. This is a massive public health undertaking with an injectable vaccine. Both safety and high coverage are critical. All the immunizations will be at a static post and no home to home immunization will be done. Ministry of Health has decided to take a phased approach. ACVIP endorses NTAGI recommendations for introducing 2nd dose measles vaccine in UIP.[15]

Measles catch-up programs are scientifically sound, highly recommended and proven effective globally. Government has already implemented the program and in many states school children are getting vaccinated where the program is in campaign mode. There is a concern that in program areas a few children especially in older age group may get additional doses as it may not be possible to screen vaccination status of every child. However, extra doses do no harm and in fact benefit miniscule of children who do not seroconvert even after 2 or 3 doses. It is also important to remember that programmatic issues always override individual interests. Many African countries nearly eliminated measles with vaccination in campaign mode and it is high time that India also eliminate measles.

RUBELLA VACCINE

Rubella per se a mild exanthematous illness but if acquired in the first trimester of pregnancy can lead to disastrous consequences in the fetus/ new born such as abortion, still birth, mental retardation, congenital heart disease, blindness and cataract. Hence the objective of vaccination against rubella is protection against congenital rubella syndrome (CRS). Developed countries have remarkably reduced the burden of CRS by universal immunization against rubella. It is essential that when immunization against rubella is instituted, more than 80% coverage is achieved. Indiscriminate use of rubella vaccine (monovalent or as a constituent of MMR) in young children through public health measure with sub-optimal coverage of the target population may be counterproductive as it may shift the epidemiology of rubella to the right with more clinical cases occurring in young adults leading to paradoxical increase in cases of CRS. This has been shown to occur using mathematical models. Direct evidence from some Latin American countries and Greece also corroborates these concerns.

There is paucity of reliable data on occurrence of CRS. WHO estimates that 100,000 cases of CRS occur in developing countries alone. Comprehensive evidence about the true burden of CRS in India is not available.[16] However, Ministry of Health estimates that around 30,000 abnormal children are being born annually because of rubella. Many experts, however, say the accurate figure would be around 200,000.[17] The 2008 estimates suggest that the highest CRS burden is in South East Asia (approximately 48%), India being a major contributor, and Africa (approximately 38%).[3,4] Other developing countries have incidence rates of 0.6–4.1 per 1000 live births.[18] In 2012 and 2013 (till 31st May) India reported 28 and 48 rubella outbreaks. Cost–benefit studies in countries with routine immunization coverage > 80% show that benefits of rubella vaccine outweigh the cost particularly when combined with measles vaccination.[19]

Vaccine

Rubella vaccine currently derived from RA 27/3 vaccine strain grown in human diploid/chick embryo cell cultures. The vaccine is available in freeze dried form that should be stored frozen or at

2–8°C and needs to be reconstituted with sterile diluent prior to use. The reconstituted vaccine must be protected from light, stored at 2–8°C and used within 6 hrs of reconstitution. The dose is 0.5 ml subcutaneously. A single dose of vaccine provides lifelong protection in 95% of the vaccinees. Apart from local side effects, a mild rash may develop in 5% of the vaccinees. Joint symptoms such as arthralgia and arthritis may occur 1–3 weeks following vaccination especially in susceptible post pubertal females but is usually mild. Immune thrombocytopenic purpura may occur in a frequency of 1 per 30,000 vaccinated children. The vaccine is contraindicated in the severely immunocompromised and in pregnancy. Pregnancy should be avoided for 3 months after vaccination but babies born to women inadvertently vaccinated in pregnancy do not exhibit an increased risk of congenital malformations. Hence accidental vaccination in pregnancy is not an indication for medical termination of pregnancy.

Recommendations for use

Individual use

ACVIP, for office practice, recommends the use of MMR vaccine instead of monovalent rubella vaccine or MR vaccine so as to provide additional protection against mumps and measles.

Public health perspectives

The NTAGI observed that since the 'disability component' of mumps is not a serious public health problem and since the addition of mumps component to UIP would result in a substantial increase (more than twice that of rubella vaccine) in cost without commensurate public health benefits, MR vaccine should be introduced instead of MMR, at the time of the second dose of measles for all children at 16–24 months of age along with DPT booster. In addition, in these states, rubella vaccine should be introduced for adolescent girls as recommended by the sub-committee. States introducing MR should also establish surveillance as recommended by the sub-committee (for monitoring the burden and trend of CRS).[14] Recently many African countries have been using MR vaccine through SIAs successfully.[6] However, ACVIP thinks mumps is also having a significant burden though not adequately reported, and not targeting mumps in the ongoing MR elimination initiative is a missed opportunity.

MMR VACCINE

Globally, most countries use MMR vaccine instead of monovalent vaccines. ACVIP feels that the combined MMR vaccine is a better option than an MR vaccine because of the following reasons: Mumps carries as much significance in terms of morbidity as rubella; complications of mumps are also many and can be profound—aseptic meningitis, encephalitis, orchitis, oophoritis, pancreatitis, deafness, transverse myelitis, facial palsy, ascending polyradiculitis and cerebellar ataxia; like rubella, mumps in a pregnant woman can also give rise to fetal damage in the form of aqueductal stenosis leading to congenital hydrocephalus.[20] The epidemiology of mumps has not been investigated in India but it is suggested that outbreaks occur every 5 to 10 years.[21] The burden of mumps has been reduced in developed countries following use of MMR vaccines. Like rubella, indiscriminate use of mumps vaccine can result in shift of epidemiology to the right and an increase in infection rates in adolescents and adults with greater complications.

Vaccine

Formulations from different manufacturers have different strains of the vaccine virus. Mumps vaccine virus strains include Leningrad-Zagreb, Leningrad-3, Jeryl Lynn, RIT 4385 or Urabe AM9 strains and are grown in chick embryo/human diploid cell cultures. MMR vaccines are supplied in lyophilized form and should be frozen for long-term storage. In the clinic these vaccines can be stored at 2 to 8°C. The vaccines should be protected from light. Reconstituted vaccine should be stored at 2–8°C, protected from light and used within 4–6 hours. The dose is 0.5 ml subcutaneously. The vaccine can be given along with all other childhood vaccines except BCG vaccine. The immunogenicity and efficacy against measles and rubella has been discussed earlier. Seroconversion rates against mumps are more than 90% but clinical efficacy and long-term protection with single dose is 60–90%; outbreaks have been noted in previously vaccinated populations. Hence two doses are needed for durable protection.

Adverse effects due to measles and rubella components have been discussed earlier. Five percent of children can get fever more than 39°C 7–12 days following vaccination and febrile seizures may occur. Aseptic meningitis can rarely occur 2–3 weeks following vaccination but is usually mild. Transient parotitis may occur. The virus does not spread from vaccine to contacts. There is now incontrovertible evidence that there is no causal relationship between MMR vaccine and autism, inflammatory bowel disease, GBS and many other neurological complications. MMR is contraindicated in patients with severe immunodeficiency, pregnancy and those with history of serious allergy to vaccine or its components. The vaccine should be given with caution after weighing risks versus benefits in patients with history of thrombocytopenic purpura and should be preferably avoided in those were thrombocytopenia followed not be given to those with history of thrombocytopenic purpura following previous vaccination with measles/ MMR. The vaccine may be safely given in those with history of egg allergy.

Recommendations for use

Public health perspectives

For the purposes of universal immunization, the vaccine should be introduced in those areas where immunization coverage is at least 80% and can be sustained on a long-term basis, failing which an epidemiologic shift and increase in CRS may occur. For this reason MMR vaccine has been introduced in those Indian states where measles coverage is at least 70%. Simultaneously a system for surveillance for CRS and catch up immunization for all adolescent girls should also be instituted. The MMR vaccine in EPI improves protection against measles by immunizing those who have missed measles vaccine or failed to seroconvert to the first dose of vaccine, should reduce burden of CRS and provides added protection against mumps.

Individual use

ACVIP recommends offering MMR vaccine to all children of parents who can afford the vaccine. This use of MMR in the private sector is unlikely to impact the epidemiology of rubella at present but must be carefully monitored. Two doses are recommended one at the age of 12–15 months and second at school entry (4–6 years) or at any time 8 weeks after the first dose. The second dose of MMR vaccine is to protect children failing to seroconvert against primarily mumps and less commonly against rubella (primary vaccine failures). In a child aged 12 months or older who has not received measles vaccine, 2 doses of MMR at 8 weeks interval suffices, monovalent measles vaccine is not required. Catch-up vaccination with two doses of the vaccine should be given to all those not previously immunized (with no upward age limit) and especially to health care workers, adolescent girls and students travelling for studies overseas. All the currently licensed preparations of MMR vaccine are safe and effective and any one may be used. Recently MMRV vaccine (Mumps Measles Rubella Varicella/Chickenpox vaccine) combining MMR and Varicella vaccine in a single shot has been introduced in the USA and a few other countries.

Government of India has reaffirmed its commitment to the resolution on measles and rubella elimination by 2020 during the 66th SEARO Regional Committee meeting in September 2013 at New Delhi. In October 2013, NTAGI Standing Technical SubCommittee decided to discuss the matter of inclusion of rubella as MR in place of measles and other operational issues related to campaigns with MR. NTAGI also decided to establish a Measles and Rubella Expert Advisory Group comprising both National and International experts to develop the strategy and monitor progress for measles elimination and rubella control by 2020 in India.

IAP perspectives on measles and rubella elimination strategies

The Academy has reviewed the recently circulated ICMR Expert Group Recommendations on rubella vaccine (2012) and also discussed this issue amongst its expert group on immunization. Following are the key summary points enlisted under different headings:

Objective of the initiative

Irrespective of the ongoing initiative by Global Measles, Rubella and CRS Elimination Initiative, SAGE and WHO recommendations, and practices of more than 100 countries in this regard, the Indian Academy of Pediatrics based on their more than 20, 000 members' clinical experience and inputs strongly support elimination of not only measles and rubella, but of mumps also. We believe that it is highly unethical to employ standalone measles vaccine today, when highly effective MR, and effective MMR vaccines available in the market at an affordable price.

We welcome the GoI stand of taking on at least two key infectious diseases, measles and rubella, though it would have been ideal if MMR is also included in this initiative.

We agree with the GoI that major concern is not rubella disease in childhood, but 'Congenital Rubella Syndrome (CRS)' in infants born to mothers who catch rubella during pregnancy. Though logistics/operational issues and global focus may be hindrance to take on two instead of three significant illnesses right now, the ultimate need of the country is to target for elimination/control of all the three diseases instead of the two. We believe, already the program managers have missed the opportunity of using at least a combined MR vaccine in previous SIAs conducted in many states.

The disease burden and country's need

The academy believes that the burden of CRS and mumps is significant. Though exact community burden of CRS is lacking, the fact that a systematic review could be conducted on the 8 multi-centric studies on the prevalence of hospital-based CRS is in itself proof of universality and existence of the problem. The documented 17% susceptibility rates among pregnant women should definitely be a cause of concern.

The burden of mumps is less specified and only sporadic outbreaks are reported.[21] However, based on the inputs and acceptance of mumps vaccination by our membership, and available data captured through our own IDSurv portal, we are confident that mumps also poses a significant burden. Based on the data available at this surveillance program, the incidence of mumps is higher than measles and almost equal to varicella. It ranks 5th amongst top 10 infectious diseases captured through this surveillance utility.[22] We believe that not only the logistics including money and human resource needs are the same, but even the adverse reactions are not expected to be more. Hence, the academy believes both CRS and mumps are eligible to target for elimination and control. At the same time, the academy urges the government/ICMR to take initiatives to strengthen ongoing rubella surveillance; preferably case based, initiate efforts to measure community-burden of CRS, and invests in starting mumps surveillance.

Why mumps is important?

Mumps carries as much significance in terms of morbidity as rubella; complications of mumps are also many and can be profound—aseptic meningitis, encephalitis, orchitis, oophoritis, pancreatitis, deafness, transverse myelitis, facial palsy, ascending polyradiculitis and cerebellar ataxia; like rubella, mumps in a pregnant woman can also give rise to fetal damage in the form of aqueductal stenosis leading to congenital hydrocephalus. Logistics also supports the use of MMR vaccine instead of MR because with the same effort, money and manpower, three common infectious diseases would be eliminated simultaneously instead of two.

The tools and timings

Fortunately we have effective and affordable vaccines to take on all the three diseases. Availability of an indigenous producer and supplier should also bolster our efforts to launch large-scale vaccination drives against them. While single dose of rubella/rubella containing vaccines is sufficient to provide almost 100% protection against the disease, two or more doses of measles and mumps vaccines are needed to accord adequate protection.

We support the suggestion that at least 80% coverage must be achieved to offset any presumed epidemiological shift of rubella (and mumps) and consequently higher incidence of congenital complications.

We think the MR/MMR vaccine should be given early to have much higher coverage than introducing it late at the time of 2nd booster of DTP. According to available evidence, both these vaccines (MR/MMR) can be given safely at different ages including at 9 months of age. Most important thing is to achieve minimum 80% coverage of childhood vaccination which will not allow virus to circulate freely and infect women of child bearing age, thus avoiding any inadvertent epidemiological shift.

Operational issues

At the time of introduction of vaccine one time campaign to vaccinate adolescent girls with rubella vaccine is a proven strategy, but we need to explore all avenues to cover all the eligible susceptible pediatric populations. So we need to have large SIAs to cover young children, school children (at entry) and adolescents. No doubt, this will pose unprecedented burden on health infrastructure and machinery, but we must remain positive and avoid speculating about the low quality/low coverage. Our experience with measles catch-up campaigns has shown it is possible to achieve very high coverage of > 80% in states.

Regarding coverage of adolescent girls and children in other age groups who are not covered with measles and rubella vaccine, apart from SIAs and school vaccination programmes, Anganwadi programs also can be a good modality. Many Kishori/adolescent girls' oriented activities are now being introduced through ICDS including iron folic acid and nutrition programs. MMR /MR vaccine can be introduced through that system.

So, in conclusion, the Academy thinks reaching all children with measles vaccine gives us an opportunity to also reach them with rubella and mumps, in a combined vaccine. Congenital rubella syndrome can be completely prevented, and the academy fully supports efforts to prevent infant and childhood disability and the associated health, social and economic costs. By preventing measles, rubella and mumps together we produce significant savings for our country and communities.

Measles

Routine vaccination:

- Minimum age: 9 months or 270 completed days.

Catch-up vaccination:

- Catch-up vaccination beyond 12 months should be MMR.

- Measles vaccine can be administered to infants aged 6 through 11 months during outbreaks. These children should be revaccinated with 2 doses of measles containing vaccines, the first at ages 12 through 15 months and at least 4 weeks after the previous dose, and the second at ages 4 through 6 years.

Measles, mumps, and rubella (MMR) vaccine

Routine vaccination

- Minimum age: 12 months

- Administer the first dose of MMR vaccine at age 12 through 18 months, and the second dose at age 4 through 6 years.

- The second dose may be administered before age 4 years, provided at least 4 weeks have elapsed since the first dose.

Catch-up vaccination

- Ensure that all school-aged children and adolescents have had 2 doses of MMR vaccine; the minimum interval between the 2 doses is 4 weeks.

- One dose if previously vaccinated with one dose.

References

1. WHO SEARO. Measles Elimination and Rubella Control 2013. Available from http://www.searo.who.int/mediacentre/events/governance/rc/66/9.pdf. (Accessed on Nov 28, 2013)

2. WHO: Measles deaths decline, but elimination progress stalls in some regions Available from http://www.who.int/mediacentre/news/notes/2013/measles_20130117/en/index.html. (Accessed on Nov 27, 2013)

3. van den Ent MM, Brown DW, Hoekstra EJ, Christie A, Cochi SL. Measles mortality reduction contributes substantially to reduction of all cause mortality among children less than five years of age, 1990–2008. J Infect Dis. 2011; 204 Suppl 1: S18–23.

4. WHO. Global Measles and Rubella. Strategic Plan 2012–2020. Available from http://www.who.int/immunization/newsroom/Measles_Rubella_StrategicPlan_2012_2020.pdf. (Accessed on Nov 27, 2013)

5. John TJ, Choudhury P. Accelerating Measles Control in India: Opportunity and Obligation to Act Now. Indian Pediatr 2009; 46: 939–943.

6. Status Report on Progress Towards Measles and Rubella Elimination. SAGE Working Group on Measles and Rubella (17 October 2013) Available from http://www.who.int/immunization/sage/meetings/2013/november/Status_Report_Measles_Rubella21Oct2013_FINAL.pdf. (Accessed on Nov 28, 2013)

7. Global Measles and Rubella Laboratory Network, January 2004–June 2005. MMWR Morb Mortal Wkly Rep. 2005: 4; 54(43): 1100–1104.

8. Gupta A. India's Universal immunization programme. GAVI Alliance Board Meeting 2012. Available from www.gavialliance.org /about/.../12.../16--- country-presentation—India.

9. Measles and Rubella Initiative. Measles deaths decline, but elimination progress stalls in some regions. Available from http://www.unicef.org/ immunization/files/Note_to_media_FINAL_17-01-13(1).pdf.

10. Sinha K. Times of India report: 47% of global measles deaths in India. 2012. Apr 24 Available from http://articles. timesofindia.indiatimes.com /2012-04-24 /science / 31392204_1_measles-vaccine-second-dose-measles-mortality. (Accessed on 28th Nov 2013)

11. UNICEF Coverage Evaluation survey, 2009 National Fact Sheet. Available from: http://www.unicef.org/india/ National_Fact_Sheet_CES_2009.pdf. (Accessed on November 28, 2013)

12. John TJ. Death of children after measles vaccination. Indian Pediatr 2008; 45: 477–478.

13. WHO. Global Vaccine Safety. Information for Health care Workers. Available from http://www.who.int/vaccine_safety/initiative/detection/ managing_AEFIs/en/index4.html. (Accessed on Nov 28, 2013)

14. Ministry of health & family Welfare. National Technical Advisory Group on Immunization, 16 June 2008. Available from http://mohfw.nic.in/ WriteReadData / l892s / 6664716297file23.pdf. (Accessed on Nov 29, 2013)

15. Vashishtha VM, Choudhury P, Bansal CP, Gupta SG. Measles control strategies in India. Position Paper of Indian Academy of Pediatrics. Indian Pediatr 2013; 50: 561–564.

16. Dewan P, Gupta P. Burden of Congenital Rubella Syndrome (CRS) in India: A Systematic Review. Indian Pediatr 2012; 49: 377–399.

17. Sinha K. Times of India report: Now, India to roll out vaccine against Rubella. May 16, 2012. Available from http://articles.timesofindia.indiatimes.com/ 2012-05-16/india/31725540_1_rubella-vaccine-congenital-rubella-syndrome-combination-vaccine. (Accessed on Nov 28, 2013)

18. Cutts FT, Robertson SE, Diaz-Ortega JL, Samuel R. Control of rubella and congenital rubella syndrome (CRS) in developing countries, Part 1: Burden of disease from CRS. Bull World Health Organ. 1997; 75(1): 55–68.

19. Investing in immunization through the GAVI Alliance. The evidence base 2011. Website: www.gavialliance.com.

20. CDC. Available from http://www.who.int /biologicals /areas/vaccines/mmr/ mumps/en. (Accessed on Nov 29, 2013)

21. John TJ. An outbreak of mumps in Thiruvananthapuram district. Indian Pediatrics 2004; 41: 298–300.

22. IDSurv, Infectious Disease Surveillance by IAP. Available at: www.idsurv.org.

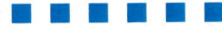

VARICELLA VACCINE

Reviewed by
Panna Choudhury, Vijay Yewale

Background

Varicella (chickenpox) is a febrile rash illness resulting from primary infection with the varicella-zoster virus (VZV). Humans are the only source of infection for this virus. Varicella severity and complications are increased among immunocompromised persons, infants, and adults. However, healthy children and adults may also develop serious complications and even die from varicella.[1] In the absence of a vaccination program, varicella affects nearly every person by mid-adulthood in most populations.

Disease Burden

The epidemiology of varicella differs between temperate and tropical climates. In tropical climates, VZV seroprevalance reflects a higher mean age of infection and higher susceptibility among adults as compared to temperate climates. There is a little data on the health burden of varicella in developing countries. However, as in tropical climates, higher proportion of varicella cases may occur among adults, varicella morbidity and mortality may be higher than that described in developed countries.[2] Seropositivity is lower in adults from tropical and subtropical areas.[3] A seroprevalence study from West Bengal reported only 42% rural adults were immune.[4]

Idsurv data: According to the academy's passive reporting system of 10 infectious diseases by the pediatricians (www.idsurv.org), a total of 816 (7.7%) cases of varicella were reported out of total 10580 cases from December 2010 to till December 11, 2013. Out of these 816 cases, 58.2% were between 5 and 18 years, 18.6% between 3 and 5 years, and 15.4% between 1 and 3 years of age. Sixty three (7.7%) cases were below 1 year of age. Only 12% were fully immunized while 74% were not immunized at all. Three percent had severe disease, needed hospitalization and there was no mortality.

Vaccine

Takahashi et al developed a live attenuated vaccine from the Oka strain in Japan in the early seventies.[5] Varicella vaccines, in use today, are all derived from the original Oka strain but the virus contents may vary from one manufacturer to another. Vaccination induces both humoral and cellular immunity.

Immunogenicity and Efficacy

Immunogenicity studies report overall seroprotection rates of 86% following single dose of the vaccine (immunogenicity reducing with increasing age) and persistence of protective antibodies for up to 10 years after vaccination. Prelicensure efficacy and postlicensure effectiveness studies have shown the efficacy of a single dose of the vaccine to range from 70 to 90% against any disease and > 95% against combined moderate and severe disease for 7–10 years after vaccination.[6–8] Administration of 2 doses three months/ 4–6 years apart improves seroprotection rates to 99% and results in higher GMT's by at least 10 fold. This translates to superior efficacy of 98.3% against any disease/ 100% against moderate/ severe disease and reduces incidence of breakthrough varicella as compared to single dose by 3.3 fold (Table 1).

Table 1. Seroconversion and efficacy of one and two doses of varicella vaccine

Parameter	1 dose	2 doses
Seroconversion	86%	99%
Efficacy—mild disease	70–90%	98.3%
Efficacy—moderate to severe disease disease	> 95%	100%

Vaccine failure and breakthrough varicella

Administration of the 2nd dose at 3 months following the first dose or at 5 years has similar efficacy. Vaccine failure with single dose is mainly 'primary' as most cases of breakthrough disease happen within 5 years of vaccination and efficacy of single dose or two doses are similar at 10 years following vaccination. The observed vaccine failure after 1 dose of vaccine may be explained in most probability as that immunized children either do not develop humoral immunity to VZV at all or that there is an initial immune "burst" of immunity that is enough to generate a positive gpELISA result but is inadequate to generate a sustained memory T cell response leading to waning of immunity over a period of time.

Breakthrough varicella is defined as varicella developing more than 42 days after immunization and usually occurs 2–5 years following vaccination. It occurs in about 1% to 4% of vaccines per year. This rate does not seem to increase with length of time after immunization.[9] Breakthrough disease in 70% of instances is typically mild, with <50 skin lesions, predominantly maculopapular rather than vesicular rash, low or no fever, and shorter (4–6 days) duration of illness.[10] It may go unnoticed/undiagnosed resulting in more opportunities to infect others due to failure to isolate these cases. Nevertheless, breakthrough varicella is contagious, may be severe, can result in outbreaks and has occasionally caused deaths in the immunocompromised. Some of the risk factors for vaccine failure and breakthrough disease include young age at vaccination (< 15 months), increasing time since vaccination, receipt of steroids within 3 months of breakthrough disease, initiation of vaccination in older children and adolescents and administration of vaccine within 28 days of MMR vaccine but not on the same day.

Safety

Adverse reactions, documented carefully in prelicensure/postlicensure studies, include local reactions such as pain, redness and swelling at vaccination site, injection site rash, fever and a systemic varicella like rash in around 5 %. Transmission of the vaccine virus from vaccines to contacts is rare especially in the absence of a vaccine related rash in the vaccines. However, vaccine recipients who develop a rash should avoid contact with persons without 'evidence of immunity' who are at high risk for severe complications. The side effect profile is similar with the 2 dose schedule.

Contraindications: The vaccine is contraindicated during pregnancy, individuals with a history of anaphylactic reactions to any component of the vaccine (including neomycin), in those with clinically manifested HIV infection and in the immuno-compromised (exceptions listed below). When used in adult females, pregnancy should be avoided for 3 months after vaccination.[10,11] Due to the theoretical risk of Reye syndrome, the use of salicylates is discouraged for 6 weeks following varicella vaccination.[8]

Risk of herpes zoster among immunized individual
Herpes zoster in vaccine recipients is known to occur due to both the vaccine virus and the wild virus; however, the overall incidence of herpes zoster in vaccinated children was noted to be much lower than unvaccinated children in prelicensure trials.

Recommendations for use

Individual use

ACVIP recommends offering the vaccine to all healthy children with no prior history of varicella with special emphasis in all children belonging to certain high-risk groups as enumerated below:

- Children with humoral immunodeficiencies.

- Children with HIV infection but with CD4 counts 15% and above the age related cut off.

- Leukemia but in remission and off chemotherapy for at least 3–6 months.

- Children on long-term salicylates. Salicylates should be avoided for at least 6 weeks after vaccination.

- Children likely to be on long-term steroid therapy. The vaccine may be given at any time if the children are on low dose steroids/ alternate day steroids but only 4 weeks after stopping steroids if the patients have received high dose steroids (> 2 mg/kg) for 14 days or more.

- In household contacts of immunocompromised children.

- Adolescents who have not had varicella in past and are known to be varicella IgG negative, especially if they are leaving home for studies in a residential school/college.

- Children with chronic lung/heart disease.

- Seronegative adolescents and adults if they are inmates of or working in the institutional set up, e.g. school teachers, day care center workers, military personnel and health care professionals.

- For post-exposure prophylaxis in susceptible healthy non-pregnant contacts preferably within 3 days of exposure (efficacy 90%) and potentially up to 5 days of exposure (efficacy 70%, against severe disease 100%).

Dosage and schedule

The recommended dose is 0.5 ml to be administered subcutaneously and the minimum infectious virus content should be 1000 Plaque Forming Units. It is available as a lyophilized vaccine, storage requirements vary with the brand and manufacturers' instructions should be followed. It should be protected from light and needs to be used within 30 minutes of reconstitution. The vaccine may be given with all other childhood vaccines. It is to be given as 2 doses.

The vaccines are licensed for age 12 months and above. However, the risk of breakthrough varicella is lower if given 15 months onwards. Hence ACVIP recommends administration of varicella vaccine in children aged 15 months or older. After a single dose of varicella vaccine, approximately 15% of vaccines remain at risk of developing a breakthrough varicella disease. These varicella infections in immunized population may raise concern regarding vaccine efficacy and a misunderstanding by physicians or parents who may lose faith in vaccination. Because immunized children who experience breakthrough disease are coinfected with both wild and vaccine strains of varicella virus, they may be at increased risk of zoster from the reactivated wild-type strain later in life, compared with vaccine recipients who do not experience breakthrough disease. Two doses of varicella vaccine offer superior individual protection as compared to a single dose. The ACVIP now recommends two doses of varicella vaccine for children of all age groups.

- For primary immunization, the first dose should be given at the age of 15 months and the second dose at 4–6 years. However, during an outbreak, the 1st dose may be administered at

12 months of age if it is ensured that the 2-dose schedule will be completed by the individual child. The second dose may be administered any time 3 months after the first dose.

- For catch-up vaccination, children below the age of 13 years should receive 2 doses 3 months apart and those aged 13 years or more should receive 2 doses at an interval of 4–8 weeks.

- All high-risk children should, however, receive two doses 4–8 weeks apart irrespective of age

A live attenuated vaccine against herpes zoster is now licensed and available in the US but not in India.

The need to implement a two-dose varicella schedule < 13 years

A two-dose schedule of varicella vaccination is now recommended along with a second-dose catch-up varicella vaccination for children and adolescents who previously had received only one dose. This is because vaccine failure has been seen to occur after a first dose. Outbreaks of varicella had been reported in populations with high coverage with one dose of vaccine.[10] A group of 148 children in the USA were tested for seroconversion after receiving 1 dose of the vaccine, using the fluorescent antibody to membrane antigen (FAMA) assay, only 76% of these children seroconverted.[12] These results were one of the reasons why a second dose of varicella vaccine was mandated in 2006 by the Centers for Disease Control and Prevention (CDC) for all children.[1] In a recent publication it has been shown that varicella incidence, hospitalizations, and outbreaks in 2 active surveillance areas declined substantially during the first 5 years of the 2-dose varicella vaccination program.[13] In India also, breakthrough varicella has been observed in children immunized with one dose, in spite of the opportunities of natural boosting. Two doses of varicella will indeed work better than one dose for the 'individuals' protection.

Rationale behind ACVIP recommendations

Why 2nd dose at 4–6 years of age?

Though the second dose can be administered after 3 months of first dose and there are many trials to support that, but why IAP ACVIP is insisting for 4–6 years is because of the following reasons:[14]

1. The recommended ages for routine first (at age 15 months) and second (at age 4–6 years) doses of varicella vaccine are harmonized with the recommendations for MMR vaccine use and intended to limit the period when children have no varicella antibody. The recommended age for the second dose is supported by the current epidemiology of varicella, with low incidence and few outbreaks among preschool-aged children and higher incidence and more outbreaks among elementary-school-aged children.

2. Although, the most studies are done when 2nd dose is given after 3 months of the first, there are a few trials where the two schedules were compared and it was concluded that among children, VZV antibody levels and GMTs after 2 doses administered 4–6 years apart were comparable to those obtained when the 2 doses were administered 3 months apart (Seroconversion: 99.2% vs 99.6%, GMTs: 212.4 vs 142.6, respectively).[15]

3. However, the CMI responses measured by mean stimulation index (SI), a marker of cell-mediated immunity were 36.9 for 2nd dose after 3 months of primary dose, and 58.6 when 2nd dose given at 4–6 years of age.[15]

Probably, the only benefit of providing 2nd dose after 3 months of first dose (given at 15 months) could be insignificant, miniscule reduction in cases of breakthrough varicella occurring in the window period of 15 months to 4 years.

Varicella Zoster Immunoglobulin (VZIG)

VZIG provided passive immunity against varicella and is indicated for postexposure prophylaxis in susceptible individuals with significant contact with varicella/ herpes zoster who are at high risk for severe disease. Susceptible individual is defined as

i. all unvaccinated children who do not have a clinical history of varicella in the past;

ii. all unvaccinated adults who are seronegative for anti-varicella IgG.

Bone marrow transplant recipients are considered susceptible even if they had disease or received vaccinations prior to transplantation. A 'significant contact' is defined as any face-to-face contact or stays within the same room for a period greater than 1 hour with a patient with infectious varicella (defined as 1–2 days before the rash till all lesions have crusted) or disseminated herpes zoster. Patients meeting these two criteria and who are at high risk of developing severe disease as enumerated below merit prophylaxis with VZIG:

- Neonates born to mothers who develop varicella 5 days before or 2 days after delivery. The risk of varicella related death in these infants as per older estimates is likely to be 30% but may be lower. Other full term healthy newborns are not at increased risk for complications and do not merit prophylaxis if exposed to varicella.

- All neonates born at less than 28 weeks of gestation/ with birth weight less than 1000 gms, exposed in the neonatal period.

- All preterm neonates born at more than 28 weeks of gestation and exposed to varicella only if their mothers are negative for anti-varicella IgG, exposed to varicella.

- Pregnant women exposed to varicella.

- All immunocompromised children especially neoplastic disease, congenital or acquired immunodeficiency or those receiving immunosuppressive therapies. Patients who received IVIG @ 400 mg/kg in the past 3 weeks are deemed protected.

Dosage and administration schedule

VZIG should be given as soon as possible but not later than 96 hours following exposure. VZIG reduces risk of disease and complications and duration of protection lasts for 3 weeks. The currently available VZIG is for intravenous use (Varitect) and is administered at a dose of 0.2 – 1ml/kg diluted in normal saline over 1 hour.

Efficacy and safety: The efficacy against death in cases where neonatal exposure has occurred is almost 100%. Side effects include allergic reactions and anaphylaxis. Since VZIG prolongs the incubation period, all exposed should be monitored for at least 28 weeks for disease manifestations.

The cost of VZIG is prohibitive. If non-affordable/ not available, other options with uncertain efficacy include IVIG @ 200 mg/kg or oral acyclovir @ 80 mg/kg/day beginning from the 7th day of exposure and given for 7–10 days.

Public health perspectives

The committee acknowledges the great burden of varicella disease and resultant morbidity on the community in India. It also admits that varicella is not entirely a benign disease and outbreaks of complicated disease and even deaths are increasingly reported especially among adolescents and adult populations. Extensive use of varicella vaccine as a routine vaccine in children will have a significant impact on the epidemiology of the disease. If sustained high coverage can be achieved, the disease may virtually disappear. If only partial coverage can be obtained, the epidemiology may shift, leading to an increase in the number of cases in older children and adults. Hence, routine childhood varicella immunization programs should emphasize high, sustained coverage.

However at the same time, the IAP ACVIP also believes that other new vaccines, such as rotavirus and pneumococcal vaccines, have the potential for a much greater public health impact, and should therefore be given priority over varicella vaccines. Hence, at the present time IAP ACVIP does not recommend the inclusion of varicella vaccination into the national immunization program of the country.

References

1. CDC. Surveillance of Varicella. Manual for the Surveillance of Vaccine-Preventable Diseases (5th Ed, 2011). Available from http://www.cdc.gov/vaccines/pubs/surv-manual/chpt17-varicella.html. (Accessed on Dec 10, 2013)

2. WHO. Varicella Vaccine. Available from http://archives.who.int/vaccines/en/varicella.shtml. (Accessed on Dec 10, 2013)

3. Ooi PL, Goh KT, Doraisingham S, Ling AE. Prevalence of varicella-zoster virus infection in Singapore. Southeast Asian J Trop Med Public Health 1992; 23: 22–25.

4. Mandal BK, Mukherjee PP, Murphy C, Mukherjee R, Naik T. Adult susceptibility to varicella in the tropics is rural phenomenon due to lack of previous exposure. J Infect Dis. 1998; 178 Suppl 1: S52–54.

5. Takahashi M. The varicella vaccine. Vaccine development. Infect Dis Clin North Am. 1996; 10(3): 469–488.

VARICELLA VACCINE

Routine vaccination:

- Minimum age: 12 months
- Administer the first dose at age 15 through 18 months, and the second dose at age 4 through 6 years.
- The second dose may be administered before age 4 years, provided at least 3 months have elapsed since the first dose. If the second dose was administered at least 4 weeks after the first dose, it can be accepted as valid.
- The risk of breakthrough varicella is lower if given 15 months onwards.

Catch-up vaccination:

- Ensure that all persons aged 7 through 18 years without 'evidence of immunity' have 2 doses of the vaccine.
- Evidence of immunity' to varicella includes any of the following:
  - ➢ documentation of age-appropriate vaccination with a varicella vaccine
  - ➢ laboratory evidence of immunity or laboratory confirmation of disease
  - ➢ diagnosis or verification of a history of varicella disease by a health-care provider
  - ➢ diagnosis or verification of a history of herpes zoster by a health-care provider
- For children aged 12 months through 12 years, the recommended minimum interval between doses is 3 months. However, if the second dose was administered at least 4 weeks after the first dose, it can be accepted as valid.
- For persons aged 13 years and older, the minimum interval between doses is 4 weeks.
- For persons without evidence of immunity, administer 2 doses if not previously vaccinated or the second dose if only 1 dose has been administered.

6. Kuter BJ, Weibel RE, Guess HA, et al. Oka/Merck varicella vaccine in healthy children: final report of a 2-year efficacy study and 7-year follow-up studies. Vaccine. 1991; 9 :643–647.

7. Skull SA, Wang EEL. Varicella vaccination— a critical review of the evidence. Arch Dis Child 2001; 85: 83–90.

8. Varicella Vaccines. WHO Position Paper. Wkly Epidemiol Rec 1998; 73: 241–248.

9. Clements DA. Modified varicella-like syndrome. Infect Dis Clin North Am. 1996; 10: 617–629.

10. Pickering LK, Orenstein WO. Active Immunization. Principles and Practice of Pediatric Infectious Diseases Revised, 3rd ed. Churchill Livingstone 2009: 48–71.

11. CDC. General recommendations on immunization: Recommendations of the Advisory Committee on Immunization Practices (ACIP). MMWR. 2011; 60(No. RR-2): 1–64.

12. Michalik DE, Steinberg SP, Larussa PS, Edwards KM, Wright PF, Arvin AM, et al. Primary vaccine failure after 1 dose of varicella vaccine in healthy children. J Infect Dis. 2008; 197: 944–949.

13. Bialek SR, Perella D, Zhang J, Mascola L, Viner K, Jackson C, et al. Impact of a routine two-dose varicella vaccination program on varicella epidemiology. Pediatrics. 2013; 132: e1134–1140.

14. Vashishtha VM. Reply. IAP Immunization Timetable 2012: Some Issues. Available from: http://www.indianpediatrics.net/dec2012/996.pdf. (Accessed on December 11, 2013)

15. MMWR, Recommendations and Reports. Prevention of Varicella. Recommendations of the Advisory Committee on Immunization Practices (ACIP). June 22, 2007/56(RR04);1-40. Available from: http://www.cdc.gov/mmwr/preview/mmwrhtml/rr5604a1.htm .

■ ■ ■ ■ ■ ■

HEPATITIS A VACCINES

Reviewed by
A.K. Patwari, Nitin Shah

Background

Hepatitis A virus (HAV) infection is a relatively benign infection in young children. As many as 85% of children below 2 years and 50% of those between 2 and 5 years infected with HAV are anicteric and may have no symptoms at all or just have non-specific symptoms like fever, malaise, diarrhea, vomiting, cough, etc. like any other viral infection. On the contrary, 70–95% of adults with hepatitis A are symptomatic with a mortality of 1%. The disease severity increases irrespective of age, in those with underlying chronic liver disease.

Burden of disease

Global burden

Based on an ongoing reassessment of the global burden of hepatitis A, preliminary WHO estimates suggest an increase in the number of acute hepatitis A cases from 117 million in 1990 to 126 million in 2005 (and increase in deaths due to hepatitis A from 30,283 in 1990 to 35,245 in 2005).[1] Increased numbers of cases were estimated to occur in the age groups 2–14 years and > 30 years.

In high-income regions the prevalence of anti-HAV antibody is very low (<50% are immune by age 30 years), but there is almost no circulation of the virus and therefore the risk of acquiring HAV infection is low. In contrast, in countries with high endemicity, most individuals acquire natural infection in childhood and therefore burden of disease including incidence of outbreaks is also low. As a shift occurs towards intermediate endemicity due to improvements in hygiene and sanitation, the population stands at a higher risk because a certain proportion of children remain susceptible till adulthood and the risk of HAV transmission continues to be high due to overall sub-optimal access to clean water and sanitation. Thus burden of symptomatic disease and incidence of outbreaks paradoxically increase despite some improvements in socioeconomic indicators.

Indian burden

India, earlier a highly endemic country, is now shifting to intermediate endemicity in some areas in cities and in higher socio-economic strata of community.[2] Seroprevalence studies show susceptibility in 30–40% of adolescents and adults belonging to the high socioeconomic class with regional differences (seropositivity in Kerala being lower than other states). Studies also show a reduction in cord blood seropositivity (indicative of young adult seronegativity) for HAV over the years.

Several outbreaks of hepatitis A in various parts of India have been recorded in the past decade; children from rural and semi-urban areas of the state of Maharashtra (2002–2004), an explosive outbreak among adults from Kerala involving 1,137 cases (2004) and over 450 cases in children and adults in Shimla (2007). An increasing contribution of hepatitis A to fulminant hepatic failure (FHF) has also been noted, especially in children. In a study from Pune, 18–50% of pediatric patients admitted for FHF either had hepatitis A alone or along with other hepatitis viruses.[3] According to the academy's passive reporting system of 10 infectious diseases by the pediatricians (www.idsurv.org), a total of 1690 (16%) cases of hepatitis A were reported out of total 10554 cases from December 2010 to till December 10, 2013.

Vaccines

Inactivated vaccines

Most of the currently available vaccines are derived from HM 175/GBM strains and grown on MRC5 human diploid cell lines. The virus is formalin inactivated and adjuvanted with aluminium hydroxide. The vaccine is stored at 2–8°C. The serologic correlate of protection is 20 mIU/ml. All hepatitis A vaccines are licensed for use in children aged 1 year or older.

A liposomal adjuvanted hepatitis A vaccine derived from the ' RG-SB strain, harvested from disrupted MRC-5 cells and inactivated by formalin is now available. The liposome adjuvant is immunopotentiating reconstituted influenza virosome (IRIV) composed of phosphatidylcholine, phosphatidylethanolamine and hemagglutinin from an H1N1 strain of influenza virus. The efficacy and safety profile is nearly similar to the other inactivated vaccines.

Combination of hepatitis A and hepatitis B vaccines are also available to be used in those who have not been vaccinated for hepatitis B previously. These are available in both adult and pediatric formulations and are discussed separately under combination vaccines. Similarly combinations of hepatitis A vaccine with Vi-polysaccharide vaccines are available internationally though not in India.

Efficacy & effectiveness: In general, 2 doses of inactivated hepatitis A vaccine induce protective efficacies of 90–95%, or more. The median predicted duration of protection has been estimated at 45.0 years.[4] The vaccine efficacy is lower in the elderly, immunocompromised, those with chronic liver disease, in transplant recipients and those with pre-existing maternal antibodies. Immunity is lifelong due to anamnestic response and no boosters are recommended at present in the immunocompetent.

A higher GMC of anti-HAV IgG was induced in the two-dose inactivated than in the one-dose inactivated and the attenuated vaccines at 12 months.[5] Compared to the classical two-dose schedule, one single dose of inactivated hepatitis A vaccines is similarly efficacious, less expensive and easier to implement. High efficacy of post-exposure prophylaxis against hepatitis A using one single dose of inactivated vaccine within 2 weeks of exposure is also documented. However, in risk groups for hepatitis A, a two-dose vaccination schedule is preferred.[4]

Dosage schedule: IAP ACVIP recommends two doses of inactivated hepatitis A vaccine given intramuscularly. Administer the second dose 6–18 months after the first.[6] Minimum age for giving hepatitis A vaccine is 12 months.

Safety: Adverse reactions are minor and usually include local pain and swelling. Cumulative global experience from the use of several hundred million doses of inactivated hepatitis A vaccines testify to their excellent overall safety profile.[4] The vaccine may be safely given with other childhood vaccines and interchange of brands is permitted though not routinely recommended.

Live attenuated vaccine

This vaccine is derived from the H2 strain of the virus attenuated after serial passage in Human Diploid Cell (KMB 17 cell line). It has been in use in China since the 1990's in mass vaccination programs. The vaccine meets WHO requirements and is now licensed and available in India. Controlled trials conducted among large numbers of children 1–15 years of age have shown up to 100% efficacy for pre-exposure prophylaxis and 95% efficacy for post-exposure prophylaxis. Anti- HAV antibodies were detected in 72–88% of the vaccines 15 years after vaccination.[4] However, live attenuated hepatitis A vaccine does not provide post-exposure protection against HAV infection during the outbreak.[7]

Dosage schedule: An overall protective rate of 100% after one dose of live attenuated hepatitis A vaccine has been reported and the long-term immunogenicity and effectiveness could last as long as 15 years.[8] In a large scale clinical trial to evaluate single dose and booster dose of live attenuated hepatitis A vaccine, 72% of children who received a single dose had detectable anti-HAV antibodies for 96 months (GMC at 96 months: 89.0 mIU/mL) and 98% children in the booster group remained anti-HAV positive at 96 months (GMC at 96 months: 262.8 mIU/mL) suggesting a booster effect of reinjection. However, results from single dose group seems not to support the need for booster doses of live attenuated hepatitis A vaccine in immunocompetent individuals.[9]

In India, a multicenteric evaluation of immunogenicity and tolerability of single dose live attenuated injectable hepatitis A vaccine was done in four centers across the country. The vaccine was, administered to 505 children aged 18 to 60 months and the evaluation was done by estimation of anti-HAV antibody titer at 6 weeks and 6 months following administration of the vaccine. At 6 weeks, 95.1 % seroconverted and at the end of 6 months, 97.9 % had seroconverted.[10] Another long-term immunogenicity study of a single dose live attenuated H2 strain hepatitis A vaccine is being conducted in healthy Indian children at KEM Hospital, Pune. 131 of the original 143 children vaccinated in 2004, were evaluated for anti-HAV antibodies 30 months post-vaccination (2007). Seroprotective antibody levels >20 mIU/mL were demonstrated in 87.8% subjects with an overall GMT of 92.02 mIU/mL. No hepatitis like illness was recorded in any of the subjects since vaccination.[11]

WHO recommends that the live attenuated vaccine is administered as a single dose.[4] However, long-term serologic data from India with single dose of live vaccine is still not available. In a significant subset of original study subjects of KEM Pune cohort,[11] there is an appreciable dip in both seroprotection levels (anti-HAV IgG < 20.0 mIU/mL) and GMTs in the eighth year of follow up despite natural boosting. The investigators are now planning to demonstrate anamenstic responses in these subjects by performing boosting with a 2nd dose of the vaccine. IAP ACVIP recommends two doses of live attenuated hepatitis A vaccine given subcutaneously in a dose of 0.5 ml subcutaneously in children 1–15 years. The second dose should be administered after 6–18 months of the first.[6] Minimum age for giving hepatitis A vaccine is 12 months.

Safety: No substantial safety concerns have been identified during vaccine trials[4] and no horizontal transmission or serious adverse effects have been noted with the live vaccine.

Recommendations for use

Individual use

The hepatitis A vaccine may be offered to all healthy children with special emphasis in risk groups as enumerated below:

- Patients with chronic liver disease
- Carriers of hepatitis B and hepatitis C
- Congenital or acquired immunodeficiency
- Transplant recipients
- Adolescents seronegative for HAV who are leaving home for residential schools
- Travellers to countries with high endemicity for hepatitis A
- Household contacts of patients with acute HAV infection within 10 days of onset of illness in the index case. It may not always be effective under such circumstances when the contact has had the same source of infection as the index patient

Which vaccine to use?

If a decision to administer the vaccine is taken, any of the licensed vaccines may be used as all have nearly similar efficacy and safety (exception, immunocompromised patients where only inactivated vaccines may be used). WHO concludes that both inactivated and live attenuated hepatitis A vaccines are safe and highly immunogenic and that in most cases, these vaccines will generate long-lasting possibly life-long protection against hepatitis A both in children and adults.[4]

Age at vaccination

Based on data suggesting a decline in the adult seropositivity rates especially in those belonging to the high socioeconomic status, it is likely that babies may be born with no maternal antibodies, thereby making a case for vaccination for hepatitis A at an earlier age. Immunogenicity studies also show that antibody titers achieved with vaccination at 12 months are comparable to those achieved at 18 months–2 years. In light of these facts, the IAP ACVIP recommends initiating hepatitis A vaccine at the age of 12 months.

Catch-up vaccination and screening for hepatitis A antibodies

In India, a very rapid socio-economic development has taken place in the last years; many high endemicity areas for HAV infection coexist with others, making a transition to intermediate endemicity. Some studies have demonstrated an epidemiological shift of the age of acquisition of the HAV infection in the community, even if the current available data do not confirm a consistent decline in childhood HAV seroprevalence rates and increased susceptibility to HAV in young adults.[12] A study from Hyderabad observed that 25% of children < 15 years remain susceptible to HAV infection.[13] Another study from Bijapur observed seropositivity in 54.4% children between 5 and 15 years.[14] Since the cost of screening to identify those susceptible to get hepatitis A infection is lower than the cost of vaccine, IAP ACVIP recommends pre-vaccination screening for hepatitis A antibody in children > 10 years of age.

Public health perspectives

According to WHO, in countries transitioning from high to intermediate endemicity, as is the case in India, large-scale hepatitis A vaccination is likely to be cost-effective and is therefore encouraged. The effectiveness of vaccination of pediatric populations at risk of hepatitis A has been demonstrated in a number of geographic regions worldwide Compared to the classical two-dose schedule, one single dose of inactivated hepatitis A vaccines is similarly efficacious, less expensive and easier to implement.[4]

Single-dose immunization

Within 2–4 weeks of the first dose of inactivated hepatitis A vaccine, up to 100% of immunocompetent children and young adults achieve anti-HAV IgG titers over 20 mIU/ml.[15] Furthermore, a single dose of this vaccine may successfully control outbreaks of hepatitis A.[4] In 2003, a randomized, double-blind trial of a single dose of inactivated hepatitis A vaccine was conducted in Nicaragua among 239 children. Protective efficacy within those 6 weeks was 85% (95% CI: 55–96%) and after 6 weeks, 100% (79.8–100%).[16]

Effectiveness of single dose in NIP: Argentina began a universal immunization program in 12-month-old children based on a single dose schedule of inactivated hepatitis A vaccine in 2005. In 2007, with vaccination coverage of 95%, the incidence of symptomatic viral hepatitis A had dropped by > 80% in all age groups.[17] Six years after implementation of this countrywide single-dose programme, no hepatitis A cases have been detected among vaccinated individuals, whereas among the unvaccinated a number of cases have occurred, confirming continued circulation of hepatitis A virus in the Argentinian Population.[4,17] The above studies demonstrate effectiveness of even a single dose of inactivated vaccine when used in large-scale programs.

Considering the uniformly high burden of the disease and effectiveness of hepatitis vaccine even in single dose, the IAP ACVIP recommends that vaccination against hepatitis A be integrated into the UIP for children aged ≥ 1 year. However, it should be part of a comprehensive plan for the prevention and control of viral hepatitis, including measures to improve hygiene and sanitation and measures for outbreak control.

Hepatitis A (Hep A) vaccine

Routine vaccination:

- Minimum age: 12 months
- Start the 2-dose hepatitis A vaccine series for children aged 12 through 23 months; separate the 2 doses by 6 to 18 months.
- Children who have received 1 dose of hepatitis A vaccine before age 24 months, should receive a second dose 6 to 18 months after the first dose.
- Two doses of both killed and live hepatitis A vaccines as of now.

Catch-up vaccination:

- Administer 2 doses at least 6 months apart to unvaccinated persons.
- For catch-up vaccination, prevaccination screening for hepatitis A antibody is recommended in children older than 10 years as at this age the estimated seropositive rates exceed 50%.
- Combination of hepatitis B and hepatitis A may be used in 0, 1, 6 schedule.

References

1. Jacobsen KH, Wiersma ST. Hepatitis A virus seroprevalence by age and world region, 1990 and 2005. Vaccine 2010; 28: 6653–6665.

2. Mathur P, Arora NK. Epidemiological transition of hepatitis A in India: Issues for vaccination in developing countries. Indian J Med Res 2008; 128: 699–704.

3. Bendre SV, Bavdekar AR, Bhave SA, Pandit AN, Chitambar SD, Arankalle VA. Fulminant hepatic failure: Etiology, viral markers and outcome. Indian Pediatr 1999; 36: 1107–1112

4. Hepatitis A Vaccine. WHO Position Paper 2012. Wkly Epidemiol Rec 2012; 87: 261–276.

5. Liu XE, Wushouer F, Gou A, Kuerban M, Li X, Sun Y, Zhang J, et al. Comparison of immunogenicity between inactivated and live attenuated hepatitis A vaccines: A single-blind, randomized, parallel-group clinical trial among children in Xinjiang Uighur Autonomous Region, China. Hum Vaccin Immunother 2013; 9(7): 1460–1465.

6. Vashishtha VM, Kalra A, Bose A, Choudhury P, Yewale VN, Bansal CP et al. Indian Academy of Pediatrics (IAP) Recommended Immunization Schedule for Children Aged 0 through 18 years—India, 2013 and Updates on Immunization. Indian Pediatr 2013; 50: 1095–1108.

7. Wang X, Ma J, Xu Z, Liu H, Zhang Y, Han C. Effectiveness of post-exposure prophylaxis using live attenuated hepatitis Alpha vaccine (H(2) strain) among school children. Zhonghua Yi Xue Za Zhi. 2002; 82: 955–957.

8. Zhuang FC, Mao ZA, Jiang LM, Wu J, Chen YQ, Jiang Q, et al. Long-term immunogenicity and effectiveness of live attenuated hepatitis A vaccine (H2-strain)-a study on the result of 15 years' follow up. Zhonghua Liu Xing Bing Xue Za Zhi. 2010; 31: 1332–1335.

9. Wang XY, Xu ZY, Ma JC, von Seidlein L, Zhang Y, Hao ZY, et al. Long-term immunogenicity after single and booster dose of a live attenuated hepatitis A vaccine: Results from 8-year follow-up. Vaccine. 2007; 25: 446–449.

10. Faridi MM, Shah N, Ghosh TK, Sankaranarayanan VS, Arankalle V, et al. Immunogenicity and safety of live attenuated hepatitis A vaccine: A multicentric study. Indian Pediatr 2009; 46: 29–34.

11. Bhave S, Bavdekar A, Sapru A, Bawangade S, Pandit A. Immunogenicity of single dose live attenuated hepatitis a vaccine. Indian Pediatr 2011; 48: 135–137.

12. Franco E, Meleleo C, Serino L, Sorbara D, Zaratti L. Hepatitis A: Epidemiology and prevention in developing countries. World J Hepatol 2012; 4: 68–73.

13. Joshi N, Yr NK, Kumar A. Age related seroprevalence of antibodies to hepatitis A virus in Hyderabad, India. Trop Gastroenterol 2000; 21: 63–65.

14. Rath CP, Akki A, Patil SV, Kalyanshettar SS. Seroprevalence of hepatitis A virus antibody in Bijapur, Karnataka. Indian Pediatr 2011; 48: 71–73.

15. Schmidtke P et al. Cell mediated and antibody immune response to inactivated hepatitis A vaccine. Vaccine, 2005, 23: 5127–5132.

16. Mayorga Pérez O et al. Efficacy of virosome hepatitis A vaccine in young children in Nicaragua: Randomized placebo-controlled trial. The Journal of Infectious Diseases, 2003, 188: 671–677.

17. Vacchino MN. Incidence of Hepatitis A in Argentina after vaccination. Journal of Viral Hepatitis, 2008, 15 Suppl 2: 47–50.

TYPHOID VACCINES

Reviewed by
Ajay Kalra, Vipin M. Vashishtha

Background

Typhoid fever is a disease of developing countries associated with poor public health and low socio-economic indices. Cases of enteric fever occurring in travellers returning to the United States and the UK suggest that it is present across the developing world but that the Indian subcontinent represents a hotspot of disease activity.

Burden of disease

Global: Globally, the disease is estimated to cause 220,000 to 600,000 deaths and 16 to 22 million illnesses per year, predominantly in children of school-age or younger in the developing world.[1–3] According to 2004 estimates, the typhoid fever caused 21,650,974 illnesses and 216,510 deaths during the year 2000, and paratyphoid fever caused 5,412,744 illnesses.[1] This estimate was based on blood culture positive cases in

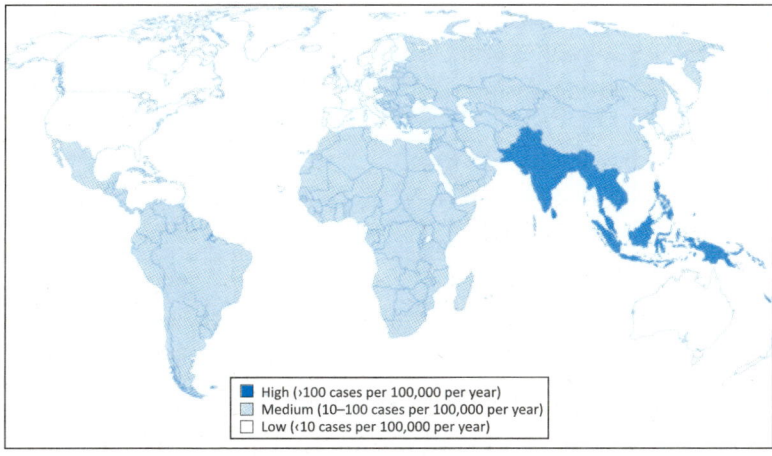

High (>100 cases per 100,000 per year)
Medium (10–100 cases per 100,000 per year)
Low (<10 cases per 100,000 per year)

Figure 1: Global burden of typhoid fever[1]

22 population-based studies. The best figures available for the global burden of enteric fever suggest that Africa (50/ 100,000) has a far lower burden of disease than Asia (274/100,000).[4] Typhoid fever is one of the most common etiological sources of bacteraemia in many developing countries, with most of the cases originating in the Indian subcontinent of South Asia (Figure-1).[1,5]

Asia and the Indian subcontinent: Typhoid fever incidence varies substantially in Asia. Very high typhoid fever incidence has been found in India and Pakistan. In comparison, typhoid fever frequency was moderate in Vietnam and China and intermediate in Indonesia.[5] However, it is the Indian subcontinent which has the highest incidence of the disease worldwide. A previous study from Pakistan in 2006 revealed an incidence rate (IR) of 170/100,000 (using blood culture), whereas a serology-based IR was 710/100,000 (using Typhidot).[6] Brooks et al. reported an overall IR of 3.9/1000 person years in an urban slum in Bangladesh.[7] In a multi-centric study in 5 Asian countries—China, India, Indonesia, Pakistan and Vietnam—it was estimated that the incidence of typhoid ranged from 15.3 per 100,000 persons/year in China to 451.7 per 100,000/year in Pakistan.[3]

In India, there have been 6 population-based studies estimating the incidence of typhoid fever in the community (Table 1).[3, 8–12] The three studies led by Chuttani were all vaccine trials, performed in the same urban slum between 1968 and 1974;[8–10] Sinha et al.

Table 1. Incidence of typhoid fever in India: Population-based studies

Study	Year	Location	Habitat	Studied population	Age group	Incidence (per 100,000 person years)	Reference
Chuttani *et al*	1971	Delhi	Urban slum	6248	<17 years	960	8
Chuttani *et al*	1973	Delhi	Urban slum	6428	1–15 years	760	9
Chuttani *et al*	1977	Delhi	Urban slum	7297	6–17 years	740	10
Sinha *et al*	1999	Delhi	Urban slum	19585	0–40 years	980	11
Ochiai *et al*	2005	Kolkata	-	57075	All ages	136.7	12
Ochiai *et al*	2008	Kolkata	Urban slum	59946	All ages	214.2	3

conducted their study in 1995–96 in a different urban slum in Delhi.[11] As is evident from the results, there has been a little change in the IR of typhoid fever in Delhi, which is in northern India. However, Ochlai et al., who conducted their surveillance in an urban slum in Kolkata in eastern India, reported a much lower incidence.[3,12] The results of these studies highlight the wide variation in incidence of disease even within the country. This could be due to various factors, including methodological differences in the studies, differences in standards of sanitation and hygiene, different geographical locations, lack of standardization among the study populations, and impact of availability of an effective vaccine in the recent studies, etc.[4]

Age distribution: In typhoid endemic areas, hospital-based data have reported most cases in children aged 5–19 years and young adults.[13–15] However, other recent population-based studies from India, Indonesia and Vietnam suggest that in some settings, typhoid fever is also common in 1–5 year old children[11, 16–18]. Ochiai et al reported that the mean age of typhoid was significantly lower in the South Asian sites (Pakistan and India) than in the South East and North East Asian sites and suggested that there was an inverse correlation between typhoid incidence and mean age of cases.[3]

Seasonality: According to one Indian study, the incidence of typhoid fever in India varied seasonally. The maximum incidence occurred during the monsoon (July–October) of 18.8 cases/1,000 person years while lower rates of 5.4 and 4.7 per 1,000 person years occurred during the summer and winter seasons respectively.[11]

Paratyphoid fever: While the 1997 Global Survey of Salmonella serotyping estimated an incidence of 1 case of paratyphoid fever for every 4 cases of typhoid fever, studies from India and Nepal suggest that in some settings, *S. Paratyphi A* can contribute up to half of all cases of enteric fever.[19–21] Population surveillance had revealed an IR of *S. Paratyphi A* of 42/100,000 persons in India, 72/100,000 in Pakistan, 13.7/100,000 in Indonesia and 27/100,000 in China.[4, 22] These figures may be due in part to the fact that current vaccines only offer protection against typhoid fever.

IDsurv data: According to the academy's passive reporting system of 10 infectious diseases by the pediatricians, a total of 2302 (22%) cases of enteric fever were reported out of total 10478 cases of 10 infectious diseases from December 2010 to till December 6, 2013.[23] There were 2261 cases of typhoid and 41 were paratyphoid cases, 10.7% were below 2 years of age and 44.6% were below 5 years, 20% cases were hospitalized, 17% were immunized with typhoid vaccine, and microbial diagnosis was established in 25% cases.[23]

Vaccines against typhoid fever

Typhoid vaccination was part of India's national immunization program till 1985 when measles vaccine was added by the government as part of UIP. There have been several vaccines against typhoid till quite recently.

Whole cell inactivated typhoid/ paratyphoid

Heat-inactivated phenol-preserved whole-cell typhoid vaccines have been available since the 1890s. The vaccine was moderately efficacious (51–88%) in children and young adults in preventing typhoid fever, and the protection persisted for up to 7 years. However, their high levels of reactogenicity; fever (up to 30% of the vaccines), headache (up to 10%), and severe local pain (up to 35%), led to the removal from public health programs in most countries.[2]

New Generation Typhoid Vaccines

The new generation current typhoid fever vaccines include oral live attenuated Ty21a vaccine, Parenteral Vi-polysaccharide and Vi-Polysaccharide Conjugate vaccines. Oral Live Attenuated Ty21a vaccine is not available in the country, hence will not be discussed further.

i. Vi-capsular polysaccharide (Vi-PS) vaccine

The vaccine contains highly purified antigenic fraction of Vi-capsular polysaccharide antigen of *S. typhi*, which is a virulence factor of the bacteria. Each dose contains 25 μg of purified polysaccharide in 0.5 ml of phenolic isotonic buffer for intramuscular or subcutaneous use. The vaccine should be stored at 2–8°C and should not be frozen. The vaccine is stable for 6 months at 37°C and for 2 years at 22°C. Since it is a pure polysaccharide vaccine, it is not immunogenic in children below 2 years of age and has no immune memory.

Efficacy: The biological marker is anti-Vi antibodies and 1 µg/ml is proposed as the serologic correlate of protection. The vaccine does not interfere with the interpretation of the Widal test. Efficacy drops over time and the cumulative efficacy at 3 years against culture confirmed typhoid fever is reported as 55%. In a recently published cluster randomized effectiveness trial conducted in over 40,000 subjects in urban slums of Kolkata, the overall effectiveness of the vaccine at 2 years follow up was 61%, and in children below 5 years was 80%.[24] Interestingly the herd protection of 44% was noted in unvaccinated children in the vaccinated cluster as compared to the control cluster.

Safety: The adverse effects are mild and include pain and swelling at injection site. The vaccine is contraindicated only in those with previous history of hypersensitivity to the vaccine and can be safely given in the immunocompromised including HIV infected.

Dosage: The Vi-polysaccharide vaccine is recommended for use as a single dose in children aged 2 years and above and can safely be given with all other childhood vaccines. Revaccination is recommended every 3 years.

Currently there are at least 3 manufacturers exporting the vaccine (Sanofi-Pastuer, GlaxoSmithKline Biologicals, and Bharat Biotech [India]) and many other companies producing for local use (e.g. Lanzhou Institute [China], Chengdu Institute [China], Finlay Institute [Cuba], DAVAC [Vietnam]). Out of these vaccines, the one from Sanofi-Pasteur is now prequalified by WHO.

ii. *Vi-capsular polysaccharide conjugate vaccines*

Vi-PS Conjugate vaccine conjugated with Pseudomonas aeruginosa exotoxin A

The limitations of the currently available typhoid vaccines include non-effectiveness below the age of 2 years, limited efficacy (of around 60%), T cell independent response which lacks immune memory and is not boostable, and finally no protection against paratyphoid fever. Conjugation of the Vi antigen with a protein carrier is hence desirable as it would induce a T cell dependent immune response.

The scientists at the US National Institute of Child Health and Disease (NICHD) have developed an improved Vi-PS conjugate typhoid vaccine by using exotoxin A of *Pseudomonas aeruginosa* as a carrier protein. This vaccine candidate underwent many human clinical trials in Vietnam. The safety and immunogenicity was evaluated in adults, 5 to 14-year-old children, and 2 to 4-year-old children. None of the recipients experienced a temperature of >38.5°C or significant local reactions after receiving an injection.[25]

A double-blind, placebo-controlled and randomized efficacy study was conducted in 2 to 5 years old children in Vietnam. 11,091 children were injected twice, 6 weeks apart, with the Vi conjugate vaccine or saline. The overall efficacy after 27 months of active surveillance followed by 19 months of passive surveillance was 89%.[18]

Lanzhou Institute in China has received this technology from US NIH and is developing this vaccine candidate, although further details are not currently available.

Vi-PS Conjugate typhoid vaccines in India: Two different Vi-PS conjugate vaccines have been licensed in India.

Vi-PS Conjugate Vaccine Conjugated with Tetanus Toxoid (Pedatyph®) by Bio-Med Pvt. Ltd.

After the initial attempt (described above) at making a conjugated typhoid vaccine, there have been many efforts to develop a conjugate typhoid vaccine by using different carrier proteins. With the technology initially transferred from US NIH, Bio-Med Pvt Ltd in India developed a conjugate vaccine using Tetanus Toxoid as the carrier protein with a dose of 5 mcg of Vi-PS antigen. This product was tested in a clinical trial in 169 subjects > 12 weeks with a comparison group (Vi) of 37 children > 2 years. The results from this study were compared with the NIH study in Vietnam and it was reported that there was 4-fold or greater rise in antibody titer (or an ELISA level higher than the threshold 1µg/ml) of each group on ELISA which was statistically equivalent to Vi-rEPA. The vaccine was well tolerated with no major local or systemic side effects. No data on duration of immunity and efficacy is available.

Based on the results of this study, this product was submitted for licensure and was licensed for more than 3 months of age in 2008 in India. This vaccine is licensed in India as two injections of 0.5 ml each at interval of 4–8 weeks in 3 months to 2 years old children; followed by booster at 2 to 2.5 years age; and as two injections at interval of 4–8 weeks in children older than 2 years of age. Booster vaccination is recommended every 10 years thereafter. The lack of detailed data before licensure was an issue[26] and hence this vaccine is currently undergoing effectiveness trial in around 2000 children in Kolkata, India.[27]

Vi-polysaccharide conjugate vaccine conjugated with Tetanus Toxoid from Bharat Biotech (Typbar-TCV®)

Typbar-TCV® is a Vi-capsular polysaccharide conjugate typhoid vaccine conjugated with tetanus toxoid. The manufacturer has used a dose of 25 µg/0.5 mL of Conjugate Vi Content polysaccharide which is the highest having been used in other trials as well on conjugate vaccine the world over.[28]

Phase IIa/IIb study revealed no difference in the GMTs between two doses (15 µg/0.5 mL) and single (25 µg/0.5 mL) dose cohorts, and a single dose of 25 µg/0.5 mL showed excellent immune response (100% seroconversion). A phase III, randomized, multi-centric, controlled trial was conducted to evaluate the immunogenicity and safety of this vaccine, Typbar-TCV® in a total of 981 healthy subjects and compared with the Typhoid Vi capsular polysaccharide vaccine of the same manufacturer (Typbar) having similar amount of antigen per dose.

The study group receiving the test vaccine (Typbar-TCV) was divided into two cohorts i.e. ≥6 months to ≤ 2 years (327 subjects) and >2 years to <45 years (654 subjects). Cohort-I was single arm open label and all the 327 subjects received single dose of the test vaccine. Cohort-II was randomized double blind trial and the subjects were recruited into two groups—one who received single dose of either test vaccine (340 subjects) or reference vaccine (314 subjects).

Immunogenicity results: In cohort-I, 98.05% subjects showed seroconversion (≥ 4-fold titre rise) on day 42, and the geometric mean titres (GMTs) on day 0 and 42 were 9.44U/mL and

1952.03 U/ml respectively. The GMTs were slightly higher in the >1–2 years than in 6 m to <1 year age group while no difference was seen in seroconversion rates. In cohort-II, 97.29% and 93.11% subjects of test and reference vaccine groups respectively, were seroconverted (≥4-fold titer rise) on day 42, whereas the GMTs on day 42 in the test and reference vaccine groups were 1301.44U and 411.11U, respectively (p = 0.00001). Both seroconversion and GMTs were higher in younger (> 2 to < 15 years) than older (15–45 years) age groups.

Long-term immunogenicity: The manufacturer has planned a 3-year follow-up for seroconversion data of phase III. So far, they have shared 18 months follow-up data which show significant waning of GMTs and seroconversion levels in both the cohorts from day 42 levels while 100% of subjects of test vaccine subjects were still seroprotected (the protective level: Vi antibody > 7.4 Elisa unit/mL). Similar trend was observed in the subgroup of cohort-II that received reference vaccine.

Safety issues: Comparative assessment of safety and tolerability of the vaccine in all subjects up to 12 weeks post vaccination. The most common local and systemic events reported were pain at injection site and fever, respectively in both the cohorts. Fever was noticed in 10.0%, 4.28%, and 2.75 % in cohort-I, test and reference vaccine groups of cohort-II, respectively. None of the enrolled subjects were withdrawn from study for vaccine-related adverse reaction. The vaccine has been licensed by the DCGI in August, 2013 for clinical use in India.

The IAP ACVIP has reviewed the pivotal trial of this new vaccine and considers it to be a promising vaccine, fulfilling the critical gap of providing protection under 2 years of age. However, before a slot is created for the vaccine in the existing IAP Immunization Timetable, the committee has shortlisted a few key issues that need to be addressed by the manufacturers.[28]

Serologic correlates of protection

Unlike many vaccine preventable diseases, serologic correlates of protection are not available for typhoid disease or typhoid vaccines. Hence, even though typically more than 90% of vaccinees achieve seroconversion after unconjugated Vi vaccine, efficacy is actually 50–70% in field efficacy trials. Different researchers have used different levels. For example, NIH estimated around 7 Elisa unit/mL as protective level of Vi antibody[18] and same group of researchers have estimated 3.52 Elisa unit/mL as protective level.[29]

Recommendations for use

Individual use

Vi-capsular polysaccharide (Vi-PS) vaccine

IAP ACVIP recommends the administration of the currently available Vi polysaccharide vaccine 0.5 ml IM every three years beginning at the age of 2 years. A child with history of suspected/confirmed enteric fever may be vaccinated 4 weeks after recovery if he/she has not received the vaccine in the past 3 years.

Vi-PS TT conjugate (Pedatyph®) by Bio-Med

IAP believes that since the immunogenicity trial assessed response to only single dose and did not assess duration of immunity, the dosing schedule seems extremely arbitrary. The extrapolation of efficacy of the vaccine from the Vietnamese trial is invalid due to fundamental differences between the two vaccines, age groups and dosing schedule. Subsequent Vietnamese trials have shown better antibody levels when the strength of the dose was increased to 12.5 mcg and 25 mcg per dose (0.5 ml).[29]

In view of these issues, the committee does not recommend the use of this conjugated vaccine at present. The committee would be able to issue its recommendations on this vaccine only after analyzing the results of the ongoing India trial.

Vi-polysaccharide conjugate vaccine conjugated with Tetanus Toxoid from Bharat Biotech (Typbar-TCV®)

Considering the typhoid epidemiology in the country and analyzing the available data of the vaccine, IAP recommends the use of new Vi-PS conjugate vaccine below one year of age, preferably between 9 and 12 months (minimum age 6 months). Since and the incompatibility data with measles vaccine is not available, there should be an interval of at least 4 weeks either before or after the former. The committee believes there is a definite need of a booster dose during second year of life; however, the available data is insufficient to specify exact timing of the same. The committee stresses the need of large-scale field effectiveness trial in real life settings to establish superiority of the product over the existing Vi-PS vaccines and to ascertain translation of higher GMTs and better seroconversion rates into superior protection.

Public health perspectives

The committee expresses its astonishment at the continued neglect of typhoid fever as a major public health problem in India by the government. There is a huge burden of the disease in almost every state of the country. Improvement in sanitary infrastructures and implementation of hygienic practices can reduce the disease burden as seen in most developed countries. However, the development of an adequate infrastructure for improved water and sanitation requires large investments, and is therefore a distant goal for the impoverished populations in the developing world

---

TYPHOID VACCINES

Routine vaccination:

- Both Vi-PS (polysaccharide) and Vi-PS conjugate vaccines are available.
- Minimum ages:
  - Vi-PS (polysaccharide) vaccines: 2 years
  - Vi-PS (Typbar-TCV®): 6 months;
- Vaccination schedule:
  - Vi-PS (polysaccharide) vaccines: Single dose at 2 years; revaccination every 3 years; (No evidence of hypo-responsiveness on repeated revaccination so far).
  - Vi-PS conjugate (Typbar-TCV®): Single dose at 9–12 months and a booster during second year of life.
- Vi-PS Conjugate vaccine (PedaTyph®): Data not sufficient to recommend for routine use.
- Greater experience and more robust data with Vi-PS polysaccharide vaccines; whereas there is limited experience with Vi-PS conjugate vaccines.

Catch-up vaccination:
- Recommended throughout the adolescent period, i.e. till 18 years.

---

including India. Basic health education such as hand washing and food handling is also known to be effective in reducing typhoid fever. Furthermore, there are licensed vaccines to prevent typhoid fever. Although typhoid fever can be effectively treated with antibiotics, growing rates of antibiotic resistance in many countries are making this treatment option increasingly more difficult and costly.

Though typhoid does not contribute significantly to the overall under-five mortality, the immense morbidity, and resultant economic burden of the disease is tremendous especially in urban and peri-urban areas of the country. With the availability of indigenous, new generation Vi-PS conjugate vaccines and a healthy pipeline of new generation conjugate typhoid vaccines, universal typhoid vaccination of Indian children must be prioritized without further delay. A few cost effectiveness studies in the past have demonstrated that administration of even a single dose of the polysaccharide vaccine in the age group of 2–15 years would be highly cost effective. The Academy strongly urges the government to include typhoid vaccination in the UIP considering the enormous burden of the disease.

References

1. Crump JA, Luby SP, Mintz ED. The global burden of typhoid fever. Bull World Health Organ. 2004; 82(5): 346–353.

2. Ivanoff B, Levine MM, Lambert PH. Vaccination against typhoid fever: Present status. Bull World Health Organ. 1994; 72(6): 957–971.

3. Ochiai RL, Acosta CJ, Danovaro-Holliday MC, et al. A study of typhoid fever in five Asian countries: Disease burden and implications for controls. Bull World Health Organ. 2008; 86(4): 260–268.

4. Kothari A, Pruthi A, Chugh TD. The burden of enteric fever. J Infect Dev Ctries 2008; 2: 253–259.

5. Kanungo S, Dutta S, Sur D. Epidemiology of typhoid and paratyphoid fever in India. J Infect Dev Ctries. 2008; 2: 454–460.

6. Siddiqui FJ, Rabbani F, Hasan R et al. Typhoid fever in children: Some epidemiological considerations from Karachi, Pakistan. Int J Infect Dis 2006; 10: 215–222.

7. Brooks WA, Hossain A, Goswami D et al. (2005) Bacteremic typhoid fever in children in an urban slum, Bangladesh. Emerg Infect Dis 2005; 11: 326–329.

8. Chuttani CS, Prakash K, Vergese A et al. Effectiveness of oral killed typhoid vaccine. Bull World Health Organ1971; 45: 445–450.

9. Chuttani CS, Prakh K, Vergese A et al. Ineffectiveness of an oral killed typhoid vaccine in a field trial. Bull World Health Organ 1973; 48: 756–757.

10, Chuttani CS, Prakash K, Gupta P et al. Controlled field trial of a high-dose oral killed typhoid vaccine in India. Bull World Health Organ 1977; 55(5): 643–644.

11. Sinha A, Sazawal S, Kumar R et al. Typhoid fever in children aged less than 5 years. Lancet 1999; 354: 734–737.

12. Ochiai RL, Wang XY, Von Siedlein L et al. *Salmonella paratyphi A* rates, Asia. Emerg Infect Dis 2005; 11: 1764–1766.

13. Sen SK, Mahakur AC. Enteric fever—a comparative study of adult and paediatric cases. Indian J Pediatr 1972; 39: 354–360.

14. Ferreccio C, Manterola A, Prenzel I et al. Benign bacteremia caused by *Salmonella typhi* and *paratyphi* in children younger than 2 years. J Pediatr 1984; 104: 899–901.

15. Mahle WT, Levine MM. *Salmonella typhi* infection in children younger than five years of age. Pediatr Infect Dis J 1993; 12: 627–631.

16. Simanjuntak CH, Paleologo FP, Punjabi NH et al. Oral immunisation against typhoid fever in Indonesia with Ty21a vaccine. Lancet 1991; 338: 1055–1059.

17. Lin FY, Vo AH, Phan VB et al. The epidemiology of typhoid fever in the Dong Thap Province, Mekong Delta region of Vietnam. Am J Trop Med Hyg 2000; 62: 644–648.

18. Lin FY, Ho VA, Khiem HB et al. The efficacy of a *Salmonella typhi* Vi conjugate vaccine in two-to-five-year-old children. N Engl J Med 2001; 344: 1263–1269.

19. Shlim DR, Schwartz E, Eaton M. Clinical importance of *Salmonella paratyphi* A infection to enteric fever in Nepal. J Travel Med 1995; 2: 165–168.

20. Sood S, Kapil A, Dash N, Das BK, Goel V, Seth P. Paratyphoid fever in India: an emerging problem. Emerg Infect Dis 1999; 5: 483–484.

21. Tankhiwale SS, Agrawal G, Jalgaonkar SV. An unusually high occurrence of *Salmonella enterica* serotype *paratyphi A* in patients with enteric fever. Indian J Med Res 2003; 117: 10–12.

22. Bhan MK, Bahl R, Bhatnagar S. Typhoid and paratyphoid fever. Lancet 2005; 366: 749–762.

23. Infectious Disease Surveillance, available at www.idsurv.org (Accessed on December 6, 2013)

24. Sur D, Ochiai RL, Bhattacharya SK, Ganguly NK, Ali M, Manna B, et al. A cluster-randomized effectiveness trial of Vi typhoid vaccine in India. N Engl J Med. 2009; 361: 335–344.

25. Kossaczka Z, Lin FY, Ho VA, et al. Safety and immunogenicity of Vi conjugate vaccines for typhoid fever in adults, teenagers, and 2- to 4-year-old children in Vietnam. Infect Immun. 1999; 67(11): 5806–5810.

26. Shah NK. Indian conjugate Vi typhoid vaccine: Do we have enough evidence?: Indian Pediatr. 2009 Feb; 46(2): 181–182.

27. India CTR. http://ctri.nic.in/Clinicaltrials/showallp. php? mid1=4714 & Enc Hid=&userName=Vi-TT.

28. Vashishtha VM, Kalra A, Bose A, Choudhury P, Yewale VN, Bansal CP et al. Indian Academy of Pediatrics (IAP) Recommended Immunization Schedule for Children Aged 0 through 18 years—India, 2013 and Updates on Immunization. Indian Pediatr 2013; 50: 1095–1108.

29. Canh DG, Lin FY, Thiem VD, et al. Effect of dosage on immunogenicity of a Vi conjugate vaccine injected twice into 2- to 5-year-old Vietnamese children. Infect Immun. 2004; 72(11): 6586–6588.

■ ■ ■ ■ ■ ■

HUMAN PAPILLOMA VIRUS (HPV) VACCINES

3.12

Reviewed by
Panna Choudhury, Rohit Agarwal

Epidemiology

HPV infections are highly transmissible and are primarily transmitted by sexual contact. Most sexually active men and women would acquire an HPV infection at some time in their lives. Whereas most HPV infections are transient, self regressing and benign, persistent genital infection with certain viral genotypes can lead to the development of anogenital precancers and cancers. Presence of oncogenic HPV-DNA has been demonstrated in 99.7% of all cervical cancer cases, the highest attributable fraction so far reported for a specific cause of major human cancer. The lag period between infection with oncogenic HPV and invasive cervical cancer is 15–20 years.[1]

Cervical cancer morbidity and mortality in India

Globally cancer of the cervix uteri is the second most common cancer among women with an estimated 529,409 new cases and 274,883 deaths in 2008. About 86% of the cases occur in developing countries, representing 13% of female cancers.[2] In many countries in sub-Saharan Africa, Central and South America, South and South-East Asia, age-standardized incidence rates of cervix cancer exceed 25 per 100,000.[3] In India, cancer of the cervix uteri is the second most important cancer in women over the past two decades. Globally Age Adjusted Incidence Rates (AAR) of cervical cancer is 15.3 per 100000, but for Indian women it is 27 per 100,000. Though the urban population based cancer registries (PBCR) at Bangalore, Bhopal, Chennai, Delhi and Mumbai have shown a significant decrease in the AARs of cervical cancer, however; since over 70 per cent of the Indian population resides in the rural areas, cancer cervix still constitutes the number one cancer. Cancer cervix is the cause for 23.5% of all cancers in women in India.[4] In 2008 it is estimated that 134,420 cases of cervical cancer cases occurred in India and of these cases there were 72826 deaths and these figure is projected to increase up to 116,171 by the year 2025.[5]

Prevention of cervical cancer: Screening or vaccination

Cervical cancer is essentially a preventable cancer as it has a long pre-invasive stage. Countries with well-organized programs to detect and treat precancerous abnormalities and early stage cervical cancer can prevent up to 80% of these cancers.[6] It has been shown that it is possible to screen and treat cervical cancer in early stages with high success even in rural India.[7] However, information on screening behaviors of Indian women related to cervical cancer is very little. In a study from Kolkata, most women reported "limited" to "no" knowledge of cervical cancer (84%) and the Pap smear test (95%).[8] Further, to implement national screening program, large investment has to be made in terms of logistics and training of healthcare personnel.

Realistically we would need human papillomavirus (HPV) vaccines to significantly reduce the health care burden currently required for cervical cancer prevention. But we also would need screening because of the limitations of current HPV vaccines both in their lack of therapeutic effect (thus not protecting women with an ongoing neoplastic processes) and in their limited number of HPV types. Thus it is imperative that we would need both vaccination as well as efficient screening schemes and rapid intervention like 'screen and treat' protocol.[9]

Pathogen

HPVs are non-enveloped, double-stranded deoxyribonucleic acid (DNA) viruses in the family of Papilloma-viridae. The HPV genome is enclosed in a capsid shell comprising major (L1) and minor (L2) structural proteins. More than 100 HPV genotypes are known. Certain HPV genotypes are associated with cell immortalization and transformation related to carcinogenesis. Of these, at least 13 may cause cervical cancer or are associated with other anogenital and oropharyngeal cancers. HPV types 16 and 18 cause about 70% of all cases of invasive cervical cancer worldwide, with type 16 having the greatest oncogenic potential. The distribution of HPV types varies among geographical regions, but the dominant oncogenic type in all regions is HPV-16.[10] The low-risk HPV types 6 and 11 are responsible for about 90% of anogenital warts and almost all recurrent respiratory papillomatosis.

In India high-risk HPV types were found in 97% of cervical cancers[11]. A meta-analysis of HPV type-distribution from India showed that in invasive cervical carcinoma(ICC), HPV-16 was the predominant type (64.8%), followed by HPV18, 45, 33, 35, 58, 59 and 31. The estimated HPV-16/18 positive fraction was 78.9% in women with ICC 61.5% with high squamous intra-epitheliaal lesion, 30.8% with low squamous intra-epithelial lesion and 3.9% in women with normal cytology/histology. There was no difference in overall HPV prevalence in cervical cancer between North and South India. However, HPV-16 and -45 appeared to be more prevalent in North India while HPV-35 appeared to be more prevalent in South India. It is estimated that HPV-16/18 vaccines will provide over 76.7% protection against ICC in South Asia.[12]

Protective immunity

Natural HPV infections do not induce a vigorous immune response as they are restricted to the intraepithelial basement layers of the mucosa. Approximately half of all women infected with HPV develop detectable serum antibodies, but these antibodies do not necessarily protect against subsequent infection by the same HPV type. They are known as 'non-neutralizing' antibodies. The neutralizing antibodies are best characterized and most type-specific HPV antibodies which are those directed against the L1 protein of the virus, which is the main capsid protein. The other L2 protein is minor and is responsible for non-oncogenic genital warts.

HPV Vaccines

Two vaccines have been licensed globally; a quadrivalent and a bivalent vaccine. Both are manufactured by recombinant DNA technology that produces non-infectious virus like particles (VLP) comprising of the HPV L1 protein. The mechanisms by which these vaccines induce protection have not been fully defined but seem to involve both cellular immunity and neutralizing immunoglobulin G antibodies. Clinical trials with both vaccines have used efficacy against cervical intraepithelial neoplasia (CIN) 2/3 and adenocarcinoma in situ (AIS) caused by HPV strains contained in the concerned vaccine as primary end points. Regulatory authorities have accepted the use of CIN grade 2 or 3 (CIN 2/3) and AIS as clinical end-points in vaccine efficacy trials instead of invasive cervical cancer.

Both vaccines do not protect against the serotype with which infection has already occurred before vaccination. Higher immune response is seen in preadolescents through 9–13 years as compared to adolescents and young adults. Both vaccines have been licensed in several countries world over. These vaccines are equally safe and both have shown nearly complete protection against precancerous and other anogenital lesions caused by the respective vaccine-related HPV-types during the 10–12 years of observation so far. The consistency of these observations strongly suggests that similar high rates of protection can be expected also against cervical cancer. However, the immune protective correlates are not known and the level of antibody titers which will be translated into clinical efficacy are ill understood.

Quadrivalent vaccine (HPV4)

Quadrivalent vaccine available in India is a mixture of L1 proteins of HPV serotypes 16, 18, 6 and 11 with aluminium containing adjuvant. Each 0.5 mL dose of this vaccine contains 20 μg of HPV-6 L1 protein, 40 μg of HPV-11 L1 protein, 40 μg of HPV-16 L1 protein and 20 μg of HPV-18 L1 protein adsorbed onto 225 μg of the AlOH.

Efficacy: The safety and efficacy of quadrivalent vaccine was assessed in a large study named FUTURE (Females United to Unilaterally Reduce Endo/Ectocervical Disease). This analysis studied 17 622 women aged 15–26 years who were enrolled in one of two randomized, placebo-controlled, efficacy trials for the HPV6/11/16/18 vaccine (first patient on December 28, 2001, and studies completed July 31, 2007). Clinical trials with three doses at 0, 2 and 6 months have shown 99% efficacy at a median follow up of 1.9 years against types 16, 18 related CIN- 2/3 and AIS in per protocol analysis (women who received all three doses of the vaccine and who remained uninfected with vaccine HPV type at onset and for 1 month after completion of the vaccine schedule). Additionally 99–100% efficacy was seen against vaccine type

IAP Guidebook on Immunization 2013–14

related genital warts, vaginal intraepithelial neoplasia (VaIN) and vulvar intraepithelial neoplasia (VIN). Reduction in HPV 16 related lesions and HPV 18 related lesions are 98% and 100%, respectively when CIN 2/3 is taken into consideration and AIS as end points. Data from two international, double blind, placebo-controlled, randomised efficacy trials of quadrivalent HPV vaccine (FUTURE I) and (FUTURE II) showed persistent protection in participants over 5 years (13, 14). The studies for 126 months (10.5 years) are still to be published and targeted studies for 14 years are being processed.

Bivalent vaccine (HPV2)

The bivalent vaccine is a mixture of L1 proteins of HPV serotypes 16 and 18 with AS04 as an adjuvant.

Efficacy and safety: The safety and efficacy of the bivalent HPV vaccine was assessed in a large study named PATRICIA (Papilloma Trial against Cancer in Young Adults). In this phase III study, prevention of vaccine-related HPV types CIN2–3 was assessed that included 18 644 healthy women aged 15–25 years at the time of first vaccination. Women were enrolled between May 2004 and June 2005. The trial was carried out at 135 centers across 14 countries worldwide, as previously described.[15]

In women with no evidence of current or previous HPV-16/18 infection (DNA negative and seronegative), Vaccine Efficacy (VE) was 90.3% (96.1% confidence interval: 87.3–92.6) against 6-month persistent infection (PI), 91.9% (84.6–96.2) against cervical intraepithelial neoplasia (CIN) 11 and 94.6% (86.3–98.4) against CIN 21 [97.7% (91.1–99.8)]. In women HPV-16/18 DNA negative but with serological evidence of previous HPV-16/18 infection (seropositive), VE was 72.3% (53.0–84.5) against 6-month PI, 67.2% (10.9–89.9) against CIN11, and 68.8% (228.3–95.0) against CIN21 [88.5% (10.8–99.8)]. In women with no evidence of current HPV-16/18 infection (DNA negative), regardless of their baseline HPV-16/18 serological status, VE was 88.7% (85.7–91.1) against 6-month PI, 89.1% (81.6–94.0) against CIN11 and 92.4% (84.0–97.0) against CIN21 [97.0% (90.6–99.5)]. In women who were DNA positive for one vaccine type, the vaccine was efficacious against the other vaccine type. The vaccine did not impact the outcome of HPV-16/18 infections present at the time of vaccination. Vaccination was generally well tolerated regardless of the woman's HPV-16/18 DNA or serological status at entry.[16] Follow-up studies in a subset of participants over 8.4 years shows no evidence of waning immunity for bivalent vaccine.

In an immunogenicity study in Nordic countries, anti-HPV IgG seropositivity was seen from 90.8% for ST 18 to 100% for ST 16 after 9 years following vaccination with bivalent vaccine.

Efficacy against genital warts:

Conventionally it is believed that HPV4 having ST 6 and 11 will prevent good efficacy against genital warts. In the FUTURE trial, 99–100% efficacy was seen against vaccine type related genital warts. In countries where this vaccine was introduced in NIP like US, reductions in HPV vaccine type prevalence of genital warts have been reported in young females. Surprisingly, in UK where Bivalent vaccine was introduced in 2008, a 13.3% to 20.8% reduction among women aged <19 years in new diagnoses of external genital warts among since the vaccine was introduced in national vaccination program.[17] Later a post hoc analysis of the phase III PATRICIA trial found efficacy against low-risk HPV types 6, 11, 74 ranged from 30.3% to 49.5%.[18]

The HPV4 vaccine was found to have good efficacy against genital warts in males also. Having an efficacy of 65% (intention to treat) and 90.4% (per protocol) against external genital lesions caused by vaccine-type in 16–26 years old males in 18 countries.[19]

Cross-protection against non-vaccine serotypes

The other serotypes phyllogenetically aligned to serotypes 16 and 18 which are responsible for about 20% of lesions are cross-protected to some extent by both the vaccines.

However, the immunity is not robust. In PATRICIA study phase three trial in four years follow up against six months persistent infections cross protection for non-vaccine ST 33, 31, 45 were seen to be 43%, 77% and 79% respectively. However, in long term follow up (LTFU) study for nine years failed to demonstrate efficacy for six months against persistent infection by the bivalent vaccine. The true cross protection for lesions non co-infected with ST 16/18 were found to be 46% for quadrivalent vaccine in FUTURE II study and 36% for bivalent vaccine in Patricia study. Whatever the cross protection concurred was less robust and less consistent.

Safety of HPV vaccines

Local adverse effects with quadrivalent vaccines reported were pain at the injection site in 83% of vaccines (mainly mild and moderate intensity) and swelling and erythema in 25%. Systemic adverse effects such as fever reported in 4% of vaccines. They are all minor adverse effects and no serious vaccine related adverse events have been reported either in trials or post-marketing surveillance studies.

Local side effects with bivalent vaccines reported were pain (mild and moderate intensity) in 90% and swelling and erythema in 40%. Systemic side effects such as fever were seen in 12%. No serious vaccine related adverse effects were observed. Both the vaccines have very good safety record. More than 175 million doses have been distributed worldwide and more countries offering the vaccine through national immunization programs. WHO's Global Advisory Committee on Vaccine Safety (GACVS) continues to be reassured by the safety profile of the available products.[20] Centre for Disease Control and Prevention (CDC) monitors HPV vaccine safety and states that there are no new or unusual patterns of adverse events to suggest a HPV vaccine safety concern. However, CDC states that syncope (fainting) can occur among adolescents following vaccination. To decrease the risk of falls and other injuries that might follow syncope, CDC's Advisory Committee on Immunization Practices (ACIP) recommends that clinicians consider observing patients for 15 minutes after vaccination.[21]

Recommendations for use

Public health perspectives

The HPV vaccines are of public health importance. WHO states that HPV vaccine should be included in national immunization programs of the countries having high burden of cervical cancer.[6] This is especially so in countries like India having considerable disease burden but without a screening program. However, introduction of vaccine in program need to take into account public awareness and programmatic feasibility. Recently, two HPV vaccination projects for operational feasibility of school-based and community-based vaccination ran into controversy.[22] The cost of vaccine is also very high though it is expected that there would be substantial cost reduction if Indian manufacturers are enabled to manufacture the vaccine and there are bulk purchases if introduced in programs. Considering above factors, ACVIP has not recommended introduction of HPV in National Immunization schedule but wishes that programmatic feasibility and cost effective studies are undertaken urgently. The efficacy with even a single dose of the vaccine such as demonstrated by the recent trial in Costa Rica[23] should facilitate favorable recommendation in future.

Individual use

The ACVIP recommends offering HPV vaccine to all females in the schedules discussed below. Since protection is seen only when the vaccine is given before infection with HPV, the vaccine should preferably be given prior to sexual debut. The vaccine should preferably be introduced to parents as a cervical cancer preventing vaccine and not as a vaccine against a sexually transmitted infection (STI). Vaccines are not 100% protective against cervical cancer and not a replacement for periodic screening. Hence screening programs should continue as per recommendations. Need for boosters and potential for serotype replacement would be known in future. The 3rd dose may be considered as booster. Both the available vaccines are equally efficacious and safe for protection against cervical cancer and precancerous lesions as of currently available data. The quadrivalent vaccine additionally protects against anogenital warts.

Currently both the vaccines are not being licensed in India, to be used in the males by the vaccine regulatory authorities and the DCGI. However, they are licensed to be used in males in some countries like Australia, New Zealand, and Austria.

Dose and Schedule

The vaccines should be stored at 2 to 8°C and must not be frozen. The dose is 0.5 ml intramuscular in deltoid. The recommended age

HUMAN PAPILLOMAVIRUS (HPV) VACCINES

Routine vaccination:

- Minimum age: 9 years

- HPV4 [Gardasil] and HPV2 [Cervarix] are licensed and available.

- Either HPV4 (0, 2, 6 months) or HPV2 (0, 1, 6 months) is recommended in a 3-dose series for females aged 11 or 12 years.

- HPV4 can also be given in a 3-dose series for males aged 11 or 12 years, but not yet licensed for use in males in India.

- The vaccine series can be started beginning at age 9 years.

- Administer the second dose 1 to 2 months after the first dose and the third dose 6 months after the first dose (at least 24 weeks after the first dose).

Catch-up vaccination:

- Administer the vaccine series to females (either HPV2 or HPV4) at age 13 through 45 years if not previously vaccinated.

- Use recommended routine dosing intervals (see above) for vaccine series catch-up.

for initiation of vaccination is 10–12 years. As of current licensing regulations in India, catch-up vaccination is permitted up to the age of 45 years. However, pre-adolescent vaccination is immunologically superior to the post-adolescent vaccination. Three doses at 0, 2 and 6 months are recommended with the quadrivalent vaccine, and 0, 1 and 6 months with the bivalent vaccine. HPV vaccines can be given simultaneously with other vaccines such as hepatitis B and Tdap. As a precaution against syncope following any vaccine in adolescents, the vaccine should be counselled prior to vaccination, vaccine be administered in a sitting/ lying down position and the patient observed for 15 minutes post-vaccination. Both vaccines are contraindicated in those with history of previous hypersensitivity to any vaccine component and should be avoided in pregnancy. The vaccines may be administered in the immunocompromised but immunogenicity and efficacy may be lower. At present there is no data to support use of boosters.

References

1. Walboomers JM, Jacobs MV, Manos MM, Bosch FX, Kummer JA, Shah KV, et al. Human papillomavirus is a necessary cause of invasive cervical cancer worldwide. J Pathol 1999; 189: 12–19.

2. Ferlay J, Shin HR, Bray F, et al (Eds.). GLOBOCAN 2008: Cancer Incidence and Mortality Worldwide. IARC Cancer Base No. 10. IARC Press: Lyon 2010.

3. Curado MP, Edwards B, Shin HR, Storm H, Ferlay J, Heanue M, Boyle P, editors. Cancer incidence in five continents, vol. IX , IARC Scientific Publications No. 160. Lyon: IARC; 2007.

4. Nandakumar A, Ramnath T, Chaturvedi N. The magnitude of cancer cervix in India. Indian J Med Res 2009;130: 219–221.

5. Human Papillomavirus and Related Cancers in India. Summary report 2010. Spain: WHO/ICO Information center on HPV and Cervical Cancer (HPV information centre); 2010Sep.4,6,7,13–15.

6. Human Papilloma Virus Vaccines. WHO Position Paper. Wkly Epidemiol Rec 2009, 84, 117–132.

7. Bhatla N, Gulati A, Mathur SR, Rani S, Anand K, Muwonge R, et al.. Evaluation of cervical screening in rural North India. Int J Gynaecol Obstet 2009 ;105(2): 145–149.

8. Roy B, Tang TS. Cervical cancer screening in Kolkata, India: beliefs and predictors of cervical cancer screening among women attending a women's health clinic in Kolkata, India. J Cancer Educ 2008; 23: 253–259.

9. Bosch FX, Castellsague X, Sanjose SD. HPV and cervical cancer: screening or vaccination? British J Cancer 2008; 98: 15–21.

10. Smith JS, Melendy A, Rana RK, Pimenta JM. Age-specific prevalence of infection with human papillomavirus in females: a global review. Journal of Adolescent Health, 2008, 43 (Suppl 4): S5.e1–S5.e62.

11. Sankaranarayanan R, Bhatla N, Gravitt PE, Basu P, Esmy PO, Ashrafunnessa KS, et al. Human papillomavirus infection and cervical cancer prevention in India, Bangladesh, Sri Lanka and Nepal. Vaccine 2008; 26 Suppl 12:M43–52.

12. Bhatla N, Lal N, Bao YP, Ng T, Qiao YL. A meta-analysis of human papillomavirus type-distribution in women from South Asia: Implications for vaccination. Vaccine. 2008; 26: 2811–2817.

13. Garland SM, Hernandez-Avila M, Wheeler CM, Perez G, Harper DM, Leodolter S, et al. Quadrivalent vaccine against human papillomavirus to prevent anogenital diseases. N Engl J Med 2007; 356:1928–1943.

14. Dillner J, Kjaer SK, Wheeler CM, Sigurdsson K, Iversen OE, Hernandez-Avila M, et al. Four year efficacy of prophylactic human papillomavirus quadrivalent vaccine against low grade cervical, vulvar, and vaginal intraepithelial neoplasia and anogenital warts: Randomised controlled trial. BMJ 2010; 341: c3493

15. Paavonen J, Naud P, Salmeron J, Wheeler CM, Chow SN, Apter D, et al. Efficacy of human papillomavirus (HPV)-16/18 AS04-adjuvanted vaccine

against cervical infection and precancer caused by oncogenic HPV types (PATRICIA): Final analysis of a double-blind, randomised study in young women. Lancet 2009; 374: 301–314.

16. A. Szarewski, WAJ Poppe, S.R. Skinner CM. Wheeler, J Paavonen, P Naud, et al. Efficacy of the human papillomavirus (HPV)-16/18 AS04- adjuvanted vaccine in women aged 15–25 years with and without serological evidence of previous exposure to HPV-16/18. Int. J Cancer 2012; 131:106–116.

17. Howell-Jones R, Soldan K, et al. Declining genital Warts in young women in England associated with HPV 16/18 vaccination: An ecological study. J Infect Dis. 2013;208:1397–1403.

18. Szarewski A, Skinner SR, et al. Efficacy of the HPV-16/18 AS04-adjuvanted vaccine against low-risk HPV types (PATRICIA randomized trial): An unexpected observation. J Infect Dis 2013;208:1391–1396.

19. Giuliano AR, Palefsky JM, et al. Efficacy of quadrivalent HPVvaccine against HPV Infection and disease in males. N Engl J Med 2011; 364:401–411.

20. WHI. Global Advisory Committee on Vaccine Safety, 12–13 June 2013. http://www.who.int/wer/2013/wer8829.pdf. (Accessed on 31st October 2013)

21. Vaccine safety. Centers for Disease Control and Prevention. http://www.cdc.gov/vaccinesafety/vaccines/HPV/Index.html (Accessed on 31st Oct 2013)

22. Choudhury P, John TJ. Human papilloma virus vaccines and current controversy. Indian Pediatr 2010: 47: 724–725.

23. Safaeian M, Porras C, Pan Y, Kreimer A, Schiller JT, Gonzalez P, et al. Durable antibody responses following one dose of the bivalent human papillomavirus l1 virus-like particle vaccine in the costa rica vaccine trial. Cancer Prev Res (Phila). 2013; 6:1242–1250.

■ ■ ■ ■ ■ ■

COMBINATION VACCINES

Reviewed by
Anuradha Bose, Panna Choudhury

Background

Combination vaccines merge into single product antigens that prevent different diseases or that protect against multiple strains of infectious agents causing the same disease. Thus, they reduce the number of injections required to prevent some diseases. These immunogens may pertain to the many antigens/ serotypes of the given pathogen (e.g. poliovirus vaccines) or of multiple pathogens (e.g. DTP vaccine). This concept differs from that of simultaneous vaccines, which, although administered concurrently, are physically separate.[1]

Combination vaccines available for many years include diphtheria and tetanus toxoids and whole-cell pertussis vaccine (DTwP); measles-mumps-rubella vaccine (MMR); and trivalent oral polio vaccine (OPV). Combinations licensed in recent years include diphtheria and tetanus toxoids and acellular pertussis vaccine (DTaP) (2-5), DTwP-*Haemophilus influenzae* type b (Hib) vaccine (DTwP-Hib), DTaP-Hib.[6] Additionally several other multivalent vaccines have been recently introduced including the Pneumococcal, Rotavirus and HPV vaccines.[3]

Advantages and disadvantages of combination vaccines

Use of combination vaccines can reduce the number of injections patients receive, alleviate the concern associated with the number of injections, improve chances of timely vaccination coverage for children who are behind the schedule, and also reduce healthcare visits. Further, the burden on cold chain and requirement of syringes and needles are also reduced. The record keeping also becomes easier. Potential disadvantages of combination vaccines include the following: 1) adverse events that might occur more frequently after administration of a combination vaccine compared with administration of separate antigens at the same visit 2) reduced immunogenicity of one or more components 3) a shorter shelf-life than the individual component vaccines.[4,5] Further discussion on combination vaccines here refers to vaccines against multiple pathogens combined in a single injection.

Dosing schedules

- Before administering a vaccine dose, verify that all previous doses were administered after the minimum age and in accordance with minimum intervals.

- Maintain intervals between doses as recommended, to the extent possible.

- Intervals that are shorter than recommended might be necessary in certain circumstances, such as impending international travel or when a person is behind schedule on vaccinations but needs rapid protection.

- Vaccine doses should not be administered at intervals less than minimum intervals or at an age that is younger than the minimum age. (Vaccine doses administered ≤4 days before the minimum interval or age are considered valid.)

Licensed combinations

A 'combination vaccine' is defined as a product containing components that can be divided equally into independently available routine vaccines.

- A dash (-) between vaccine products indicates that products are supplied in their final form by the manufacturer and do not require mixing or reconstitution by the user.

- A slash (/) indicates that the products must be mixed or reconstituted by the user.

The use of a combination vaccine generally is preferred over separate injections of the equivalent component vaccines. It is preferable to use the same combination vaccine to complete the series for a child but where the same brand of vaccine is not available, the course may be completed with any available brand.

Combination vaccines currently licensed in India

The traditional combination vaccines which have been available for many years in India are:

- Diphtheria, Pertussis, Tetanus (DPT)
- Measles, Mumps, Rubella (MMR)
- Injectable Polio Vaccine (IPV)
- Oral Polio Vaccine (OPV)

The more recently available vaccines are:

i.   *DTwP+ Hib*

ii. *DTwP+ Hep B*

iii. *DTwP+Hib+ Hep B*

These are available in two forms.

1) As ready to use liquid preparations: DTwP+Hep B, DTwP+Hib, DTwP+Hep B+Hib and

2) lyophilized Hib needs to be reconstituted with DTwP/ DTwP+Hep B from the same manufacturer.

The antibody response to Hib is reduced in these combination vaccines as compared to separate administration, most subjects attain the seroprotective level of 1 µg/ml and there is no reduced efficacy against Hib disease. The antibody responses to diphtheria, pertussis, tetanus and hepatitis B are unchanged. The liquid and the lyophilized formulations have similar immunogenicity and safety for both primary and booster immunization.[6]

Combinations with DTaP (Acellular Pertussis)

DTaP+Hib, DTaP+Hib+IPV

Currently the DTaP/Hib is available as lyophilized Hib which needs to be reconstituted with liquid DTaP just prior to administration. DTaP (2 component)+Hib+IPV is available as a ready to use formulation. Antibody responses to diphtheria, pertussis, tetanus and (if applicable) polio are satisfactory and comparable to those obtained after administration as separate doses. There is a reduction in Hib immunogenicity as with the aforementioned combination vaccines.

This reduction in Hib immunogenicity is not noted when these vaccines are used for booster vaccination even in subjects who had been administered combination vaccines for primary immunization. The reduction in Hib antibody titers was noted across all studies with different formulations of DTaP (exception Canadian five component DTaP vaccine) and different Hib conjugate vaccines and was more significant when vaccination was administered earlier in life and in premature babies. Studies with the five component Canadian vaccine combination vaccine with Hib did not show reduced Hib immunogenicity. Hence DTaP+ Hib combination vaccines were initially licensed in Europe for both primary and booster immunization but in the USA only for booster vaccination. An increased incidence of Hib disease was noted in the UK but not in other European countries following shift to DTaP+ Hib combination vaccines. This was initially attributed to the lower immunogenicity of the combination vaccine but later conclusively attributed to other factors mainly non-administration of a booster dose at 18 months. The US FDA and ACIP has approved DTaP (5 components) + IPV + Hib combination vaccine for primary immunization.[7] The DTaP-IPV/PRP-T vaccine, given concomitantly with monovalent hepatitis B vaccine, was found to be highly immunogenic at 6, 10 and 14 weeks of age in infants in India. The vaccine was well tolerated.[8] Booster dose of the vaccine given at 18–19 months of age was well tolerated and induced strong antibody responses.[9]

DTaP/Hepatitis B

This combination vaccine is given at the 2, 4, 6 months schedule versus the currently recommended schedules— hepatitis B at birth, 1 and 6 months and DPT at 6, 10 and 14 weeks. Similar or higher antibody responses for every component of the combined vaccine except hepatitis B were found. Hepatitis B had lower titres. However, 98% had titres greater than 10IU/L, which are protective.

Hepatitis A+ Hepatitis B

Available in both adult and pediatric formulations. The recommended schedule is three doses at 0, 1 and 6 months. These combination vaccines show acceptable and comparable immune response against hepatitis A and hepatitis B as compared to separate administration. A rapid immunization schedule particularly suitable for travellers at 0, 7 and 21 days has acceptable short and long-term efficacy. The adult formulation may also be used effectively in children aged 1–15 years as two doses at 0 and 6 months.

Internationally available combination vaccines

DTwP+IPV, DTwP+IPV+Hib

These vaccines are available internationally and show acceptable immunogenicity (against all components) and safety. These vaccines are potentially of immense importance in the Indian EPI to facilitate a shift from OPV to IPV during the end game period of global polio eradication.

DTaP+IPV, DTaP+Hep B, DTaP+IPV+Hep B, DTaP+Hib+Hep B, DTaP+IPV+Hep B+Hib

These quadrivalent, pentavalent and hexavalent combination vaccines show acceptable and comparable immunogenicity against diphtheria, pertussis, tetanus and polio. The responses against Hib are lower as discussed earlier. The hepatitis B antibody titers following primary immunization are also lower than when hepatitis B is administered separately which is believed to be due to close spacing of the doses at 1 month interval rather than immune interference. The hexavalent vaccines are available internationally in two different formulations; one is lyophilized Hib which needs to be reconstituted with liquid DTaP + IPV + Hep B and the other as a ready to use liquid vaccine.

Other formulations

Hepatitis B/Hepatitis A: However, this combination can be administered only after one year of age in children who have not been immunized earlier.

Hepatitis A/Typhoid: New hepatitis A/typhoid combined vaccine as well as traditional vaccine induced high levels of protective antibodies,[28] but the combined vaccine has higher incidence of local reactions.

Hepatitis A + typhoid: These vaccines particularly for use in travellers to endemic countries show comparable immunogenicity and safety as compared to separate administration of vaccines.

Hepatitis B+Hib: These vaccines show acceptable immunogenicity against Hib and hepatitis B as compared to separate administration of vaccines.

MMRV vaccine

A combination of MMR and Varicella vaccine was licensed in the USA in 2005 for healthy children aged 12 months to 12 years. The antigen content of varicella is higher than single antigen varicella vaccine. The vaccine demonstrates comparable immunogenicity and efficacy against all components but greater side effects of fever and rash as compared to separate administration of the vaccines. Post-marketing surveillance reports indicate an increased (double) risk of febrile seizures following the receipt of this vaccine as compared to separate MMR and varicella vaccines.[10]

Another combination MMRV vaccine licensed in Europe is with comparable immunogenicity and efficacy but an increased risk of fever as compared to separate administration of vaccines.

Recommendations for use

ACVIP concludes that all currently licensed combination vaccines in India have an immunogenicity, efficacy and safety profile comparable to separately administered vaccines as of currently available data. However, the manufacturer's recommendation for mixing the vaccines in the same syringe should be strictly followed.

References

1. Dodd D. Benefits of combination vaccines: Effective vaccination on a simplified schedule. Am J Manag Care. 2003; 9(1 Suppl): S6−12.

2. Decker MD, Edwards KM, Bogaerts HH. Combination vaccines. In Plotkin S, Orenstien W, Offit P (Editors) Vaccine fifth edition, Philadelphia, Saunders Elsevier 2008, pp 1069.

3. Offit PA, Quarles J, Gerber MA, et al: Addressing parents' concerns: Do multiple vaccines overwhelm or weaken the infant's immune system? Pediatrics 2002; 109: 124−129.

4. Dagan R, Eskola J, Leclerc C, Leroy O. Reduced response to multiple vaccines sharing common protein epitopes that are administered simultaneously to infants. Infect Immun 1998; 66: 2093−2098.

5. Gatchalian S, Reyes M, Bernal N, Lefevre I, David MP, Han HH, et al. A new DTPw-HBV/Hib vaccine is immunogenic and safe when administered according to the EPI (Expanded Programme for Immunization) schedule and following hepatitis B vaccination at birth. Human Vaccines 2005; 1:e6−e11.

6.   Combination vaccines for childhood immunization. MMWR 1999/(48) RR05; 1–15. Available from http://www.cdc.gov/mmwr/preview/mmwrhtml/rr4805a1.htm (Accessed on Dec 11, 2013)

7.   CDC. Licensure of a Diphtheria and Tetanus Toxoids and Acellular Pertussis Adsorbed, Inactivated Poliovirus, and Haemophilus b Conjugate Vaccine and Guidance for Use in Infants and Children. MMWR. 2008/57 (39); 1079–1080 Available from http://www.cdc.gov/mmwr/preview/mmwrhtml/mm5739a5.htm (Accessed on Dec 11, 2013)

8.   Dutta AK, Verghese VP, Pemde HK, Mathew LG, and Ortiz E. Immunogenicity and safety of a pentavalent diphtheria, tetanus, acellular pertusis, inactivated poliovirus, *Haemophilus influenzae* type b conjugate combination vaccine (Pentaxim) with hepatitis B vaccine. Indian Pediatr 2009; 46: 975–982.

9.   Dutta AK, Verghese VP, Pemde HK, Mathew LG, and Ortiz E. Immunogenicity and safety of a DTaP-IPV/PRP-T vaccine (Pentaxim) booster dose during the second year of life in Indian children primed with the same vaccine. Indian Pediatr 2012; 49 : 793 –798.

10.   CDC. Use of Combination Measles, Mumps, Rubella, and Varicella Vaccine. MMWR. 2010/59(RR03); 1–12. Available from http://www.cdc.gov/mmwr/preview/mmwrhtml/rr5903a1.htm (Accessed on Dec 11, 2011)

■ ■ ■ ■ ■ ■

INFLUENZA VACCINES

Reviewed by
Panna Choudhury, Vipin M. Vashishtha

Background

Pathogen

The influenza virus, an orthomyxovirus, is a single stranded RNA virus. It is capable of causing disease in humans, birds and animals. There are three types of influenza viruses A, B and C. The subtypes of type A influenza virus is determined by hemagglutinin and neuraminidase. The influenza type A causes moderate to severe illness in all age groups in humans and other animals. The illness caused by type B is usually a milder disease in humans only and primarily affects children. The illness by type C influenza virus is rarely reported in humans and it does not cause epidemics. The nomenclature of influenza virus is in order of virus type, geographic origin, strain no, year of isolation and virus subtype. Therefore, the nomenclature of the pandemic influenza virus is A/California/7/2009/H1N1.

Influenza virus is characterized by frequent mutations — antigenic drifts (minor antigenic change, both A and B) and antigenic shifts (major antigenic change, only A). The human pandemic A/H1N1 is an example of antigenic shift. Vaccines elicit a relatively strain specific humoral response, have reduced efficacy against antigenically drifted viruses and are ineffective against unrelated strains. It is of utmost importance therefore that vaccine should incorporate the current strain prevalent during that time. The influenza vaccine is therefore unique as the precise composition has to be changed periodically in anticipation of the prevalent influenza strain expected to circulate in a given year. To ensure optimal vaccine efficacy against prevailing strains in both the northern and southern hemispheres, the antigenic composition of the vaccines is revised twice annually and adjusted to the antigenic characteristics of circulating influenza viruses obtained within the WHO global influenza surveillance and response system (GISRS). This gives the vaccine manufacturer's 4–6 months to manufacture the vaccine in time for the flu season for the respective hemisphere.[1]

Historical perspectives

The 20th century pandemics were in 1918 due to H1N1 (Spanish flu), 1957 due toH2N2 (Asian flu) and 1968 due to H3N2 (Hong Kong flu). Of these pandemics, the 1918 pandemic was the most severe, causing an estimated 20–40 million or more deaths worldwide.

The new virus tends to replace endemic/seasonal influenza viruses and post-pandemic, it continues to circulate as the new seasonal virus. Thereafter it would exhibit antigenic drift; thus more than one drifted variant may co-circulate. H1N1 virus circulated globally from 1918 till 1957 and was replaced by H2N2 virus; in 1968, H3N2 virus replaced H2N2. The seasonal H3N2 viruses that continue to be isolated globally are descendants of the 1968 pandemic virus. In 1977 a descendant of the 1918 pandemic H1N1 virus reappeared in northern hemisphere; it might have been accidentally released from a laboratory. It slowly established circulation globally; subsequently endemic/seasonal viruses in both hemispheres are H3N2 and H1N1. In 2009, global outbreaks caused by the A (H1N1) strain designated as A(H1N1)pdm09 attained pandemic proportions although it gradually evolved into a seasonal pattern in 2010.

Disease burden

Seasonal influenza

Global: Influenza occurs globally with an annual attack rate estimated at 5%–10% in adults and 20%–30% in children.[1] Children, particularly below 2 years of age, have a high burden of influenza. In 2008 there were 90 million (95%, CI 49–162 million) new cases of seasonal influenza, 20 million (95%, CI 13–32 million) cases of influenza-associated acute lower respiratory infections (ALRI), and 1–2 million cases of influenza associated severe ALRI, including 28,000–111,500 deaths.[2] The incidence of influenza episodes and associated ALRI is significantly higher in developing countries as compared to developed countries.[2] A systematic review of seasonal influenza epidemiology in sub-Saharan Africa showed that influenza accounted for about 10% of all outpatient visits and for about 6.5% of hospital admissions for acute respiratory infections in children.[3]

India: Adequate data on the prevalence and burden of influenza in India is lacking. According to published data, it contributes to around 5–10% of all acute respiratory infections (ARI). The reported incidence of influenza URI was found to be 10/ 100 child years and that of ALRI to be only 0.4/100 child years. According to an Indian review, influenza virus was responsible for about 1.5% to 14.5% of all ARIs episodes.[4] A community-based study from north India estimated incidence of influenza episodes among children with ARI around 180 and 178 per 1000 children per year, amongst children below 1 and 2 years, respectively. Similarly, the incidence of influenza associated ALRI was calculated as 33 and 44 per 1000 children per year.[2, 5] It is estimated that around 24,179 influenza-associated ALRI mean deaths are occurring per year based on verbal autopsy confirmed ALRI deaths in the community in children younger than 5 years.[6] Though burden of ILI was highest in children <5 years, the isolation rate for lab confirmed influenza was highest for individuals aged >46 years.[6]

Swine flu or A (H1N1)

Globally, between 151,700 and 575,400 people died from 2009 H1N1 virus infection during the first year the virus circulated according to a new study from CDC Influenza Division. A disproportionate number of deaths occurred in Southeast Asia and Africa, where access to prevention and treatment resources are more likely to be limited.[7] According to the data from Government of India, 22.8% of the samples out of the total samples from 202,790 persons who had been tested have been found positive for A (H1N1). In the majority, the illness was self-limited with recovery within a week. Among those tested 94% cases recovered and 2,728 deaths were reported till December 2010.[8]

Influenza Vaccines

Most of the current seasonal influenza vaccines include 2 influenza A strains and 1 influenza B strain. Globally, trivalent inactivated vaccines (TIV) and live attenuated influenza vaccines (LAIV) are available. In order to enhance immunogenicity, some current formulations of trivalent vaccines include adjuvants such as oil-in-water adjuvants or virosomes. Adjuvanted trivalent influenza vaccines (aTIVs) show enhanced priming and boosting, as well as efficacy in infants, although need for two doses remains. The development of Quadrivalent Influenza Vaccine (QIV) formulation for seasonal influenza is of interest in providing comprehensive protection against influenza B viruses.

Inactivated Influenza Vaccines

The inactivated influenza vaccines are produced from virus growth in embryonated hen's eggs and are of three types: Whole virus, split product, subunit surface—antigen formulations. Whole virus vaccines are associated with increased adverse reactions, especially in children and are currently not used. Most influenza vaccines are split-product vaccines, produced from detergent treated, highly purified influenza virus, or surface antigen vaccines containing purified hemagglutinin and neuraminidase. Table 1 provides a list of available influenza vaccines in Indian market. All currently available trivalent vaccines now have the influenza strain that is antigenically similar to 2009 pandemic swine flu strain, i.e. A(H1N1)pdm09. Hence, there is no need to go for separate 'swine flu' vaccine. The trivalent vaccines contain 15 g of each of WHO recommended two influenza A strains (H1N1 and H3N2) and one influenza B strain. Vaccines are licensed for use in children aged 6 months and older.

WHO recommendations on composition of influenza vaccines: For the 2013–14 influenza season (northern hemisphere) it is recommended that TIVs for use contain the following: An A/California/7/2009 (H1N1)pdm09-like virus; an A(H3N2) virus antigenically like the cell-propagated prototype virus A/Victoria/361/2011; a B/Massachusetts/2/2012-like virus.[9] For the Southern hemisphere trivalent vaccines for use in will contain the following: An A/California/7/2009 (H1N1)pdm09-like virus; an A/Texas/50/2012 (H3N2)-like virus; a B/Massachusetts/2/2012-like virus.[10]

Table 1: Influenza vaccines licensed in India

Brand names	Manufacturer	Type of vaccine	Composition
Vaxigrip	Sanofi Pasteur India Private Limited	Split-Virion, inactivated	TIV (both SH & NH)*
Agrippal	Chiron Panacea (Panacea Biotec Ltd)	Surface Antigen, inactivated	TIV (NH)
Influgen	Lupin Laboratories Ltd	Split-Virion, inactivated	TIV (NH)
Influvac	Solvay Pharma India Pvt Ltd (Abott)	Split-Virion, inactivated	TIV (NH)
Fluarix	GlaxoSmithKline Pharmaceuticals Ltd.	Split-Virion, inactivated	TIV (NH)
Vaxiflu	Zydus Cadila	Purified H1N1 Monovalent inactivated	TIV (NH)
Nasovac	Serum Institute of India Ltd	Live attenuated monovalent	LAIV (A/H1N1pdm)

SH: Southern Hemisphere; NH: Northern Hemisphere

Dosage and schedule: The dosage schedule is provided in Table 2. Revaccination is recommended with a single annual dose irrespective of age.

Table 2: Dosage and schedule of TIVs

Age	6–35 months	3–8 years	from 9 years of age
Dose	0.25 ml	0.5 ml	0.5 ml
No. of doses	1 or 2*	1 or 2*	1

For children who have not previously been vaccinated a second dose should be given after an interval of at least 4 weeks.

Efficacy and effectiveness of Trivalent Influenza vaccines

The reported efficacy/effectiveness of influenza vaccines varies substantially with factors such as the case definition (e.g. laboratory-confirmed influenza disease or the less specific influenza-like illness), the 'match' between the vaccine strains and prevailing influenza strains, vaccine preparation, dose, prior antigenic experience, and age or underlying disease conditions of an individual.[1] There is no data on efficacy/ effectiveness of influenza vaccines from India.

Duration of protection: Following vaccination, anti-HA antibody titers peak 2–4 weeks post-vaccination in primed individuals but may peak 4 weeks or later in unprimed individuals or older adults. Serum antibody titers may fall by 50% or more by 6 months after vaccination, with the degree of reduction being proportional to the peak titers achieved. Vaccine induced serum antibody titers then remains stable for two to three years. Evidence from clinical trials suggests that protection against viruses that are similar antigenically to those contained in the vaccine extends for at least 6–8 months.[11]

Safety of Trivalent Influenza Vaccines

Transient local reactions at the injection site occur frequently (>1/100), and fever, malaise, myalgia, and other systemic adverse events may affect persons without previous exposure to the influenza vaccine antigens, trivalent influenza vaccines are generally considered safe.[1] During some influenza seasons, TIVs have been associated with a slight increase in the risk of Guillain-Barré syndrome. However, time-series analysis demonstrated no evidence of seasonality and revealed no statistically significant increase in hospital admissions because of GBS after the introduction of the universal influenza immunization program.[12]

However, the vaccine should preferably be avoided in patients with history of GBS and who are not at high risk of severe influenza-related complications. A brand of seasonal TIVs from M/s CSL 2010 batch, Fluzone was associated with febrile seizures in children < 5 years of age in Australia and US. Detailed analysis concluded that the risk was only present among 6–23 month olds when TIV was given along with PCV13.[13] The vaccine should be administered with caution in patients with history of severe egg allergy only if expected benefits outweigh risks.

Live Attenuated Influenza Vaccines (LAIV)

Live attenuated influenza vaccine provides broader and higher levels of protection than trivalent inactivated vaccines in healthy children aged 2–5 years of age. A Cochrane review of RCTs evaluating live vaccines in healthy children aged >2 years found an overall efficacy against laboratory confirmed influenza of 82% (95%, CI 71–89%) and an effectiveness against influenza-like illness (ILI) of 33% (95%, CI 28–38%). Inactivated vaccines had a lower efficacy of 59% (95%, CI 41–71%) but similar effectiveness at 36% (95%, CI 24–46%).[14] A quadrivalent live attenuated vaccine for intranasal application containing 2 influenza A strains and 2 influenza B strains was licensed in the USA in 2012.[1] Live attenuated vaccine is not recommended below 2 years of age, in high-risk individuals and in pregnant women. Non-pregnant individuals aged 2–49 years may receive either TIV or LAIV in accordance with national policy.

Recommendations for use

Individual use

Whom to give?

IAP has recommended seasonal influenza vaccine (including the earlier monovalent A (H1N1) vaccine) only for the category of 'high-risk children'.[13] This category contains the following:

- Chronic cardiac, pulmonary (excluding asthma), hematologic and renal (including nephritic syndrome) condition, chronic liver diseases, and diabetes mellitus

- Congenital or acquired immunodeficiency (including HIV infection)

- Children on long-term salicylates therapy

- Laboratory personnel and healthcare workers

Vaccination against 'swine flu' (A (H1N1)pdm)

It is expected to have A (H1N1) infections slightly more severe with higher mortality than seasonal influenza caused by other co-circulating strains. Considering the fact that the available influenza vaccines are going to have much better effectiveness against the circulating A(H1N1)pdm09 strain than other influenza viruses owing to more 'complete match' between the strain circulating in the community and the strain contained in the vaccines, IAP justifies its earlier recommendation of using the influenza vaccine in all children with risk factors as mentioned above and also wherein the vaccine is desired/ requested by parents.[15]

'Target group prioritization' for seasonal influenza vaccination:

IAP ACVIP believes that influenza vaccination should aim primarily at protecting vulnerable high-risk groups against severe influenza-associated disease and death. However, there is lack of effectiveness data in a few categories of individuals and in different age groups. The suggested prioritization (Box 1 and Table 3) is based on following attributes: Contribution of risk group to the overall influenza disease burden in population, disease severity within individual risk group, and vaccine effectiveness in different age groups and categories. Elderly individuals, pregnant women, and children with underlying chronic medical conditions should be given highest priority.[13] WHO position paper states that pregnant women have increased risk of severe disease and death from influenza; the infection may also lead to complications such as stillbirth, neonatal death, preterm delivery, and decreased birth weight.[1] Pregnant women should be vaccinated with TIV at any stage of pregnancy. This recommendation is based on evidence of a substantial risk of severe disease in this group and evidence that seasonal influenza vaccine is safe throughout pregnancy and effective in preventing influenza in the women as well as in their young infants, in whom the disease burden is also high.

Box 1: IAP recommendations on 'target group prioritization' for seasonal influenza vaccination[13]

Prioritization of target groups
(1-Highest priority, 4-Lowest priority)

1. Elderly individuals (> 65 years) and nursing-home residents (the elderly or disabled)

2. Individuals with chronic medical conditions including individuals with HIV/AIDS, and pregnant women (especially to protect infants 0–6 months)

3. Other groups: Health care workers including professionals, individuals with asthma, and children from ages 6 months to 2 years.

4. Children aged 2–5 years and 6–18 years, and healthy young adults.

Table 3: Summary of disease burden, efficacy / effectiveness of TIVs, and prioritization of influenza vaccination in different age groups and categories of target population

Age group/ category	Burden of disease	Fatalities/ severe disease	Effectiveness/ efficacy of vaccine	Level of evidence	Prioritiz- ation
0–6 months	High (+++)	Very high (++++)	Not eligible	NA	2*
6–23 months	High (+++)	High (+++)	Not effective/ very low	Moderate	3
2–5 years	Substantial (++)	Moderate (++)	Moderate	Limited	4
6–64 years	Low (+)	Low (+)	Moderate to high	Moderate	4
> 65 years	High (+++)	Very high (++++)	Low	Low	1
Pregnant women	Substantial (++)	High (+++)	Moderate**	Limited to high*	2
Individuals with asthma	Not known	Moderate (++)	Not effective	Limited	3
Individuals with HIV/AIDS	Not known	High (+++)	Moderate	Low	2
Individuals with other underlying medical conditions	Not known	High (+++)	Low	Limited	2
Healthcare workers	Substantial (++)	Moderate (++)	High	High	3

Amongst pediatric population, apart from the children with chronic medical conditions (see above), the children below 2 years of age should be considered a target group for influenza immunization because of a high burden of severe disease in this group.

Which vaccine to give?

In those who with underlying risk factors only the inactivated vaccines should be used. In healthy individuals aged 2 years to 49 years either the inactivated or live attenuated vaccines may be used. In India, since the LAIV is currently not available, hence only TIVs should be used.

When to give ?

As far as the influenza virus circulation in India is concerned, the data since 2004 suggests a clear peaking of circulation during the rainy season across the country— 'June to August' in north (Delhi), west (Pune) and east (Kolkata), and 'October to December' in south (Chennai).[16] This data is also consistent with the WHO circulation patterns for 2010 and 2011 for India which also shows a clear peak coinciding with the rainy season across the country. These data illustrate the difficulty in having effective uniform vaccination timing for a vast country like India and have implications when formulating vaccination policies. The evidence of antigenic drifts of circulating influenza viruses in India, together with the temporal peaks in seasonality of influenza in different parts of the country; illustrate the need for a staggered approach in vaccination timing. Hence, the best time for offering vaccine for individuals residing in southern states would be just before the onset of rainy season, i.e. before October while for rest of the country, it should be before June. Though, the committee acknowledges that this issue is still contentious and unresolved. This is to be noted that WHO convenes two meetings to provide recommendations for the usage of influenza vaccine in February and September each year. The vaccine for the February recommendations (Northern hemisphere) and September recommendations (Southern hemisphere) becomes available after 6 months of each recommendation. In addition to this, WHO classifies India under the 'South Asia' transmission zone of influenza circulation. This strongly points India's alignment with the availability of Southern hemisphere vaccine (March–April) to ensure we have the latest available strains for early vaccination to prevent the peak of circulation of influenza in the rainy season across the country.[13,16]

Public health perspectives

IAP ACVIP has not yet recommended introduction of influenza vaccine into UIP for several reasons. Sufficient data to estimate precisely the contribution of influenza to childhood mortality in India is not available. Data on morbidity and mortality of influenza in India is very limited and current status does not justify the prioritization of strategies for influenza prevention and control. The risk groups for influenza in low and middle-income countries including India are less well defined, still, based on global estimates for developing and low- and middle-income group countries, IAP believes that influenza vaccination should aim primarily at protecting vulnerable high-risk groups against severe influenza-associated disease and death. The attack rates of seasonal influenza is although greatest in young children, the highest mortality and morbidity are observed in the elderly, individuals with certain underlying chronic health conditions, pregnant women, and health care workers.

One estimate shows 6·5% of all pediatric ALRI deaths in India were associated with influenza in 2006–08 and also showed substantial yearly variation in magnitude of influenza epidemic activity and associated ALRI deaths.[6] Thus there is need for a more extensive region-specific surveillance. Further, there is a little evidence regarding effectiveness of influenza vaccines in children below 2 years of age even from industrialized countries.[14] Data are limited on the effectiveness of TIVs in tropical regions including India. There are also issues related to vaccine availability, timing and suitability which preclude routine recommendation of influenza vaccine in children.[13]

INFLUENZA VACCINE

Routine vaccination:

- Minimum age: 6 months for trivalent inactivated influenza vaccine (TIV)
- Recommended only for the vaccination of persons with certain high-risk conditions.
- First time vaccination: 6 months to below 9 years: Two doses 1 month apart; 9 years and above: Single dose
- Annual revaccination with single dose.
- Dosage (TIV) : Aged 6–35 months 0.25 ml; 3 years and above: 0.5 ml
- For children Aged 6 months through 8 years: For the 2012–13 season, administer 2 doses (separated by at least 4 weeks) to children who are receiving influenza vaccine for the first time.
- All the currently available TIVs in the country contain the 'Swine flu' or 'A (H1N1)' antigen; no need to vaccinate separately.
- Best time to vaccinate:
  - ➢ As soon as the new vaccine is released and available in the market
  - ➢ Just before the onset of rainy season.

References

1. WHO. Vaccines against influenza WHO position paper—November 2012. Wkly Epidemiol Rec. 2012 23; 87(47): 461–476.

2. Nair H, Brooks WA, Katz M, Roca A, Berkley JA, Madhi SA, et al. Global burden of respiratory infections due to seasonal influenza in young children: A systematic review and meta-analysis. Lancet. 2011; 378: 1917–1930.

3. Gessner BD, Shindo N, Briand S. Seasonal influenza epidemiology in sub-Saharan Africa: A systematic review. Lancet Infect Dis. 2011; 11: 223–235.

4. Mathew JL. Influenza vaccination of children in India. Indian Pediatr. 2009; 46: 304–307.

5. Broor S, Parveen S, Bharaj P, Prasad VS, Srinivasulu KN, Sumanth KM, et al. A prospective three-year cohort study of the epidemiology and virology of acute respiratory infections of children in rural India. PLoS ONE 2007; 2: e491.

6. Chadha MS, Broor S, Gunassekaran CP, Krishnan A, Chawla-Sarkar M, et al. (2011) Multi-site virological influenza surveillance in India: 2004–2008. Influenza Other Respir Viruses. 2012; 6: 196–203.

7. CDC. First Global Estimates of 2009 H1N1 Pandemic Mortality Released by CDC-Led Collaboration. Available from http://www.cdc.gov/flu/spotlights/pandemic-global-estimates.htm. (Accessed on Dec 2, 2013)

8. Ministry of Health & Family Welfare, Government of India. Pandemic influenza, A H1N1, Available from: http://www.mohfw-h1n1.nic.in/ (Accessed on Dec 2, 2013)

9. WHO. Recommended composition of influenza virus vaccines for use in the 2013–14 northern hemisphere influenza season. Available from http://www.who.int /influenza/vaccines/ virus/recommendations/ 2013_14_north/en/index.html (Accessed on Dec 3, 2013)

10. WHO. Recommended composition of influenza virus vaccines for use in the 2014 southern hemisphere influenza season. Available from http://www.who.int /influenza/vaccines /virus/recommendations/ 2014_south/en/index.html (Accessed on Dec 3, 2013)

11. Fiore AE, Uyeki TM, Broder K, Finelli L, Euler GL, Singleton JA, et al. Prevention and control of influenza with vaccines: Recommendations of the Advisory Committee on Immunization Practices (ACIP), 2010. MMWR Recomm Rep. 2010; 59: 1–62.

12. Juurlink DN, Stukel TA, Kwong J, Kopp A, McGeer A, Upshur RE, et al. Guillain-Barré syndrome after influenza vaccination in adults: A population-based study. Arch Intern Med. 2006; 166(20): 2217–2221.

13. Vashishtha VM, Kalra A, Choudhury P. Influenza Vaccination in India: Position Paper of Indian Academy of Pediatrics, 2013. Indian Pediatr 2013; 50: 867–874.

14. Jefferson T, Rivetti A, Harnden A, Di Pietrantonj C, Demicheli V. Vaccines for preventing influenza in healthy children. Cochrane Database Syst Rev. 2008; 16: CD004879.

15. Influenza vaccines. In: Yewale V, Choudhury P, Thacker N, eds. IAP Guide Book on Immunization. Indian Academy of Pediatrics 2009; 10: 123–130.

16. Indian Academy of Pediatrics Committee on Immunization. Consensus recommendations on immunization and IAP immunization timetable 2012. Indian Pediatr 2012; 49(7): 549–564.

JAPANESE ENCEPHALITIS VACCINES

Reviewed by
Vipin M. Vashishtha

Background

Japanese encephalitis, a mosquito borne flavivirus disease, is a leading form of viral encephalitis in Asia in children below 15 years of age. The JEV has shown a tendency to extend to other geographic regions. Case fatality averages 30% and a high percentage of the survivors are left with permanent neuropsychiatric sequelae[1].

Global burden

Japanese encephalitis (JE) is one of the most important causes of viral encephalitis in Asia. During 2006–2009, JE-endemic countries reported 27,059 cases of JE (annual range: 4502–9459; average: 6765) to WHO. Fully 86% of these (23,176 cases; average: 5,794 cases per year) were reported from China and India; 16 countries reported a total of 3,883 cases (annual average: 971); and 5 countries reported no cases[2]. According to WHO, nearly 50,000 cases of JE occur worldwide per year and 15,000 of them die.[3] In endemic areas, the annual incidence of disease ranges from 10–100 per 1,00,000 population. Japan, South Korea, North Korea, Taiwan, Vietnam, Thailand, and the Peoples Republic of China (PRC) practice routine childhood immunization against JE. The results of the most recent study[2] suggest that the actual incidence of JE is nearly 10 times higher than reflected in recent reports to WHO.

Indian burden

JE has been reported from all states and union territories in India except Arunachal, Dadra, Daman, Diu, Gujarat, Himachal, Jammu, Kashmir, Lakshadweep, Meghalaya, Nagar Haveli, Orissa, Punjab, Rajasthan, and Sikkim. Highly endemic states include West Bengal, Bihar, Karnataka, Tamil Nadu, Andhra

Pradesh, Assam, Uttar Pradesh, Manipur, and Goa. The risk is highest in children aged 1–15 years, in rural areas and in the monsoon/post-monsoon season.

Seasonality

Patterns of JE transmission vary within individual countries and from year to year. In endemic areas, sporadic cases occur throughout the year. In North temperate area (Japan, Taiwan, Nepal, Northern India), large epidemics occur from May to October. In Southern tropical areas (South India, Indonesia, Sri Lanka), the disease is endemic but peak starts after rains that is from July to December. Within India it is seen from July to December in North India. It occurs during May to October in Goa, October to January in Tamil Nadu, August to December in Karnataka, September to December in Andhra Pradesh, and July to December in Northern States.[4] Urban cases have been reported from Lucknow.

Outbreaks of JE in India

In India JE was first diagnosed in Vellore in 1955 and the first major outbreak took place in West Bengal in 1973. Presently highly endemic areas are Andhra Pradesh, Tamil Nadu, Karnataka, and Uttar Pradesh.[2] In 2005, Uttar Pradesh faced a devastating epidemic of JE mostly confined to Gorakhpur district affecting 6061 cases with 1500 deaths followed by another outbreak in 2006 with 2320 cases and 528 deaths. Similarly JE cases in Uttar Pradesh were confined predominantly in Gorakhpur during 2007 reporting 3024 cases and 645 deaths.[5] The reported mortality rate

Table 1: AES/JE cases and deaths, India 2007–12

AES/JE Cases and deaths in the country since 2007

S. No.	Affected States/UTs	2007		2008		2009		2010		2011 (P)		2012 (P)	
		Cases	Deaths	Cases	Deaths	Cases	Deaths	Cases	Deaths	Cases	Deaths	Cases	Deaths
1	Andhra Pradesh	22	0	6	0	14	0	139	7	73	1	64	0
2	Assam	424	133	319	99	462	92	469	117	1319	250	1343	229
3	Bihar	336	164	203	45	325	95	50	7	821	197	745	275
4	Delhi	0	0	0	0	0	0	0	0	9	0	0	0
5	Goa	70	0	39	0	66	3	80	0	91	1	66	0
6	Haryana	85	46	13	3	12	10	1	1	90	14	5	0
7	Jharkhand	0	0	0	0	0	0	18	2	303	19	16	0
8	Karnataka	15	3	3	0	246	8	143	1	397	0	189	1
9	Kerala	2	0	2	0	3	0	19	5	88	6	29	6
10	Maharashtra	2	0	24	0	1	0	24	17	35	9	37	20
11	Manipur	65	0	4	0	6	0	116	15	11	0	2	0
12	Nagaland	7	1	0	0	9	2	11	6	44	6	21	2
13	Punjab	0	0	0	0	0	0	2	0	0	0	0	0
14	Uttrakhand	0	0	12	0	0	0	7	0	0	0	174	2
15	Tamil Nadu	42	1	144	0	265	8	466	7	762	29	804	53
16	Uttar Pradesh	3024	645	3012	537	3073	556	3540	494	3492	579	3145	450
17	West Bengal	16	2	50	0	0	0	70	0	714	58	675	32
	Total	4110	995	3048	684	4482	774	5167	679	8249	1169	7315	1070

As per the reports received from state till October 2012

varies between 8.5% and 72%.[6,7] Table 1 summarizes total cases of AES/JE during the later years.

The Case Fatality Rate (CFR) due to acute encephalitis syndrome (AES)/JE in India has been around 17% with wide variations in states.

Vaccines

World over, following vaccines are available for use against JE:

- Mouse Brain derived inactivated JE vaccine (JE –VAX)
- Inactivated Primary Hamster Kidney cells-P3 –China
- Live Attenuated, Cell culture-derived SA 14-14-2
- Newer JE vaccines:
    - ➢ Inactivated SA-14-14-2 vaccine (IC51) (IXIARO® by Intercel & JEEV® by Biological Evans India Ltd.)
    - ➢ Inactivated Vero cell culture-derived Kolar strain, 821564XY, JE vaccine (JENVAC® by Bharat Biotech)
    - ➢ Live attenuated recombinant SA 14-14-2 Chimeric Vaccine (JE-CV, IMOJEV® by Sanofi Pasteur)
    - ➢ Inactivated vero-cell derived JE vaccine (Beijing-1 JE strain by Biken & Kaketsuken, Japan)

Owing to many drawbacks (high cost, complicated dosing schedule, requirement of numerous doses and boosters, concerns about side-effects and reliance neurological tissue for production) and availability of better vaccines, the first two vaccines, i.e. mouse brain-derived and Primary Hamster Kidney cells-P3 are no longer being produced, hence will not be discussed further.

Live attenuated Cell culture derived SA-14-14-2 vaccine

This vaccine is based on the genetically stable, neuro-attenuated SA 14-14-2 strain of the JE virus, which elicits broad immunity against heterologous JE viruses. Reversion to neurovirulence is considered highly unlikely. WHO technical specifications have been established for the vaccine production.[8] Chengdu Institute of Biological Products is the only manufacturer authorized to export this vaccine from China.

The live attenuated vaccine was licensed in China in 1989. Since then, more than 300 million doses have been produced and more than 200 million children have been vaccinated. Currently, more than 50 million doses of this vaccine are produced annually.[3] Extensive use of this and other vaccines has significantly contributed to reducing the burden of JE in China from 2.5/100,000 in 1990 to <0.5/100,000 in 2004. This vaccine is also licensed for use in Nepal (since 1999); South Korea (since 2001); India (since 2006); Thailand (since 2007) and Sri Lanka.[3] The price per dose of the vaccine is comparable to the EPI measles vaccine.

Dosage and administration: In China, the vaccine is licensed for 0.5-mL dose to be administered subcutaneously to children at 8 months of age and a second opportunity again at 2 years. In some areas, a booster dose is given at 7 years. Measles has been given concurrently.[9] It should not be used as an "outbreak response vaccine". It can also be offered to all susceptible children up to 15 years as catch -up vaccination.[3]

Stability: The infectious titer of the vaccine is not appreciably changed after storage at 37°C for 7–10 days, at room temperature for 4 months, or at 2 to 8°C for at least 1.5 years.[9]

Immunogenicity and correlate of protection: After a single dose, antibody responses are produced in 85 to 100% of nonimmune 1- to 12-year-old children. A neutralization antibody titer of more than 1:10 is generally accepted as evidence of protection and post-vaccination seroconversion.[9]

Efficacy and effectiveness

Efficacy in China: A case-control study performed in 1993 in Sichuan Province China in children < 15 years measured effectiveness of routinely delivered SA 14-14-2 vaccine at 80% (CI 44–93%) for a single dose and 97.5% (CI 86–99.6%) for two doses given at a one year interval.[10]

Five major efficacy trials of SA 14-14-2 vaccine, completed in China from 1988 to 1999 in 1 to 10 year-old, consistently yielded high protection rates, above 98%.[9] Case control studies and numerous large-scale field trials in China have consistently shown an efficacy of at least 95% following 2 doses administered at an interval of 1 year.[3]

Efficacy in Nepal: In a field trial in Nepal in 1999, involving more than 160,000 subjects 1 to 15 years of age, reported efficacy of a single dose of 99.3% in the same year and 98.5% one year later.[11, 12] At 5 years the protective efficacy was 96.2%.[13] Vaccine in this study contained 105.8 PFU/0.5 mL. The study provides evidence that SA 14-14-2 will be useful to combat epidemics.

Indian experience: In India, one dose of SA-14-14-2 imported from China is being used in many states including Eastern Uttar Pradesh, Bihar, and Assam since 2006 and children between the age group of 1 and 15 years were vaccinated with a single dose of the vaccine.[14] Following the campaigns targeting all children in the age group of 1–15 years in the high-risk districts, the vaccine is integrated into the UIP of endemic districts. Children at 16–24 months of age (with DPT/OPV booster) are targeted for one dose of this vaccine in select endemic districts after the campaign.[15]

A small case-control study from Lucknow, India found an efficacy of 94.5% (95% CI, 81.5 to 98.9) after a single dose of this vaccine within 6 months after its administration.[16] However, data from post-marketing surveillance (PMS) in India (ICMR unpublished study) showed that protective efficacy of the vaccine in India is not as high as that seen in Nepal. PMS study showed that virus neutralizing antibodies were seen in 45.7% of children before vaccination. Seroconversion against Indian strains 28 days after vaccination was 73.9% and 67.2% in all individuals and in those who were nonimmune pre-vaccination, respectively. The protective efficacy of the vaccine at one year was 43.1% overall and 35% for those who were non-immune pre-vaccination, respectively.[17]

Preliminary results of a recent case control study carried out by ICMR on impact of JE vaccine shows an unadjusted protective effect of 62.5% in those with any report of vaccination. According to this report, the JE vaccine efficacy has been around 60% in Uttar Pradesh and around 70% in Assam. Following this report, the ICMR has recommended a study on the impact of 2 doses vs. single dose of SA-14-14-2 vaccine in Assam.[17]

Boosters: Conventionally, boosters are unlikely to be required as with most live, attenuated vaccines, one dose will provide lifelong protection. Studies have already documented ongoing protection from a single dose for a minimum of 5 years in a JE-endemic area.[3] However, after analyzing recent Indian efficacy/effectiveness data, the academy thinks there is need of a second dose of the vaccine to provide more complete and more sustained protection. Government of India has also recommended 2 doses of the vaccine to be used in UIP since 2013.

Safety: An estimated 300 million children have been immunized with this vaccine without apparent complication.[9] WHO's Global Advisory Committee on Vaccine Safety acknowledged the vaccine's "excellent" safety profile. Transient fever may occur in 5–10%, local reactions, rash, or irritability in 1–3%. Neither acute encephalitis nor hypersensitivity reactions have been associated with the use of this vaccine.[18]

Inactivated Vero cell culture-derived SA 14-14-2 JE vaccine (JE-VC), IXIARO® by Intercel & JEEV® by Biological E. Ltd

IXIARO® by Intercell AG

This is an inactivated vaccine (JE-VC) derived from the attenuated SA 14-14-2 JEV strain propagated in Vero cells. This vaccine has been evaluated in several clinical trials conducted in India and abroad in both adults and children.[19-21] IXIARO® has now been approved by US FDA and EU for use in children from the age of 2 months onwards.[22,23] There is no efficacy data for IXIARO®, and the vaccine has been licensed in pediatric age group especially for travellers to Asian countries on the basis of a phase III RCT conducted in the Philippines,[24] and favourable interim data from a second Phase III trial in EU, U.S. and Australia.[25] The safety profile of the test vaccine was good, and its local tolerability profile was more favorable than that of the mouse brain vaccines.

Indian trial: A half-dose given to young children (1 to 3 years of age) has the excellent immunogenicity and the safety profile comparable to that of adults taking the full adult dosage. A phase II trial investigated the safety and immunogenicity of JE-VC in healthy children aged 1 and 2 years in India, using a standard (6-µg) or half (3-µg) dose[19]. Children in both groups received 2 doses of JE-VC administered 28 days apart. A third group of children received 3 doses of a JE-MB vaccine (JenceVac) on days 0, 7 and

28. At 56 days after the vaccination series was complete, seroconversion rates in the 6-µg (n = 21) and 3-µg (n = 23) JE-VC recipient groups and the JE-MB vaccine group (n = 11) were 95%, 96%, and 91%, and PRNT50 GMTs were 218 (95% confidence interval [CI] = 121–395), 201 (CI = 106–380), and 230 (CI = 68–784), respectively. The corresponding figures at 28 days were 71.4% (15/21), 65.2% (15/23), and 63.6% (7/11). None of the differences in seroconversion rates or GMTs was statistically significant.[19]

JEEV®— the Indian variant of IC51, IXIARO by Biological E. Ltd

Biological E. Ltd. has launched a vaccine for the endemic markets under the trade name JEEV® based on Intercell's technology and has already been WHO prequalified. In 2011, the BE Ltd. India conducted a multi-centric open label randomized controlled phase II/III study to evaluate safety and immunogenicity of JEEV® vaccine in ~450 children (≥ 1 to <3-year old) and compared to control Korean Green Cross Mouse Brain Inactivated (KGCC) vaccine.[26] This study demonstrated seroconversion (SCR) of 56.28% on day 28 and 92.42% on day 56 in JEEV® vaccinated group. Non-inferiority of JEEV® established against control in terms of proportion of subjects seroconverted. GMTs in JEEV® group were significantly higher than GMTs achieved in KGCC-JE vaccine group (218 vs 126). There was no significant difference between the groups in proportion of subjects' seroprotected, and in proportion of subjects reporting adverse events between groups. JEEV® has been licensed by DCGI for use in prevention of JE virus infection in children and adult population on the basis of its ability to induce JEV neutralizing antibodies as a surrogate for protection.[26]

Inactivated Vero cell culture-derived Kolar strain, 821564XY, JE vaccine (JENVAC®)

JENVAC® is a Vero cell culture derived, inactivated, adjuvanted and thiomersal containing vaccine developed by Bharat Biotech International Limited (BBIL). The original virus strain used in the vaccine was isolated from a patient in the endemic zone in Kolar, Karnataka, India by National Institute of Virology (NIV), Pune and later transferred to BBIL for vaccine development.

A phase II/III, randomized, single blinded, active controlled study to evaluate the immunogenicity and safety of the vaccine was conducted among 644 healthy subjects. Out of 644 subjects, 212 were between the age of ≤ 50 and >18 years, 201 subjects were between the age of ≤18 and > 6 years and 231 subjects were between the age of ≤ 6 and >1 years. Subjects received two doses of the test vaccine or a single dose of a reference vaccine (Live attenuated, SA 14-14-2 Chinese vaccine) as the first dose and a placebo as the second dose.

The results revealed that even a single dose of the test vaccine was sufficient to elicit the immune response. On 28th day, the subjects who had received a single dose were 98.67% seroprotected and 93.14% seroconverted (4 fold) for ≤ 50 – ≥ 1 years, whereas the corresponding figures for the reference vaccine were 77.56% and 57.69%, respectively (p-value <0.001). There was no statistically significant difference in all the 3 groups. The seroconversion (93.14% and 96.90%) and seroprotection (98.67% and 99.78%) percentages on the 28th and 56th day were not significantly different and similarly, no statistically significant difference in these rates was noted amongst different age groups. Higher GMTs were achieved in younger age groups. After the second dose of the test vaccine, the GMTs increased exponentially from day 28 (145) to day 56 (460.5) in ≤50 – ≥1 years. However, there was waning of both seroconversion and GMTs in both the test vaccine and reference vaccine groups at 18 months. All the subjects were followed up for 56±2 days. There was no serious adverse event or adverse event of any special interest noted in the study.

Live attenuated recombinant SA 14-14-2 Chimeric Vaccine (JE-CV, IMOJEV® by Sanofi Pasteur)

A promising new genetic approach is adopted in the construction of a chimeric live attenuated vaccine comprising neutralizing antigen-coding sequences of the SA 14-14-2 strain of the JE virus inserted into the genome of the 17 D yellow fever vaccine strain. The resulting recombinant virus is cultivated on Vero cells.[27] This novel, live, recombinant vaccine, was previously known as ChimeriVax-JE and developed initially by Acambis. It is a safe, highly immunogenic and capable of inducing long-lasting immunity in both preclinical and clinical trials. A single dose was sufficient to induce protective immunity, similar to that induced in adults by three doses of JE-VAX® with a seroconversion rate of > 97% (after single dose).[3] This vaccine has been licensed in Australia and is under review in Thailand.[28] The clinical development of this vaccine (IMOJEV) is currently on hold in India due to severe delays in authorization of the Phase III study.

Inactivated Vero-cell derived JE vaccine (Beijing-1 JE strain by Biken & Kaketsuken, Japan)

This is an inactivated vaccine derived from the Beijing-1 JE virus strain grown on Vero cells. The vaccine was licensed in Japan in 2008 and is targeted currently for the Japanese market only. This vaccine is not available in India.

Recommendations for use

Individual use

The vaccination against JE is not recommended for routine use, but only for individuals living in endemic areas. Though occasional cases have been reported from urban areas in a few districts, JE is exclusively a disease of rural areas. Hence, even in endemic areas, the children residing only in rural areas should be targeted for vaccination. Government of India has identified around 180 districts to be endemic for JE in India so far. JE vaccine is also recommended for travellers to JE endemic areas provided they are expected to stay for a minimum of 4 weeks in rural areas in the JE season.

Live attenuated SA-14-14-2 vaccine: After analyzing the recent Indian efficacy/effectiveness data, the academy thinks there is a need of a second dose of the vaccine to provide more complete and sustained protection. First dose of the vaccine can be administered at 9 months along with measles vaccine and second at 16 to 18 months at the time of 1st booster of DTP vaccine.[26]

JEEV® by Biological E. Ltd: The committee believes that although Biological E. India Ltd. has used the same strain, adjuvant and technology in production of JEEV® as used by Intercell AG in development of IXIARO®, the two vaccines cannot be treated as the same product. Considering the proven efficacy and safety profile of its parent vaccine in many countries over past many years, and demonstration of good seroprotection in Indian trial, the committee endorses use of this vaccine in India and recommends a primary schedule of 2 doses of 0.25 ml for children aged ≥ 1 – ≤ 3 years and 2 doses of 0.5 mL for children > 3 years, adolescents and adults administered intramuscularly on days 0 and 28. However, the long-term persistence of protective efficacy and need of boosters are still undetermined.[26] In February 2011, ACIP approved recommendations for a booster dose of JE-VC (IXIARO®) in adults.

JENVAC® by BBIL: The committee reviewed the data provided by the manufacturer on the clinical trials of JENVAC® in India. Although it lacks the experience of multinational trials of IXIARO® in different country, nevertheless the results of a pivotal phase II/III study conducted in India appear satisfactory for issuing recommendations for clinical use. The committee recommends two doses of the vaccine (0.5 mL each) administered intramuscularly at 4 weeks interval for the primary immunization series for office practice starting from 1 year of age. Since appreciable waning was noted in both seroconversion and seroprotection rates, and GMTs were also waned significantly, there is definitely a need of booster dose at later stage. The exact timing of the booster along with feasibility of single dose for primary series can be determined only after obtaining the long- term follow-up data.[26]

Public health perspectives

Vaccination of humans is the method of choice for prevention of JE. The consensus statement from all the Global JE meetings over the years (1995, 1998 and 2002) has been that human vaccination is the only effective long-term control measure against JE. All at-risk population should receive a safe and efficacious vaccine as part of their national immunization program.

ACVIP supports the government's decision to include JE vaccine in its UIP program in endemic districts only. Large scale JE vaccination is required because there is a large population which is susceptible to JE, ratio of asymptomatic to symptomatic infection is high, disease has a high mortality and morbidity and other control measures are not effective. Vaccination of the susceptible population has been demonstrated to be cost effective strategy in

China, Nepal, Japan and Thailand. After introduction of mass vaccination in high-risk areas of Andhra Pradesh (population of 75 million) cases of JE decreased from 300 cases in 2002 to 25 in 2003.[19] However, there is need to undertake periodic assessment of the effectiveness of the employed JE vaccine.

JE campaigns in India: In India though JE is primarily a disease that affects children living in rural areas, there have also been reports of cases from urban areas. Therefore, a decision has been made to vaccinate all target children in both rural and urban areas of the operational districts to have the maximum impact of the program.

Following the massive outbreak of JE in 2005 in the districts of Eastern Uttar Pradesh and the adjoining districts of Bihar, vaccination campaigns were carried out in 11 of the highest risk districts of the country in 2006, 27 districts in 2007, 22 districts in 2008 and 30 districts in 2009. Children between the age group of 1 and 15 years were vaccinated with a single dose of SA14-14-2 vaccine. Mass vaccinations will continue to cover all the 109 endemic districts. Following the mass campaign, the vaccination will continue in the Routine Immunization (RI) Program to cover the new cohort.

As mentioned above, Government of India has identified around 180 districts to be endemic for JE in India so far.

Campaigns in adults: Following mass vaccination of campaigns with Chinese SA-14-14-2 vaccine among pediatric age group, adult JE cases have outnumbered pediatric cases in some JE endemic states including Assam. This has become a cause of concern for public health program, researchers, and medical practitioners in India. This led Government of Assam to conduct SIAs of JE vaccines in adults (> 15 years) in the most affected districts like Sivasagar in Assam. The exact reason behind this shift in age group is not well understood.

JE vaccine should not be used as an "outbreak response vaccine". With the availability of two quality inactivated vaccines in India, the academy urges the government to introduce one of these products in the UIP program of affected districts based on cost effective analysis. The performance of the current live attenuated Chinese vaccine, SA-14-14-2 has not been very satisfactory in high burden states.

JAPANESE ENCEPHALITIS (JE) VACCINES

Routine vaccination:

- Recommended only for individuals living in the rural areas of endemic districts

- Three types of new generation JE vaccines are licensed in India: One, live attenuated, cell culture-derived SA-14-14-2, two inactivated JE vaccines, namely 'vero cell culture-derived SA 14-14-2 JE vaccine' (JEEV® by BE India) and three 'vero cell culture-derived, 821564XY, JE vaccine' (JENVAC® by Bharat Biotech)

- **Live attenuated, cell culture-derived SA-14-14-2:**
  - ➢ Minimum age: 8 months;
  - ➢ Two dose schedule, first dose at 9 months along with measles vaccine and second at 16 to 18 months along with DTP booster
  - ➢ Not available in private market for office use

- **Inactivated cell culture-derived SA-14-14-2 (JEEV® by BE India) :**
  - ➢ Minimum age: 1 year (US-FDA: 2 months)
  - ➢ Primary immunization schedule: 2 doses of 0.25 mL each administered intramuscularly on days 0 and 28 for children aged ≥ 1 to ≤ 3 years
  - ➢ 2 doses of 0.5 ml for children > 3 years and adults aged ≥ 18 years
  - ➢ Need of boosters still undetermined

- **Inactivated Vero cell culture-derived Kolar strain, 821564XY, JE vaccine (JENVAC® by Bharat Biotech)**
  - ➢ Minimum age: 1 year
  - ➢ Primary immunization schedule: 2 doses of 0.5 mL each administered intramuscularly at 4 weeks interval
  - ➢ Need of boosters still undetermined.

Catch-up vaccination:

All susceptible children up to 15 years should be administered during disease outbreak/ahead of anticipated outbreak in campaigns.

References

1. Tiwari S, Singh RK, Tiwari R, Dhole TN. Japanese encephalitis: A review of the Indian perspective. Braz J Infect Dis. 2012;16:564–573.

2. Campbell GL, Hills SL, Fischer M, Jacobson JA, Hoke CH, Hombach JM, et al. Estimated global incidence of Japanese encephalitis: A systematic review. Bull World Health Organ 2011; 89:766–774.

3. World Health Organization. Japanese encephalitis vaccines. Wkly Epidemiol Rec 2006;81:331–340.

4. Tiroumourougane SV, Raghava P, Srinivasan S. Japanese viral encephalitis. Postgrad Med J 2002; 78:205–215.

5. Arunachalam N, Samuel PP, Paramasivan R, Balasubramanian A, Tyagi BK. Japanese encephalitis in Gorakhpur Division, Uttar Pradesh. Indian J Med Res. 2008 Dec;128(6):775–777.

6. Gourie-Devi M. Clinical aspects and experience in the management of Japanese encephalitis patients. Proceedings of the national conference on Japanese encephalitis, 1984. New Delhi: Indian Council of Medical Research, 1984: 25–29.

7. Kumar R, Mathur A, Kumar A. Clinical features and prognostic indicators of Japanese encephalitis in children in Lucknow (India). Indian J Med Res 1990;91:321–327.

8. WHO Expert Committee on Biological Standardization. Fifty-first report. Geneva, World Health Organization, 2002 (WHO Technical Report Series, No. 910). Available at : http://www.who.int/biologicals/publications/trs/51/en/index.html.

9. Halstead SB, Jacobson J. Japanese Encephalitis Vaccines. In: Plotkins SA, Orenstein WA, Offit PA. Vaccines, 5th ed. Philadelphia: Saunders Elsevier; 2008, pp 311–352.

10. Hennessy S, Zhengle L, Tsai TF, et al: Effectiveness of live-attenuated Japanese encephalititis vaccine (SA14-14-2): A case control study. Lancet 1996; 347:1583–1671.

11. Bista MB, Banerjee MK, Shin SH, et al: Efficacy of single-dose SA 14-14-2 vaccine against Japanese encephalitis: A case control study. Lancet 2001; 358:791–795.

12. Ohrr H, Tandan JB, Sohn YM, et al: Effect of single dose of SA 14-14-2 vaccine 1 year after immunisation in Nepalese children with Japanese encephalitis: A case-control study. Lancet 2005; 366:1375–1378.

13. Andan JB, Ohrr HC, Sohn YM, et al: Single dose of SA14-14-2 vaccine provides long-term protection against Japanese encephalitis: A case-control study in Nepalese children five years after immunization. Vaccine 2007; 25(27): 5041–5045.

14. Operational Guide Japanese Encephalitis Vaccination in India, Immunization Division Department of Family Welfare Ministry of Health and Family Welfare Government of India, September 2010, pp 13–15.

15. Immunization Handbook for Medical Officers, Revised 2011, MOHFW, New Delhi, 2011. Available from:http:// www.searo.who.int/india/topics/routine_immunization/Immunization_Handbook_for_Health_Workers_English_2011.pdf Accessed on August 11, 2013.

16. Kumar R, Tripathi P, Rizvi A. Effectiveness of one dose of SA 14-14-2 vaccine against Japanese encephalitis. N Engl J Med. 2009; 360:1465–1466.

17. Indian Council of Medical Research. Minutes of the meeting of the Core Committee on Vaccines. Available from: http://www.icmr.nic.in/minutes/Minutes%20Core%20Committee%20on%20Vaccines.pdf.

18. WHO. Global Advisory Committee on Vaccine Safety, 9-10 June 2005. Wkly Epidemiol Rec 2005;80: 242–243.

19. Kaltenbock A, Dubischar-Kastner K, Schuller E, Datla M, Klade C, Kishore T. Immunogenicity and safety of IXIARO (IC51) in a Phase II study in healthy Indian children between 1 and 3 years of age. Vaccine 2010; 28: 834–839.

20. Schuller E, Jilma B, Voicu V, Golor G, Kollaritsch H, Kaltenböck A, et al. Long-term immunogenicity of the new Vero cell-derived, inactivated Japanese encephalitis virus vaccine IC51 Six and 12 month results of a multicenter follow-up phase 3 study. Vaccine 2008; 26:4382–4386.

21. Dubischar-Kastner K, Eder S, Kaltenboeck A, Klade C, Schuller E, Wolfl G. Long-term immunity following vaccination with the inactivated Japanese encephalitis vaccine IXIARO and neutralizing antibody response to a booster dose. 11th Conference of the International Society of Travel Medicine; May 24–28, 2009, Budapest, Hungary.

22. Intercell Announces Pediatric Approval of its Japanese Encephalitis Vaccine in the U.S. Available from: http://www.vaccines.mil/documents/1624_2013-05-21 _ JEV _ pediatric_US_ENG_final.pdf

23. ACIP Unanimously Votes to Extend the Recommendations for Use of IXIARO(R) Vaccine. Available from:http:/ / www.reuters.com/article/2013/06/21/idUSnHUGd8N0+72+ONE201306

24. Dubischar-Kastner K, Eder S, Kaltenboeck A, Klade C, Schuller E, Wolfl G. Safety and Immunogenicity of the Inactivated Japanese Encephalitis Vaccine IXIARO®, IC51, in Filipino Children aged 2 months to < 18 years. Presented at the 4th Northern European Conference on Travel Medicine, June 2012, Abstract P.9. Available at http://nectm.com/wp-content /uploads / BookofAbstracts.pdf

25. Dubischar-Kastner K, Eder S, Kaltenboeck A, Klade C, Schuller E, Wolfl G. Interim Safety and Immunogenicity Data for the Inactivated Japanese Encephalitis Vaccine IXIARO®, IC51, in Children from JE non-endemic countries. Presented at the 4th Northern European Conference on Travel Medicine, June 2012, Abstract P.9. Available at http://nectm.com/wp-content / uploads / BookofAbstracts.pdf

26. Vashishtha VM, Kalra A, Bose A, Choudhury P, Yewale VN, Bansal CP et al. Indian Academy of Pediatrics (IAP) Recommended Immunization Schedule for Children Aged 0 through 18 years– India, 2013 and Updates on Immunization. Indian Pediatr 2013; 50: 1095–1108.

27. Appaiahgari MB, Vrati S. IMOJEV®: A Yellow fever virus-based novel Japanese encephalitis vaccine. Expert Rev Vaccines 2010; 9:1371–1384.

28. Halstead SB, Thomas SJ. New Japanese encephalitis vaccines: Alternatives to production in mouse brain. Expert Rev Vaccines 2011; 10:355–364.

■ ■ ■ ■ ■

MENINGOCOCCAL VACCINES

Reviewed by
Vipin M. Vashishtha, Vijay N. Yewale, MMA Faridi

Background

Meningococcal disease is caused by gram-negative bacterium *Neisseria meningitides*, which is a diplococcus and appears bean-shaped lying with flat surfaces adjacent to each other in a polysaccharide capsule. The meningococci are usually found as commensal organisms in the upper respiratory tract of about 10% of the population at any one time. Humans are the only natural reservoir. Meningococcal disease generally manifests as acute illness but chronic course with a mean duration of 6–8 weeks is also known.[1] The disease spectrum includes meningitis, septicemia, pneumonia, myocarditis, pericarditis, arthritis, and conjunctivitis, and occasionally may present as shock referred to as Waterhouse-Friderichsen syndrome with high risk of mortality.

There are 13 known serogroups but 90% of the disease causing isolates belong to serogroups A, B, C, Y and W-135. The burden of meningococcal disease is greatest in the African meningitis belt. In these areas, disease occurs endemically in the dry season and also as epidemics every 7–14 years and is usually due to serogroups A and W-135. Disease outbreaks in Hajj Pilgrims have been attributed to A and W-135. Disease in industrialized countries is primarily due to B, C and Y.[2] There is lack of information of serogroup responsible for endemic meningococcal disease in India. In one study from Postgraduate Institute of Medical Education and Research in Chandigarh, out of 12 isolates, eight were found to be serogroup A and four were serogroup C. However, Group A Meningococci is the cause of all the major investigated Indian epidemics Surat, Gujarat (1985–87), areas adjoining Delhi (1966–1985) and (2004–2005) and more recently in Meghalaya and Tripura in (2008–2009). (The most complete data available for this period is taken from an unpublished National Institute of Communicable Disease Report 2009)

Epidemiology of Meningococcal Disease

Global

In most countries, *Neisseria meningitidis* is recognized as a leading cause of meningitis and fulminant septicemia and a significant public health problem. Endemic disease mostly afflicts young children; older children, adolescents and young adults mainly suffer during epidemics. In developing countries the background incidence of meningococcal disease is 15–20 cases per 100,000 peoples per year. When three or more cases of meningococcal disease occur in a 3-month period in the same locality, amounting to at least 10 cases per 100,000 persons suffering from the disease, the situation is referred as outbreak. However, in sub-Saharan Africa disease is hyperendemic due to unknown reasons and is considered to have the highest annual incidence (10–25/100,000 population) of meningococcal disease in the world. In the African meningitis belt, the WHO definition of a meningococcal epidemic is >100 cases/100,000 population/year. In endemic regions, an incidence of >10 cases, 2–10 cases, and <2 cases per 100,000 population in a year characterizes high, moderate, and low endemicity, respectively.[3]

India

The data available on the background incidence of meningococcal disease in India are suggestive of low incidence of meningococcal disease. Hence routine childhood vaccination with meningococcal vaccine is unlikely to be a priority. As per the review by Sinclair et al,[4] which is a comprehensive study of epidemiology of Meningococcal disease in India, prevalence of meningitis is 1.5–3.3% of all acute hospital admissions in children. *N. meningitidis* is the third most common cause of bacterial meningitis in India in children less than 5 years of age and is responsible for an estimated 1.9% of all cases regardless of age.[4] Prevalence of septicemia according to one study is 2.8% of all hospital admissions.

As far as the epidemic disease is concerned, the outbreaks have occurred at a periodicity of 20 years. Since 2005, there has been an increase in the number of meningococcal disease outbreaks reported throughout India: New Delhi (2005–2009), Meghalaya (2008–2009) and Tripura (2009). Outbreaks have been reported more in temperate northern than tropical southern regions of the country. Large cities of North and coastal areas like Mumbai, Kolkata are being affected sparing the southern and central regions. The important contributing factors in major outbreaks may be overcrowding or vulnerability to importation of new strain or a suitable climatic condition.

The epidemic period coincides with dry season of November – March and the cases reduce with onset of monsoon and again increase November onwards. The outbreaks occur when season is dry and temperature is low. The seasonal cycle is similar to that seen in Africa where outbreaks peak in hot dry season and subside during monsoon. The mechanism of this seasonal association is not exactly known. This happens probably because during dry period there is damage to natural mucosal barrier of the nasopharynx increasing the chance of invasion of viral infection. Most of the epidemics in India are reported from the drier northern parts of the country than the more humid south is supportive of the current view of seasonal effect of the disease.

The existence of endemic disease is recognized, but much of the epidemiological data that are available are collected during outbreaks. Unlike *Haemophilus influenzae* type b (Hib), *N. meningitidis* affects adults, as well as children. Endemic disease occurs primarily in infants and children with highest attack rates in infants aged 3–12 months. The disease is found more in males than females. During an epidemic condition, the disease is found in children; however, shift is noted from young children to adolescents and young adults later. Overall carriage rates are lower in India than other similar settings. High carriage rates are found in close household contacts which justifies chemoprophylaxis. High carrier rates are also found among the military recruits.

Severe meningococcal disease is associated with high case-fatality rates (5–15%) even where adequate medical facilities are available and permanent disability occurs in about 19% survivors. Chemoprophylactic measures are in general insufficient for the control of epidemics because secondary cases comprise only 1–2% of all meningococcal cases.

Vaccines

Two types of meningococcal vaccines have been developed but all are not available everywhere (Table 1). They include:

*   Meningococcal polysaccharide vaccines (MPSV).

*   Meningococcal polysaccharide-protein conjugate vaccines (MCV).

Table 1: Licensed meningococcal vaccine in India

Type	Valency/strains covered	Brand/ manufacturer	Nature and diluent	Dose and schedule
Polysaccharide (MPSV: Meningococcal polysaccharide vaccine)	**Quadrivalent** (serogroups A, C, W-135 & Y; contains individual capsular polysaccharides 50 µg each)	Mencevac, GSK; QuadriMening, BioMed	Lyophilized, sterile distilled water	0.5ml by SC or IM, recommended in children > 2 years[#], revaccination after 3–5 years in high-risk children and adolescents
	Bivalent (serogroups A and C contains individual capsular polysaccharides 50 µg each)	MPV A+C, GSK; BiMeningo, BioMed		
MCV: Meningococcal conjugate vaccine	Quadrivalent (serogroups A, C, W135 & Y; contains 4 µg each of A, C, Y and W-135 polysaccharide conjugated to 48 µg of diphtheria toxoid)	Menactra, Sanofi Pasteur	Lyophilized, sterile distilled water	0.5 ml by deep IM, revaccination after 3–5 years in high-risk children and adolescents
	*Monovalent (Serogroup A: 10 µg of group A polysaccharide conjugated to 10–33 µg tetanus toxoid, with alum as adjuvant and thiomersal as preservative)	Serum Institute of India, Ltd	Lyophilized vaccine	0.5 ml intramuscular single administration for individuals 1–29 years of age

*   Going to be available very soon in Indian market.

\#   In infants aged 3 months to 2 years, MPSV may be given if risk for meningococcal disease is high, e.g. outbreaks/ close household contacts: 2 doses 3 months apart.

Meningococcal polysaccharide vaccines (MPSV)

These are either bivalent (A+C) or quadrivalent (A, C, Y, W-135) and contain 50 µg of each of the individual polysaccharides, available in lyophilized form, reconstituted with sterile water and stored at 2 to 8°C. These "T cell independent" vaccines do not induce immunological memory and the response in children younger than two years is poor. Hence these are indicated for adults and children older than 2 years (only under special circumstances in children three months to two years of age).

Immunogenicity and efficacy: The antibody responses to each of the four polysaccharides in the quadrivalent vaccine are serogroup-specific and independent. Protective antibody levels are usually achieved within 10–14 days of vaccination. The serogroup A polysaccharide induces antibody in some children as young as 3 months of age, although a response comparable with that occurring in adults is not achieved until age 4–5 years. The serogroup C component is poorly immunogenic in children less than 2 years. The serogroup A and C vaccines have good immunogenicity, with clinical efficacy rates of 85% or higher among children 5 years of age or older and adults. Serogroup Y and W-135 polysaccharides are safe and immunogenic in older children and adults; although clinical protection has not been documented.

Duration of protection: In infants and young children aged < 5 years, measurable levels of antibodies against serogroup A and C polysaccharides, as well as clinical efficacy, decrease substantially during the first 3 years after a single dose of the vaccine administration. Antibody levels also decrease in healthy adults, but antibodies are still detectable up to 10 years after immunization. Multiple doses of serogroup A and C polysaccharides are known to cause immunologic hyporesponsiveness (impact on clinical efficacy has not been demonstrated). Vaccines are safe and most common side effects are local pain and redness at site of injection.

Meningococcal conjugate vaccines (MCVs)

Currently two different types of meningococcal conjugate vaccines (MCVs) are licensed in India. The first which is now readily available in private market also, is a quadrivalent vaccine Menactra® from Sanofi Pasteur, and another a monovalent serogroup A vaccine from Serum Institute of India (SII).

Quadrivalent Meningococcal Polysaccharide-protein Conjugate vaccine (MenACWY-D, Menactra®, manufactured by Sanofi Pasteur)

This is a quadrivalent (A, C, W-135, Y) meningococcal conjugate vaccine using diphtheria toxin as carrier protein (A, C, W-135, Y-D), and was licensed in the US in 2005. However, it is licensed in India only in 2012 for use among persons aged 2 through 55 years. In 2011, ACIP recommended a two-dose series of this vaccine for use in children aged 9–23 months. This vaccine contains 4 µg each of A, C, Y and W-135 polysaccharide conjugated to 48 µg of diphtheria toxoid. A single dose of 0.5 ml IM is recommended. This vaccine had comparable immunogenicity to the previously used polysaccharide vaccine.

Recent estimates of the effectiveness of MenACWY-D, the first licensed quadrivalent vaccine suggest that within 3 to 4 years after vaccination, effectiveness is 80% to 85% (5, 6). There is higher level of evidence for protection of children against meningococcal disease in children > 12 months to < 5 years of age than in individuals aged ≥ 5 years.[6]

It is associated with minor local side effects such as pain, and swelling. Guillain-Barré Syndrome (GBS) was noted as a possible but unproven risk in some adolescents following immunization with quadrivalent MCV. As a precaution, people who have previously been diagnosed with GBS should not receive this vaccine unless they are at increased risk of meningococcal disease. Interference with PCV13 immune responses was noted when MenACWY-D and PCV13 were administered simultaneously in patients with asplenia. Hence, CDC ACIP has now recommended that at least one month interval should be kept between PCV13 and MenACWY-D, and PCV13 should be administered first.[7]

A safety and immunogenicity open label non-randomized multi-centric phase III trial (unpublished) of the vaccine has also been conducted amongst Indian children, adolescents and adults, and preliminary results on the safety has been found to be similar to US trials. However, no data on immunogenicity is available so far.

Monovalent serogroup A conjugate vaccine (PsA–TT, MenAfriVac®, manufactured by SII)

Meningococcal Group A Conjugate Vaccine is a lyophilized vaccine of purified meningococcal A polysaccharide covalently bound to tetanus toxoid (TT) which acts as a carrier protein. It contains 10 µg of group A polysaccharide conjugated to 10–33 µg tetanus toxoid, with alum as adjuvant and thiomersal as preservative.[3] The vaccine is licensed in India since 2009 and prequalified by WHO in 2010, but the company has not launched this inexpensive vaccine (costing around half a cent to African nations) in India so far. It has been used in large campaigns in Burkina Faso, Mali, and Niger and is being progressively introduced in other countries of the African meningitis belt.[3]

It should be administered as a single intramuscular injection of 0.5 mL to individuals 1–29 years of age.[3] The possible need for a booster dose has not yet been established. Persons who have previously received a meningococcal A polysaccharide-containing vaccine can be vaccinated with the conjugate vaccine.

The single intramuscular dose induces functional antibody titres against meningococcal serogroup A which are significantly higher and more persistent than those induced by a corresponding polysaccharide vaccine.[8-10] The immune response seems to persist for a long time. The vaccine has also got a very good safety profile. There is moderate level of evidence for protection of children against Group A meningococcal disease in both children >12 months to < 5 years, and in individuals ≥ 5 years old.[11] Furthermore, the vaccine has demonstrated a great effectiveness when used in Africa in campaigns.

Three characteristics of conjugate vaccines are believed to be important for establishing long-term protection against a bacterial pathogen: Memory response, herd immunity, and circulating antibody. Recent data from the United Kingdom indicate that although vaccination primes the immune system, the memory response after exposure might not be rapid enough to protect against meningococcal disease. After initial priming with a serogroup C meningococcal conjugate vaccine, a memory response after a booster dose was not measurable until 5–7 days later. The incubation period for meningococcal disease usually is less than

3 days. In the UK, to date no evidence of herd immunity has been observed. Therefore, circulating bactericidal antibody is critical for protection against meningococcal disease.

There is sufficient evidence to indicate that approximately 50% of persons vaccinated 5 years earlier had bactericidal antibody levels protective against meningococcal disease. Therefore, more than 50% of persons immunized at age 11 or 12 years might not be protected when they are at higher risk at ages 16 through 21 years. This is the reason why ACIP has now recommended revaccination with MCV in individual previously vaccinated with either conjugated or polysaccharide vaccine who are at increased risk for meningococcal disease. Those who are vaccinated at age greater than 7 years should be vaccinated 5 years after their previous meningococcal vaccine and those vaccinated at ages 2–6 years should be revaccinated 3 years after their previous meningococcal vaccine. Persons who remain in one of these increase risk group indefinitely should continue to be revaccinated at 5 year interval.

Recommendations for use

Individual use

The current epidemiology and burden of meningococcal diseases in India do not justify routine use of meningococcal vaccines. Meningococcal vaccines are recommended only for certain high-risk conditions and situations as enumerated below in children aged 2 years or more (3 months or older if risk of meningococcal disease is high, e.g. outbreaks/ close household contact). Conjugate vaccines are preferred over polysaccharide vaccines due to their potential for herd protection and their increased immunogenicity, particularly in children < 2 years of age.

IAP recommendations on dosage in different categories[12]

IAP now recommends the use of MCVs in different categories as per following description:

A. During disease outbreaks

Due to the limited efficacy of polysaccharide vaccines in children < 2 years of age, conjugate vaccines should be used for protection of those aged 12–24 months, particularly for Men A disease. Since majority of documented outbreaks in India are caused by Men A, monovalent MCV, like PsA-TT should be employed in mass vaccination.

B. *Vaccination of persons with high-risk conditions/situations*

i. *Children with terminal complement component deficiencies:* A two-dose primary series of MCV administered 8–12 weeks apart is recommended for persons aged 24 months through 55 years with persistent deficiencies of the late complement component pathway. A booster dose should be administered every 5 years. Children who receive the primary series before their seventh birthday should receive the first booster dose in 3 years and subsequent doses every 5 years.

ii. *Children with functional/anatomic asplenia/hyposplenia (including sickle cell disease):* Administer 2 primary doses of either MCV with at least 8 weeks between doses for individuals aged 24 months through 55 years. Vaccination should ideally be started two weeks prior to splenectomy.

iii. *Persons with Human Immunodeficiency Virus:* Administer two doses at least eight weeks interval.

iv. *Laboratory personnel and healthcare workers:* Who are exposed routinely to *Neisseria meningitides* in solutions that may be aerosolized should be considered for vaccination. A single dose of MCV is recommended. A booster dose should be administered every 5 years if exposure is ongoing.

v. *Adjunct to chemoprophylaxis:* In close contacts of patients with meningococcal disease (healthcare workers in contact with secretions, household contacts, day care contacts) single dose of appropriate group MCV is recommended.

C. *International travellers*

i. *Students going for study abroad:* Some institutions have policies requiring vaccination against meningococcal disease as a condition of enrolment (mandatory in most universities in the USA). Persons aged ≤21 years should have documentation of receipt of a MCV not more than 5 years before enrolment. In the US, ACIP recommends routine vaccination of all adolescents with single dose of MCV4 at age 11–12 years, with a booster dose at age 16 years (available online at http://www.cdc.gov/vaccines/pubs/acip-list.htm). For further details, follow the catch-up recommendations for meningococcal vaccination of the destination country.

ii. *Hajj pilgrims:* Vaccination in the 3 years before the date of travel is required for all travellers to Mecca during the annual Hajj. The quadrivalent vaccine is preferred for Hajj pilgrims and international travellers as it provides added protection against emerging W-135 and Y disease in these areas. A single dose 0.5 ml IM is recommended in age group 2–55 years.

iii. *Travellers to countries in the African meningitis belt:* A single dose of monovalent or quadrivalent vaccine is recommended. Conjugate vaccine is preferred to polysaccharide vaccine. A booster dose of MCV is needed if the last dose was administered 5 or more years previously.

Public health perspectives

Sporadic outbreaks of meningococcal disease have been recorded for last many decades in India. These outbreaks, particularly the larger epidemics have almost universally been caused by serogroup A meningococci.[4] The committee believes that the new affordable serogroup A containing monovalent conjugate vaccine manufactured by SII should have a critical role in containing future epidemics. The Academy urges the Indian manufacturer to make this vaccine available in the country also. The quadrivalent MenACWY-D should be employed in individuals having certain high-risk conditions and situations and amongst international travellers (mentioned above).

Conjugated meningococcal vaccines are more expensive than polysaccharide vaccines. Based on results on the cost effectiveness of use of MCVs in Australia, Canada, Netherlands, Portugal, Switzerland and United Kingdom, it was found that one dose in the second year of life was more cost-effective than a 3-dose infant schedule. The most cost-effective strategy was routine vaccination of children at 12 months of age combined with a catch-up campaign for all children and adolescents < 18 years of age.[13] No studies on the cost-effectiveness of meningococcal vaccination have yet been reported from India.

Decision to Vaccinate

If ≥ 3 cases of meningococcal disease have occurred in either an organization or a community-based outbreak during <3 months (starting at the time of the first confirmed or probable case), a primary attack rate should be calculated. Attack rate per 100,000 = (number of primary confirmed or probable cases during a 3-months period)/ (number of population at risk) x 100,000.

If the attack rate of the meningococcal disease exceeds 10 cases per 100,000 persons, then vaccination of the population at risk should be considered keeping following factors in sight.[2]

Outbreak identification and management

A decision to carry out mass vaccination is based on following conditions:

- Completeness of case reporting and number of possible cases of meningococcal disease for which bacteriologic confirmation or serogroup data are not available.

- Occurrence of additional cases of meningococcal disease after recognition of a suspected outbreak (e.g., if the outbreak occurred 2 months before and if no additional cases have occurred, in which case vaccination might be unlikely to prevent additional cases of meningococcal disease).

- Logistic and financial considerations. Because available vaccines are not effective against *N. meningitdis* serogroup B, vaccination should not be given during serogroup B outbreaks.

- Age consideration. Meningococcal disease outbreaks occur predominantly among persons aged < 30 years. If the calculated attack rate remains > 10 cases/100,000 persons, then vaccination should be considered for part or all of the population at risk.

- In infants aged 3 months to 2 years, meningococcal conjugate vaccine is preferred.

- If MCVs are not available, two doses of meningococcal polysachharide vaccine (MPSV) given 3 months apart may be administered if the risk for meningococcal disease is high, e.g. outbreaks/ close household contacts.

- Close child contacts of a patient with invasive meningococcal disease are at increased risk of secondary disease. Most secondary cases occur within the first 72 hours after presentation of the index case; risk of secondary disease decreases to near baseline by 10–14 days.[5] Meningococcal vaccines may be given to pregnant women during epidemics.

When there is an outbreak, immediate action is taken by the government. However, in remote areas of the country, more time may be needed before remedial action can be expected. A rapid response team typically composed of an epidemiologist, medical professionals and a microbiologist is deployed to identify individuals exposed to meningococcal disease and to assist in the management of those who are ill. If diagnostic facilities are not available locally, as is typical for remote areas of the country, patient samples are sent to the NCDC for diagnostic testing. During the recent outbreaks, microscopy, culture and latex agglutination tests were employed for diagnosis PCR was also used to investigate the epidemic in New Delhi.

Outbreak prevention and control actions in India

Following actions should be urgently taken after confirmation of an outbreak:

- Active case surveillance
- Early diagnosis and prompt treatment
- Chemoprophylaxis of close contacts (household members, healthcare professionals)
- Fostering disease awareness within the community, including the need to seek medical help and to avoid crowded places
- Respiratory isolation of patients for 72 hours
- Reactive vaccination of high-risk groups

> ## MENINGOCOCCAL VACCINE
>
> - Recommended only for certain high-risk group of children, during outbreaks, and international travellers, including students going for study abroad and travellers to Hajj and sub-Sahara Africa.
>
> - Both Meningococcal conjugate vaccines (Quadrivalent MenACWY-D, Menactra® by Sanofi Pasteur and monovalent group A, PsA–TT, MenAfriVac® by Serum Institute of India) and polysaccharide vaccines (bi- and quadrivalent) are licensed in India. PsA–TT is not freely available in market.
>
> - Conjugate vaccines are preferred over polysaccharide vaccines due to their potential for herd protection and their increased immunogenicity, particularly in children < 2 years of age.
>
> - As of today, quadrivalent conjugate and polysaccharide vaccines are recommended only for children 2 years and above.
>
> - Monovalent group A conjugate vaccine, PsA–TT can be used in children above 1 year of age.

References

1. Granoff DM, Gilsdorf JR. *Neisseria meningitidis*. In Kleigman RM, Stanto BFn, St Geme JW, Schor NF, Behrman RE (Eds). Nelson textbook of Pediatrics, 19th Edition. Pliladelphia: Elsevier Saunders. 2012, p 929–933.

2. Centres for Disease Control and Prevention. Meningococcal disease. Available from: http://wwwnc.cdc.gov/travel/yellowbook/2014/chapter-3-infectious-diseases-related-to-travel/meningococcal-disease.

3. Meningococcal vaccines: WHO position paper, November 2011. Wkly Epidemiol Rec. 2011; 86:521–539.

4. Sinclair D, Preziosi MP, Jacob John T, Greenwood B. The epidemiology of meningococcal disease in India. Trop Med Int Health. 2010;15: 1421–1435.

5. Macneil J R. Early estimate of the effectiveness of quadrivalent meningococcal conjugate vaccine. The pediatric infectious disease journal, 2011, 30:451–455.

6. Grading of scientific evidence– Table VI a & b (efficacy of quadrivalent meningococcal conjugate vaccines). Available at http://www.who.int/entity/immunization/meningococcal_grad_efficacy.pdf

7. Kroger A. General Recommendations on Immunization. ACIP Presentation Slides: February 2013 Meeting. Available from: http://www.cdc.gov/vaccines/acip/meetings/downloads/slides-feb-2013/02-GenRecs-Kroger.pdf

8. Kshirsagar N, Mur N, Thatte U, Gogtay N, Viviani S, Préziosi MP, et al. Safety, immunogenicity, and antibody persistence of a new meningococcal group A conjugate vaccine in healthy Indian adults. Vaccine 2007; 25 (Suppl 1): A101–7.

9. Sow SO, Okoko BJ, Diallo A, Viviani S, Borrow R, Carlone G, et al. Immunogenicity and safety of a meningococcal A conjugate vaccine in Africans. N Engl J Med 2011; 364: 2293–2304.

10. Hirve S, Bavdekar A, Pandit A, Juvekar S, Patil M, Preziosi MP, et al. Immunogenicity and safety of a new meningococcal A conjugate vaccine in Indian children aged 2–10 years: A phase II/III double-blind randomized controlled trial. Vaccine. 2012; 30: 6456–6460.

11. Grading of scientific evidence — Table IV a and b (efficacy of MenA conjugate vaccine). Available from: http://www.who.int/entity/immunization/meningococcalA_grad_efficacity. Pdf

12. Vashishtha VM, Kalra A, Bose A, Choudhury P, Yewale VN, Bansal CP et al. Indian Academy of Pediatrics (IAP) Recommended Immunization Schedule for Children Aged 0 through 18 years — India, 2013 and Updates on Immunization. Indian Pediatr 2013; 50: 1095–1108.

13. Welte R, Trotter CL, Edmunds WJ, Postma MJ, Beutels P. The role of economic evaluation in vaccine decision making: Focus on meningococcal group C conjugate vaccine. Pharmacoeconomics. 2005; 23(9): 855–874.

14. Zalmanovici Trestioreanu A, Fraser A, Gafter-Gvili A, Paul M, Leibovici L. Antibiotics for preventing meningococcal infections. Cochrane Database Syst Rev. 2011 Aug 10; (8): CD004785.

■ ■ ■ ■ ■ ■

RABIES VACCINES

3.17

Reviewed by
Anuradha Bose, Panna Choudhury

Background

Rabies is a viral zoonosis and is transmitted by bites, scratches, and licks on mucous membrane or non-intact skin by a rabid animal. Human-to-human transmission occurs almost exclusively as a result of organ or tissue transplantation (including cornea). The incubation period usually averages 4–6 weeks but can range from five days to 6 years. The disease is uniformly fatal and only 6 survivors have been reported in world literature.

In India the most common transmitting animal is dog, accounting for more than 96% cases. As per the national multicentric rabies survey done in 2003,[1] about 17 million animal bites occur annually out of which 20,000 human rabies deaths occur in India. About 35% of these are in children.[2]

Analysis of Million Death Study by verbal autopsy in 2005, estimated that there were 12,700 (99% CI 10,000 to 15,500) symptomatically identifiable furious rabies deaths in India. Most rabies deaths were in males (62%), in rural areas (91%), and in children below the age of 15 years (50%). The overall rabies mortality rate was 1.1 deaths per 100,000 population (99%CI 0.9 to 1.4). As verbal autopsy is not likely to identify atypical or paralytic forms of rabies, figure of 12,700 deaths due to classic and clinically identifiable furious rabies underestimates the total number of deaths due to this virus. One third of the national rabies deaths were found in Uttar Pradesh (4,300) and nearly three quarters (8,900) were in 7 central and south-eastern states: Chhattisgarh, Uttar Pradesh, Odisha, Andhra Pradesh, Bihar, Assam, and Madhya Pradesh.[3]

Care of animal bite wounds

The first step is thorough cleansing of the wound with soap and flushing under running water for 10 minutes. This should be followed by irrigation with a virucidal agent such as 70% alcohol or povidone iodine. Antimicrobials and tetanus toxoid should be given if indicated. Rabies immunoglobulin (RIG) should be infiltrated in and around the wound in category 3 bites (for information on exposure categories, see post-exposure prophylaxis below). Any suturing of wound should be avoided. When suturing is unavoidable for purpose of hemostasis, it must be ensured that RIG has been infiltrated in the wound prior to suturing.

Passive Immunization

Rabies immunoglobulin (RIG)

Dosage: It contains specific anti-rabies antibodies that neutralize the rabies virus and provide passive protection till active immunity is generated. There are 2 types of RIG:

(1) Human rabies immunoglobulin (HRIG— dose is 20 U/kg body weight, maximum dose 1500 IU); and

(2) Equine rabies immunoglobulin (ERIG—dose is 40 U/kg, maximum dose 3000 IU).

HRIG is preferred, but if not available/ unaffordable ERIG may be used. Most of the new ERIG preparations are potent, safe, highly purified and less expensive as compared to HRIG but do carry a small risk of anaphylaxis. As per latest recommendations from WHO, skin testing prior to ERIG administration is not recommended as skin tests do not accurately predict anaphylaxis risk and ERIG should be given whatever the result of the test.[4]

Administration: RIG is indicated in all cases of category 3 wounds where it should be infiltrated thoroughly into and around the wound. The remaining part if any is to be injected IM into the deltoid region or anterolateral aspect of thigh away from the site of vaccine administration to avoid vaccine neutralization. In case RIG dose (quantity) is insufficient for adequate infiltration of extensive or multiple wound, it may be diluted with equal volume of normal saline so that all the wounds can be thoroughly infiltrated.

If RIG could not be given when antirabies vaccination was began, it should be administered as early as possible but no later than the seventh day after the first dose of vaccine was given. From the eight day onwards, RIG is not indicated since an antibody response to the vaccine is presumed to have occurred. RIG is also not indicated in individuals who have received pre-exposure prophylaxis/ post-exposure prophylaxis in the past.[5]

Adverse reactions: Include tenderness/stiffness at the injection site, low-grade fever; sensitization may occur after repeated injections.

Active Immunization

Rabies vaccines

Vaccines are the mainstay for prevention of development of rabies. The nerve tissue vaccines, used earlier, are no longer available due to poor efficacy and life threatening adverse effect of neuroparalytic reactions.

The currently available vaccines are:

*   the Cell Culture Vaccines (CCV) and include Purified Chick Embryo Cell Vaccine (PCECV), Human Diploid Cell Vaccine (HDCV), Purified Vero Cell Vaccine (PVRV);

*   Purified Duck Embryo Vaccine (PDEV).

It is to be noted that all CCVs and PDEV should have potency (antigen content) greater than 2.5 IU per intramuscular dose irrespective of whether it is 0.5 mL or 1.0 mL vaccine by volume.

Efficacy & effectiveness: The vaccines are available in lyophilized form with sterile water as diluent, are stable for 3 years at 2 to 8°C and should be used within 6 hours of reconstitution. All CCVs have almost equal efficacy and any one of these can be used. These vaccines induce protective antibodies in more than 99% of vaccinees following pre-/ post-exposure prophylaxis. Studies from many countries in South-East Asia have established the effectiveness of CCVs for both pre-exposure and post-exposure prophylaxis. In both pre-exposure and post-exposure use, these vaccines induce an adequate antibody response in almost all individuals. Prompt post-exposure use of CCVs combined with proper wound management and simultaneous administration of

RIG is almost invariably effective in preventing rabies, even following high-risk exposure. However, delays in starting or failure to complete correct prophylaxis may result in death, particularly following bites in highly innervated regions, such as the head, neck or hands, or following multiple wounds.[2]

Duration of immunity: The current CCVs possess immunological memory after vaccination, and individuals who had received their primary series 5–21 years previously showed good anamnestic responses after booster vaccination even when antibodies are no longer detectable.[2]

Adverse effects: The main adverse effects are local pain, swelling and redness and less commonly fever, headache, dizziness and gastrointestinal side effects. Systemic hypersensitivity reactions in vaccines have been reported with HDCV particularly following booster injections but not with PCEC/ PVRV. Intradermal vaccination may cause more local irritation as compared to the intramuscular route.[2]

Post-exposure prophylaxis (PEP)

Post-exposure prophylaxis is a medical urgency and is indicated following a significant contact (discussed in detail below) with any warm-blooded animal. These include dogs, cats, cows, buffaloes, sheep, goats, pigs, donkeys, horses, camels, foxes, jackals, monkeys, mongoose, bears and others. In case of bites by pet animals, PEP may be deferred only if the pet at the origin of exposure is more than a year old and has a vaccination certificate indicating that it has received at least 2 doses of a potent vaccine, the first not earlier than 3 months of age and the second within 6 to 12 months of the first dose and in the past 1 year. If vaccination is deferred, the pet should be observed for 10 days; if the dog shows any sign of illness during the observation period, the patient should receive full rabies post-exposure prophylaxis urgently. Rabies due to rodent bites has not been reported in India till date and post-exposure prophylaxis is not normally recommended for these bites. Post-exposure prophylaxis should be initiated as soon as possible and should not be delayed till results of lab tests or animal observation is available.

Because rabies is a lethal disease there are no contraindications for post-exposure prophylaxis including infants, pregnant and lactating women. Persons presenting several days/ months/ years after the bite should be managed in a similar manner as a person who has been bitten recently (with RIG if indicated) as rabies may have a long incubation period and the window of opportunity for prevention remains. Rabies exposure may be classified as per WHO into three categories (Table 1).[2]

Table 1: Categories of rabies exposure and recommended post-exposure prophylaxis

Category	Type of contact	Type of exposure	Recommended post-exposure prophylaxis (PEP)
I	Touching or feeding of animals. Licks on intact skin.	None	None, if reliable case history is available
II	Nibbling of uncovered skin. Minor scratches or abrasions without bleeding.	Minor	Wound management + Anti-rabies vaccine
III	Single or multiple transdermal bites or scratches, licks on broken skin. Contamination of mucous membrane with saliva (i.e. licks)	Severe	Wound management + Rabies immunoglobulin + Anti-rabies vaccine

NB. Bites from unidentified animal is classified as category III

Schedule of vaccination

The standard schedule (Essen protocol) is five doses on days 0, 3, 7, 14 and 30, with day '0' being the day of commencement of vaccination. A regimen of 5 one-mL doses of HDCV or PCECV should be administered IM to previously unvaccinated persons. The first dose of the 5-dose course should be administered as soon as possible after exposure. This date is then considered day 0 of the post-exposure prophylaxis series. Additional doses should then be administered on days 3, 7, 14, and 28 after the first vaccination.

A reduced, four-dose vaccine schedule (1-1-1-1-0) for healthy people is supported by the peer-reviewed literature, unpublished data, epidemiological reviews and expert opinion. This shortened Essen regimen, consisting of one dose on each of days 0, 3, 7 and 14, may be used as an alternative for healthy, fully immune competent, exposed people provided they receive wound care plus rabies immunoglobulin in category III as well as in category II exposures and a WHO-prequalified rabies vaccine.[6]

Most interruptions in the vaccine schedule do not require re-initiation of the entire series. For most minor deviations from the schedule, vaccination can be resumed as though the patient were on schedule. For example, if a patient misses the dose scheduled for day 7 and presents for vaccination on day 10, the day 7 dose should be administered that day and the schedule resumed, maintaining the same interval between doses. In this scenario, the remaining doses would be administered on days 17 and 31. The dose is same at all ages and is 1 ml IM for HDCV, PCEV, PDEV and 0.5 ml for PVRV.

Alternative 4 day schedule, if an accelerated response is considered necessary

As an alternative, the 2-1-1 regimen (Zagreb schedule) may be used. Two doses are given on day 0 in the deltoid muscle, right and left arm. In addition one dose in the deltoid muscle on day 7 and one on day 21 are administered. This schedule is, however, not approved for use in India.

Any of the CCVs may be used intramuscularly in anterolateral thigh or the deltoid. Rabies vaccine should never be injected in the gluteal region. Interchange of vaccines is permitted only in special circumstances but should not be done routinely. If RIG is not available, then two doses of the vaccine may be given on day 0 (this is, however, not a substitute for RIG). If the animal remains healthy over a 10 days observation period, further vaccination may be discontinued. It is, however, desirable to administer one more dose on day 28 in order to convert to the pre-exposure prophylaxis schedule.

Intradermal vaccination

Intradermal vaccination is cost effective alternative to intramuscular vaccination as the dose required is only 0.1 ml. Only two of the three WHO prequalified vaccines—purified Vero cell rabies vaccine and purified Chick Embryo cell vaccine—have been shown to be safe and effective when administered intradermally at a dose of 0.1 ml in a WHO-recommended pre- or post-exposure prophylaxis regimen.[7] The intradermal schedules have been used successfully in Thailand, Philippines and Sri Lanka.[8–10] The unit dose of 0.1 ml for ID should have at least 0.25 units.[11]

Based on the recommendations of the expert group as well as WHO, the Drug Controller General of India (DCGI) has recently decided to allow ID route administration of tissue culture based anti-rabies vaccine for post-exposure prophylaxis in a phased manner in certain government anti-rabies centers. The schedules permitted in the 1st phase include the Thai Red Cross Regimen (2-2-2-0-1-1, two intradermal doses on the deltoid on days 0, 3, 7 and 1 dose on day 30 and 90) and the Updated Thai Red Cross Regimen (2-2-2-0-2-0, two doses on days 0, 3, 7 and 30). Another schedule not currently approved by DCGI is the 8 site regimen (8-0-4-0-1-1, 8 intradermal doses on each upper arm, each lateral lower abdominal quadrant, each thighs and each suprascapular regions on day 0, 4 doses on day 7 on each thigh and upper arm and 1 dose on day 30 and 90 on upper arm). Vaccines currently recommended for ID route administration in India are purified Vero cell rabies vaccine and purified Chick Embryo cell vaccine. The intradermal route should not be used for immunocompromised patients and those on chloroquine therapy.

The criteria for selection of anti-rabies center for ID use are:

a) Attendance of minimum 50 patients per day for post-exposure prophylaxis

b) Has adequately trained staff to give ID inoculation

c) Can maintain cold chain and ensure adequate supply of disposable syringes and needles.

Intradermal administration is not recommended in individual practice. Also it does not make economic sense to practice it for individual cases.

Post-exposure prophylaxis of immunocompromised patients

Several studies of patients with HIV/AIDS have reported that those with low CD4 (< 200 counts) will mount a significantly lower or no detectable neutralizing antibody response to rabies. In such patients and those in whom the presence of immunological memory is no longer assured as a result of other causes, proper and thorough wound management and antisepsis accompanied by local infiltration of RIG followed by anti-rabies vaccination are of utmost importance. Even immune compromised patients with category II exposures should receive RIG in addition to a full post-exposure vaccination. Preferably, if the facilities are available, anti-rabies antibody estimation should be done 10 days after the completion of course of vaccination.

Post-exposure prophylaxis in previously vaccinated children: Children who have received previously full rabies post-exposure prophylaxis or pre-exposure vaccination (either IM or ID route) with CCV/PDEV should be given only two booster doses, either intramuscularly (0.5 ml/1 ml) or intra-dermally (0.1 ml at a single site only, using ID compliant vaccine) on days 0 and 3. This is given irrespective of the duration of previous vaccination. In these situations treatment with RIG is not necessary. As always proper wound toilet should be done. In case of travellers who cannot come for the second visit, a single visit 4 site (0.1 mL X 4 ID sites, two deltoids and two suprascapular or thighs) ID booster may be given as per WHO recommendation.[2]

Pre-exposure prophylaxis

Pre-exposure prophylaxis is particularly important where the exposure may be unrecognized (lab) or unreported (children). Pre-exposure prophylaxis eliminates need for RIG (awareness, cost and availability of RIG is a problem). It also reduces post-exposure prophylaxis to two doses only. Pre-exposure prophylaxis is recommended for certain high-risk groups enumerated below.

- ***Continuous exposure:*** Lab personnel involved with rabies research and production of rabies biologics. Source and exposure may be unrecognized.

- ***Frequent exposure:*** Veterinarians, laboratory personnel involved with rabies diagnosis, medical and paramedical staff treating rabies patients, dog catchers, zoo keepers, and forest staff.

- ***Infrequent exposure***
  - Postmen, policemen, courier boys
  - Travellers to rabies endemic countries particularly those who intend to backpack/ trek.

Most Indian children are at risk for rabies. Therefore, ACVIP recommends offering pre-exposure prophylaxis to children at high risk of rabies exposure after discussion with parents.

Any of the tissue culture vaccines can be given for this purpose. Three doses are given intramuscularly in deltoid/ anterolateral thigh on days 0, 7 and 28 (day 21 may be used if time is limited but day 28 preferred). The intradermal schedule is 0.1 ml of any vaccine by the intradermal route on day 0, 7 and 21/28.

Routine assessment of anti-rabies antibody titer after completion of vaccination is not recommended unless the person is immunocompromised. It is desirable to monitor antibody titers every 6 months in those with continuous exposure and every year in those with frequent exposure. A booster is recommended if antibody levels fall below 0.5 IU/ml. When serologic testing is not available booster vaccination every 5 years is an acceptable alternative. For re-exposure at any point of time after completed (and documented) pre- or post-exposure prophylaxis, two doses are given on days 0 and 3. RIG should not be used as it may inhibit the relative strength or rapidity of an expected anamnestic response.

Public Health perspective

Rabies is not a notifiable disease and the deaths reported by national authorities represent mainly the deaths reported from hospitals. Further atypical paralytic cases are likely to remain undiagnosed. As such number of deaths due to rabies may be many times more than the reported numbers. Rabies is endemic in all states of India except Andaman, Nicobar and Lakshadweep Island. Although all age groups are susceptible, rabies is most common in children aged < 15 years.[2] Children are also at high risk, as they likely to have contact with stray or community-owned animals while playing outside and may not be able to ward off aggressive animals as easily as an adult.

There are no estimates of number of dogs and cats in India. In an epidemiological study about 17% of households reported having a pet/domesticated dog and the pet dog: man ratio was 1: 36. Pet dog care/management practices were not satisfactory with a low veterinary consultation (35.5%) and vaccination (32.9%). A high proportion of bite victims did not wash their wounds with soap and water (39.5%). The recourse to indigenous treatment (45.3%) and local application to wound (36.8%/) was quite prevalent.[12]

Currently a few activities are underway to prevent rabies occurrence in humans and to control rabies in dogs, even when the

---

RABIES VACCINES

- Only modern tissue culture vaccines (MTCVs) and IM routes are recommended for both 'post-exposure' and 'pre-exposure' prophylaxis in office practice.

- Post-exposure prophylaxis is recommended following a significant contact with dogs, cats, cows, buffaloes, sheep, goats, pigs, donkeys, horses, camels, foxes, jackals, monkeys, mongoose, bears and others. Rodent bites do not require post-exposure prophylaxis in India.

- *Post-exposure prophylaxis:*
  - ➤ MTCVs are recommended for all category II and III bites.
  - ➤ Dose: 1.0 ml intramuscular (IM) in antero-lateral thigh or deltoid (never in gluteal region) for Human Diploid Cell Vaccine (HDCV), Purified Chick Embryo Cell (PCEC) vaccine, Purified Duck Embryo Vaccine (PDEV); 0.5 ml for Purified Vero Cell Vaccine (PVRV). Intradermal (ID) administration is not recommended in individual practice.
  - ➤ Schedule: 0, 3, 7, 14, and 30 with day '0' being the day of commencement of vaccination. A sixth dose on day 90 is optional and may be offered to patients with severe debility or those who are immunosuppressed.
  - ➤ Rabies immunoglobin (RIG) along with rabies vaccines are recommended in all category III bites.
  - ➤ Equine rabies immunoglobin (ERIG) (dose 40 U/kg) can be used if human rabies immunoglobin is not available.

- *Pre-exposure prophylaxis:*
  - ➤ Three doses are given intramuscularly in deltoid/ anterolateral thigh on days 0, 7 and 28 (day 21 may be used if time is limited but day 28 preferred).
  - ➤ For re-exposure at any point of time after completed (and documented) pre- or post-exposure prophylaxis, two doses are given on days 0 and 3.
  - ➤ RIG should not be used during re-exposure therapy.

IAP Guidebook on Immunization 2013–14

number of human deaths, especially involving children is high. Further, most of the patients do not receive the necessary rabies immunoglobulin because of a perennial global shortage and because of its high price, so that it is unaffordable and not easily available at all places.

Canine rabies can be eliminated, as demonstrated in North America, western Europe, Japan and many areas of South America and parts of Asia. It is, however, still widespread, occurring in over 80 countries and territories, predominantly in the developing world.[7] In the current scenario it is unlikely that in India, national dog rabies control would be instituted in foreseeable future.

Mass vaccination of dogs is the singlemost cost-effective intervention to control and eliminate canine rabies. However, successful rabies control also depends on measures such as managing the dog population, mainly by promoting responsible dog ownership; compulsory notification of rabies in humans and animals; ensuring the availability of reliable diagnostic procedures; conducting postmortem examinations to confirm the cause of death in people suspected to have been infected with rabies, etc.[2] These pre-requisites are not feasible to fulfil by public health department of the country which is non-existent in almost all states. Hence, this is not a doable option, and under the circumstance, ACVIP is of the opinion that universal pre-exposure vaccination especially for children could reduce the number of human rabies dramatically. Use of intradermal vaccination would bring down the vaccine cost for the program substantially.

References

1. Assessing Burden of Rabies in India, WHO sponsored national multi-centric rabies survey. Association for Prevention and Control of Rabies in India. May 2004, Available from http://rabies.org.in/rabies/wp-content/uploads/2009/11/whosurvey.pdf. (Accessed on Dec 11, 2013)

2. Rabies vaccines. WHO position paper. Wkly Epidemiol Record, 2010; 85: 309–320.

3. Suraweera W, Morris SK, Kumar R, Warrell DA, Warrell MJ, et al. (2012) Deaths from Symptomatically Identifiable Furious Rabies in India: A Nationally Representative Mortality Survey. PLoS Negl Trop Dis 6(10): e1847. doi:10.1371/journal.pntd. 0001847 Available from http://www.plosntds.org/article/info%3Adoi%2F10.1371%2Fjournal.pntd.0001847 (Accessed on Dec 13, 2013)

4. WHO Expert Consultation on Rabies: first report. Geneva, World Health Organization, 2005 (WHO Technical Report Series, No. 931; http://whqlibdoc.who.int/trs/ WHO_TRS_931_eng.pdf).

5. Manual on RIG administration. Association for prevention and control of rabies in India. Bangalore, 2009. Available from http://rabies.org.in/rabies/ wp-content/uploads/2009/11/Manual-on-Rabies-Immunoglobulin-Administration.pdf. (Accessed on Dec 11, 2013)

6. Rupprecht CE, Briggs D, Brown CM, Franka R, Katz SL, Kerr HD et al. Use of a reduced (4-dose) vaccine schedule for postexposure prophylaxis to prevent human rabies: recommendations of the advisory committee on immunization practices. MMWR Recomm Rep. 2010; 59(RR-2): 1–9.

7. WHO Technical Report Series 982. WHO Expert Consultation on Rabies. Second report 2013. Available from http://apps.who.int/iris/bitstream/ 10665/85346/1/9789241209823_eng.pdf. (Accessed on Dec 13, 2013)

8. Briggs DJ, Banzhoff A, Nicolay U, Sirikwin S, Dumavibhat B, Tongswas S, et al. Antibody response of patients after postexposure rabies vaccination with small intradermal doses of purified chick embryo cell vaccine or purified Vero cell rabies vaccine. Bull World Health Organization 2000; 78: 693–698.

9. Quiambao BP, Dimaano EM, Ambas C, Davis R, Banzhoff A, Malerczyk C. Reducing the cost of post-exposure rabies prophylaxis: efficacy of 0.1 ml PCEC rabies vaccine administered intradermally using the Thai Red Cross post-exposure regimen in patients severely exposed to laboratory-confirmed rabid animals. Vaccine 2005; 23: 1709–1714.

10. Madhusudana SN, Sanjay TV, Mahendra BJ, Sudarshan MK, Narayana DH, Giri A, et al. Comparison of safety and immunogenicity of purified chick embryo cell rabies vaccine (PCECV) and purified vero cell rabies vaccine (PVRV) using the Thai Red Cross intradermal regimen at a dose of 0.1 ML. Hum Vaccin. 2006 ;2(5):200–204.

11. Human and dog rabies prevention and control: Report of the WHO/Bill & Melinda Gates Foundation consultation, Annecy, France, 7–9 October 2009. Geneva, World Health Organization. (WHO/HTM/NTD/NZD/2010.1); http://whqlibdoc.who.int/hq/2010/WHO_HTM_NTD_NZD_2010.1_eng. pdf.). (Accessed on Dec 11, 2013)

12. Sudarshan MK, Mahendra BJ, Madhusudana SN, Ashwoath Narayana DH, Rahman A, Rao NS, et al. An epidemiological study of animal bites in India: results of a WHO sponsored national multi-centric rabies survey. J Commun Dis 2006; 38: 32–39.

■ ■ ■ ■ ■ ■

CHOLERA VACCINES

3.18

Reviewed by
Ajay Kalra, Panna Choudhury

Background

Cholera is an important public health problem in developing countries with poor sanitation and hygiene as well as in displaced populations. It occurs over a wider geographic area in India than was previously recognized.

The predominant strain is *V. cholerae* O1 (classical and El tor biotype); while *V. cholerae* O139 is an emerging strain. As per WHO estimates, the annual burden of cholera is estimated to be 3–5 million cases with 100,000–130,000 deaths.[1] Cholera is endemic in India where only 25% of the population has access to piped water supply and sanitation. A recent meta analysis reports 22,000 cases a year in India (probably a gross underestimate) of which most is *V. cholerae* O1 El tor biotype.[2] In a longitudinal community base surveillance study in urban slums of Kolkata, the overall incidence was around 1.6/1000 person years with the highest incidence seen in children below the age of 2 years (8.6/1000 per year) followed 6.2 in the age group 2–5 years and 1.2 in those aged above 5 years.[3]

As a WHO collaborating Center for Diarrhoeal Diseases Research and Training, the National Institute of Cholera and Enteric Diseases (NICED) received during 1990–2007, a total of 16,624 strains of *Vibrio cholerae* from 24 states, of which 7,225 strains of *V. cholerae* were included for phage typing study. The states which sent strains for consecutive three years in any block were Andhra Pradesh, Delhi, Goa, Gujarat, Karnataka, Madhya Pradesh, Maharashtra, Punjab, Rajasthan, Tamil Nadu and West Bengal. Highest numbers of strains were received from Maharashtra, followed by West Bengal, and the pathogen was isolated every year during the study period. No strains were submitted from Puducherry in this period. From 2004 onwards, the new states entering in the cholera map were Kerala and Sikkim. Of the total strains received, 96.5 per cent strains were serotyped as Ogawa and the remaining 3.5 per cent were Inaba. Periodic shifts in the occurrence of Ogawa and Inaba serotypes in a given area are usual phenomenon and are thought to be a consequence of population-level immunity patterns.[4]

Vaccines

The parenteral killed vaccine which had a 3-month efficacy of 45% is no longer recommended. The WC-rBS vaccine available internationally as Dukoral oral vaccine and widely used in travellers is a vaccine comprising of killed *V. cholerae* O1 with recombinant b subunit of cholera toxoid. Because of similarity in the structure and functions of the cholera toxin B, this vaccine provides cross protection against enterotoxigenic *E. Coli*. However, this vaccine is no longer marketed in India and not produced any more.[5]

The variant WC-rBS vaccine first developed and licensed in Vietnam comprises only killed whole cell *V. cholerae* O1 (classical and El Tor) and *V. cholerae* O139. There is no recombinant beta subunit toxoid and will therefore not protect against enterotoxigenic *E. Coli*. This inexpensive oral vaccine is administered as 2 doses 2 weeks apart and protection starts about 1 week after the last scheduled dose. A booster dose is recommended after 2 years. The vaccine has been demonstrated to have 50% efficacy for up to 3 years after vaccination. This vaccine (Shanchol-TM) is now manufactured and licensed in India for children above the age of 1 year. It is provided in a single dose vials and does not require a buffer or water for administration although water may be given. The vaccine has a shelf life of 2 years at 2–8°C.[1] The vaccine has a good safety profile.[6]

Efficacy and effectiveness: A randomized double blind immunogenicity trial with this vaccine in Kolkata demonstrated 4-fold rise in titers in 53% of adults and 80% of children with response to O139 being lesser than O1. Subsequently a very large cluster randomized double blind placebo-controlled trial in Kolkata demonstrated that the average per protocol efficacy of the vaccine to be 67% across all ages for up to 2 years after vaccination and 3 year efficacy is 65%. Subsequent study by the same authors has also shown that the cumulative efficacy at 5 years is also 65%.[7] No adverse effects were noted.

Recommendations for use

Public health perspectives

The ideal method for cholera control is improvement in water supply and sanitation. As recommended by the WHO cholera vaccines should be used preemptively in endemic areas and in crises situations and not as outbreak control measure. The inclusion of new killed whole cell oral cholera vaccine in the national immunization schedule is being considered by the policy makers in those areas where cholera is highly endemic, particularly the states of West Bengal and Orissa. Cost effectiveness analysis studies have demonstrated that vaccination of the 1–14 year old population would be highly cost effective.

Individual use

IAP ACVIP has included the cholera vaccine in the category of vaccines to be used under special circumstances only. These include travel to or residence in a highly endemic area and circumstances where there is risk of an outbreak such as during pilgrimages like Kumbh Mela, etc. Protection starts 2 weeks after receipt of the 2nd dose.

Cholera Vaccine

- Minimum age: One year [killed whole cell *Vibrio cholerae* (Shanchol)]

- Not recommended for routine use in healthy individuals; recommended only for the vaccination of persons residing in highly endemic areas and travelling to areas where risk of transmission is very high like Kumbh Mela, etc.

- Two doses 2 weeks apart for > 1 year old.

References

1. Cholera vaccines. WHO Position Paper 2010. Wkly Epidemiol Record 2010, 85, 117–128. Available from http:/ /www.who.int /wer /2010/wer8513.pdf. (Accessed on Dec 12, 2013)

2. Verma R, Khanna P, Chawla S. Cholera vaccine: New preventive tool for endemic countries. Hum Vaccin Immunother 2012; 8: 682–684.

3. Deen JL, von Seidlein L, Sur D, Agtini M, Lucas ME, Lopez AL et al. The high burden of cholera in children: Comparison of incidence from endemic areas in Asia and Africa. PLoS Negl Trop Dis 2008; 2(2): e173.

4. Sarkar BL, Kanungo S, Nair GB. How endemic is cholera in India? Indian J Med Res. 2012; 135: 246–248.

5. Lopez Al, Clemens JD, Deen J, Jodar L. Cholera Vaccines for the developing world. Hum Vaccine 2008; 4: 165–169.

6. Mahalanabis D, Lopez AL, Sur D, Deen J, Manna B, Kanungo S et al. A randomized, placebo-controlled trial of the bivalent killed, whole-cell, oral cholera vaccine in adults and children in a cholera endemic area in Kolkata, India. PLoS One 2008; 3: e2323.

7. Bhattacharya SK, Sur D, Ali M, Kanungo S, You YA, Manna B, et al. 5 year efficacy of a bivalent killed whole-cell oral cholera vaccine in Kolkata, India: A cluster-randomised, double-blind, placebo-controlled trial. Lancet Infect Dis 2013; 13: 1050–1056.

■ ■ ■ ■ ■ ■

YELLOW FEVER VACCINE

3.19

Reviewed by
Panna Choudhury, Abhay K. Shah

Background

Yellow fever is caused by Yellow fever virus (YFV), a single-stranded RNA virus that belongs to the genus Flavivirus. Vector-borne transmission occurs via the bite of an infected mosquito; primarily Aedes or Haemagogus spp. Humans infected with YFV experience the highest levels of viremia and can transmit the virus to mosquitoes shortly before onset of fever and for the first 3–5 days of illness.

Yellow fever (YF) is confined to certain countries in sub-Saharan Africa and Central/ South America and varies in severity from influenza like illness to severe hepatitis and hemorrhagic fever. Though yellow fever does not exist in India, conditions are conducive for its spread in the country due to the widespread presence of the mosquito vector *Aedes aegypti* and favorable environmental conditions. Therefore, the Government of India has strict regulations in place to restrict the entry of susceptible and unvaccinated individuals from yellow fever endemic countries.

Epidemiology and risk for travellers

Yellow fever (YF) is endemic and intermittently epidemic in sub-Saharan Africa and tropical South America. The growth of air travel has diminished the barriers to the spread of yellow fever, posing a threat to regions that have not previously been reached by the disease but are considered receptive, including the Middle East, coastal East Africa, the Indian subcontinent, Asia and Australia. The risk for travellers to endemic areas of Africa has been estimated as 23.8/100,000/week, in epidemic areas 357/100,000/week.[1] Data from US travellers produced an estimate of 0.4 to 4.3 cases/million travellers to yellow fever endemic areas.[2] Each year, approximately 9 million tourists travel to countries where yellow fever is endemic.[3] A traveller's risk for acquiring yellow fever is determined by various factors, including immunization status, location of travel, season, duration of exposure, occupational and recreational activities while travelling, and local rate of virus transmission at the time of travel. For a 2-week stay, the risks for illness and death due to yellow fever for an unvaccinated traveller travelling to an endemic area is as follows:[4]

- West Africa are 50 per 100,000 and 10 per 100,000, respectively
- South America are 5 per 100,000 and 1 per 100,000, respectively

CDC, WHO, and other yellow fever experts recently completed a comprehensive review of available data and revised the criteria and global maps designating the risk of YFV transmission. The new criteria establish 4 categories of risk for YFV transmission that apply to all geographic areas:

- endemic
- transitional
- low potential for exposure
- No risk.

Yellow fever (YF) vaccination is recommended for travel to endemic and transitional areas. Although vaccination is generally not recommended for travel to areas with low potential for exposure, it might be considered for a small subset of travellers whose itinerary could place them at increased risk for exposure to YFV (such as prolonged travel, heavy exposure to mosquitoes, or inability to avoid mosquito bites).

Based on the revised criteria for yellow fever risk classification, the current maps and country-specific information (Yellow Fever and Malaria Information, by Country) designate 3 levels of yellow fever vaccine recommendations: Recommended, generally not recommended, and not recommended.[5]

Vaccine

It is a live attenuated vaccine derived from 17D strain of the virus grown in chick 140 embryo cells. The 17D live yellow fever vaccine has been widely acknowledged as one of the most effective and safe vaccines in use and is the only commercially available yellow fever vaccine.[6]

The vaccine is available as a freeze dried preparation in single/multidose vials that should be stored at 2 to 8°C (must not be frozen) along with sterile saline as diluent. The reconstituted vaccine is heat labile, must be stored at 2 to 8°C and discarded within 1 hour of reconstitution. The dose is 0.5 ml subcutaneously. It can be safely given along with all other childhood vaccines.

Immunogenicity and efficacy are greater than 90%. Immunogenicity is lower in pregnancy and immunocompromised. Protective immunity is attained by 10th day of vaccination and lasts for at least 10 years. The International Health Regulations (IHR) published by the World Health Organization (WHO) requires revaccination at 10-year intervals.

Vaccine Safety and Adverse Reactions

10–30% of vaccines report mild systemic adverse events like low-grade fever, headache, and myalgias that begin within days after vaccination and last 5–10 days. Severe adverse reactions are rare and include immediate hypersensitivity reactions, characterized by rash, urticaria, bronchospasm, or a combination of these. Anaphylaxis after yellow fever vaccine is reported to occur at a rate of 1.8 cases per 100,000 doses administered.

Serious adverse events following immunization (AEFI) with YF vaccine fall into 3 categories:

1. Immediate severe hypersensitivity or anaphylactic reactions. Anaphylactic reactions have been estimated to occur in 0.8 per 100,000 vaccinations, most commonly in people with allergies to eggs or gelatine.

2. *Yellow fever vaccine-associated neurologic disease (YEL-AND):* YEL-AND represents a conglomerate of different clinical syndromes, including meningoencephalitis, Guillain-Barré syndrome, acute disseminated encephalomyelitis, bulbar palsy, and Bell palsy. The onset of illness for documented cases is 3–28 days after vaccination, and almost all cases were in first-time vaccine recipients. YEL-AND is rarely fatal. The incidence of YEL-AND in the United States is

0.8 per 100,000 doses administered. The rate is higher in people aged ≥60 years, with a rate of 1.6 per 100,000 doses in people aged 60–69 and 2.3 per 100,000 doses in people aged ≥ 70 years.

3. *Yellow fever vaccine-associated viscerotropic disease (YEL-AVD):* YEL-AVD is a severe illness similar to wild-type disease, with vaccine virus proliferating in multiple organs and often leading to multisystem organ failure and death. Since the initial cases of YEL-AVD were published in 2001, more than 50 confirmed and suspected cases have been reported throughout the world. YEL-AVD appears to occur after the first dose of yellow fever vaccine, rather than with booster doses. The onset of illness for YEL-AVD cases averaged 3 days (range, 1–8 days) after vaccination. The case-fatality ratio for reported YEL-AVD cases is 65%. The incidence of YEL-AVD in the United States is 0.4 cases per 100,000 doses of vaccine administered. The rate is higher for people aged ≥ 60 years, with a rate of 1.0 per 100,000 doses in people aged 60–69 years and 2.3 per 100,000 doses in people aged ≥ 70 years.[5,7,8]

The risk of neurologic and viscerotropic disease is higher and hence the vaccine is contraindicated in infants below the age of 6 months, those with history of thymus disease and the severely immunocompromised including HIV with severe immunosuppression (CD4 count < 15% of age-related cutoff) and

Table 1: Contraindications and precautions to yellow fever vaccine administration

CONTRAINDICATIONS	PRECAUTIONS
• Allergy to vaccine component • Age < 6 months • Symptomatic HIV infection or CD4 T-lymphocytes < 200/mm³ (or < 15% of total in children aged < 6 years)[1] • Thymus disorder associated with abnormal immune-cell function • Primary immunodeficiencies • Malignant neoplasms • Transplantation • Immunosuppressive and immunomodulatory therapies	• Age 6–8 months • Age ≥ 60 years • Asymptomatic HIV infection and CD4 T-lymphocytes 200–499/mm³ (or 15–24% of total in children aged < 6 years)[1] • Pregnancy • Breastfeeding

those with history of serious egg allergy. The vaccine is preferably avoided in infants aged 6–9 months, individuals aged > 65 years and in pregnant and lactating women. The contraindications and precautions to yellow fever vaccine is given in Table 1.

Recommendations for use

The vaccine is mandatory for all travellers to YF endemic zones as per International Health Regulations. All vaccinees receive an international certificate for vaccination duly dated, stamped and signed by the center administering the vaccine.

Dosage and administration: YF vaccines are given as a single dose (0.5 ml) and the manufacturers recommend that the vaccine be injected either subcutaneously or intramuscularly. The vaccination site is usually the lateral aspect of the upper part of the arm or the anterolateral aspect of the thigh in babies and very young children.[9]

Endemic countries: In these countries, YF vaccine is given to children at age 9–12 months at the same time as the measles vaccine. Vaccination should be provided to everyone aged ≥ 9 months in any area with reported cases.[9]

Travellers to endemic countries: Vaccine should be offered to all unvaccinated travellers aged > 9 months, travelling to and from at-risk areas, unless they belong to the group of individuals for whom YF vaccination is contraindicated.[9]

The vaccine is contraindicated in children aged < 6 months and is not recommended for those aged 6–8 months, except during epidemics when the risk of infection with the YF virus may be very high.[9]

International certificate of vaccination of prophylaxis (ICVP)

Travellers need to check with the destination country's embassy or consulate before departure. Under the revised IHR (2005), effective December 15, 2007, all state parties (countries) are required to issue a new ICVP. People who received a yellow fever vaccination after December 15, 2007, must provide proof of vaccination on the new ICVP. If the person received the vaccine before December 15, 2007, the original ICV card is still valid, provided that the vaccination was given < 10 years previously.

Failure to secure validations can cause a traveller to be quarantined, denied entry, or possibly revaccinated at the point of entry to a country. Revaccination at the point of entry is not a recommended option for the traveller.

This certificate of vaccination is valid for a period of 10 years, beginning 10 days after the date of vaccination. When a booster dose of the vaccine is given within this 10-year period, the certificate is considered valid from the date of revaccination. For medical contraindications, a physician who has decided to issue a waiver should fill out and sign the Medical Contraindications to Vaccination section of the ICVP. The traveller should be advised that issuance of a waiver does not guarantee its acceptance by the destination country. On arrival at the destination, the traveller may be faced with quarantine, refusal of entry, or vaccination on site.

India

Any traveller (except infants <9 months old) arriving by air or sea without a certificate is detained in isolation for up to 6 days if that person:

1) arrives within 6 days of departure from an area with risk of YFV transmission,

2) has been in such an area in transit (except those passengers and members of flight crews who, while in transit through an airport in an area with risk of YFV transmission, remained in the airport during their entire stay and the health officer agrees to such an exemption),

3) arrives on a ship that started from or touched at any port in an area with risk of YFV transmission up to 30 days before its arrival in India, unless such a ship has been disinsected in accordance with the procedure recommended by WHO, or

4) arrives on an aircraft that has been in an area with risk of YFV transmission and has not been disinsected in accordance with the Indian Aircraft Public Health Rules, 1954, or as recommended by WHO.

The following countries and areas are regarded as having risk of YFV transmission:

Africa: Angola, Bénin, Burkina Faso, Burundi, Cameroon, Central African Republic, Chad, Congo, Côte d'Ivoire, Democratic Republic of the Congo, Equatorial Guinea, Ethiopia, Gabon, The Gambia, Ghana, Guinea, Guinea-Bissau, Kenya, Liberia, Mali, Niger, Nigeria, Rwanda, Senegal, Sierra Leone, Sudan, Togo, and Uganda.

Americas: Bolivia, Brazil, Colombia, Ecuador, French Guiana, Guyana, Panama, Peru, Suriname, Trinidad and Tobago, and Venezuela.

Yellow Fever Vaccine

- Not for routine vaccination in India

- Only needed for those individuals travelling to sub-Saharan Africa and few tropical South American countries

- Live attenuated, single dose vaccine sufficient to confer sustained life-long protection

- Dose: 0.5 ml subcutaneously or intramuscularly in lateral aspect of the upper arm or the anterolateral thigh

- Minimum age: 9 months

References

1. Khromava AY, Barwick Eidex R, Weld LH, Kohl KS, Bradshaw RD, Chen RT, et al. Yellow fever vaccine: An updated assessment of advanced age as a risk factor for serious adverse events. Vaccine 2005; 23: 3256–3263.

2. Centers for Disease Control Prevention. Health information for international travel 2003–2004. Atlanta: U.S. Department of Health and Human Services, Public Health Service; 2003.

3. Barnett ED, Wilder-Smith A, Wilson ME. Yellow fever vaccines and international travelers. Expert Rev Vaccines 2008; 7: 579–587.

4. CDC. Yellow Fever Vaccine. MMWR 2010/59(RR07); 1-27. Available from http: //www.cdc.gov/mmwr/preview/mmwrhtml/rr5907a1.htm. (Accessed on Dec 15, 2013)

5. CDC. Infectious Diseases Related to Travel. Available from http://wwwnc.cdc.gov/travel/yellowbook/2014/chapter-3-infectious-diseases-related-to-travel/yellow-fever. (Accessed on Dec 15, 2013)

6. Kay A, Chen LH, Sisti M, Monath TP. Yellow fever vaccine seroconversion in travelers. Am J Trop Med Hyg. 2011; 85: 748–749.

7. Thomas RE, Lorenzetti DL, Spragins W, Jackson D, Williamson T. Reporting rates of yellow fever vaccine 17D or 17DD associated serious adverse events in pharmacovigilance data bases: systematic review. Curr Drug Saf. 2011; 6: 145–154.

8. Silva ML, Espírito-Santo LR, Martins MA, Silveira-Lemos D, Peruhype-Magalhães V, Caminha RC, et al. Clinical and Immunological Insights on Severe, Adverse Neurotropic and Viscerotropic Disease following 17D Yellow Fever Vaccination. Clinical and Vaccine Immunology 2010 ; 17 : 118–126.

9. Vaccines and vaccination against yellow fever; WHO Position Paper — June 2013. Wkly Epidemiol Rec 2013; 88, 269–284.

■ ■ ■ ■ ■ ■

SECTION
IV

Vaccination of
Special Groups

IMMUNIZATION OF ADOLESCENTS

Reviewed by
Panna Choudhury

Immune protection induced by vaccines given during infancy wanes over the years.[1, 2] This leads to higher than expected incidence of vaccine-preventable diseases in adolescents and young adults. Now vaccines have been developed suitable for administering at adolescent age giving protection against many diseases. Important adolescent vaccines related to pertussis, human papillomavirus and meningococcal vaccines are available in many countries including India.[3] IAP recommended vaccines for adolescents are given in Figure 1 and Table 1.

Table 1: IAP recommended vaccines for Adolescents (10 years to 18 years)

Vaccine	Schedule
Tadp/Td*	10 years
HPV^	10 to 12 years

* Tdap preferred to Td, followed by repeat Td every 10 years (Tdap to be used once only)
^ Only females, three doses at 0, 1 or 2 (depending on the vaccine used) and 6 months

Pertussis vaccination

Pertussis vaccination in adolescents is of particular interest, as it is known that the humoral and cellular immunity evoked by vaccines tends to wane after some years, and this has been confirmed by immunological and clinical studies in recent years.[4, 5] Many factors determine the speed at which the immunity wanes like vaccination schedule and the type of vaccine. Acellular pertussis vaccine have shown to provide shorter-lasting protection than wP vaccine.[6] Waning of protection has led to increase in incidence of pertussis in older children and adolescents worldwide. In fact, adolescents have become the main cause of the spread of pertussis in the community and the persistently high incidence of disease infants, who are at the greatest risk of severe disease because they are not fully vaccinated.[7] Pertussis vaccination in adolescents has many advantages including significant lowering of new cases among vaccinated subjects. A retrospective analysis of pertussis cases reported in the USA between 1990 and 2009 showed that the introduction of TdaP for adolescents in 2005 was associated with a considerable decrease in the number of cases involving subjects aged 11–18 years.[8] It is also expected that unvaccinated or partially vaccinated infants may benefit from herd effect due to reduction of circulation of pertussis organism. In Australia, where TdaP was administered to all high school students during the 2008–2009 epidemic, there was a decrease in pertussis case reports involving adolescents and infants aged <6 months.[9] Adolescents vaccination is also highly cost effective: Vaccination of all in 10–19 years age group in the USA in 2005 may prevent 0.4–1.8 million cases of pertussis and lead to 10-year savings of $0.3–1.6 billion.[10] A detailed account on pertussis immunization through all ages is available in a recent publication.[11]

HPV vaccine

HPV vaccination in adolescents also deserves special attention as HPV infection is the most common sexually transmitted infection in humans; HPV is closely associated with the development various anogenital and oropharyngeal cancers, of which cervical cancer is the most frequent; and most infections are acquired very early during adolescence, at the time of initial sexual activities.[12] HPV-related diseases are mainly due to a few types of HPV and two vaccines have been developed for use in many countries. One contains types 16 and 18 (mainly responsible for cervical cancer) and is known as bivalent HPV vaccine, and the other one has additionally types 6 and 11 (responsible for anogenital warts), known as qudrivalent HPV vaccine. Extensive trials have shown that both the vaccines are safe and efficacious against pre-cancerous lesions due to types 16 and 18 of HPV in 90–100% of cases.[13] Regarding the time of administration, it is generally agreed that HPV vaccines should be administered to adolescents before they start to engage in sexual activity.[14] This is due to the fact that HPV vaccines are inactive against the types of HPV previously acquired by a vaccine recipient and because antibody responses are highest between the ages of nine and 15 years. There are national differences in the recommendations the subjects to whom HPV vaccine should be administered. The most recent recommendation in the USA considers that adolescents of both sexes should be vaccinated at the age of 11–12 years. Either bivalent or quadrivalent vaccine may be used for females, but only qudrivalent vaccine for males. American experts strongly support the vaccination of males because they think that it provides a direct benefit for the vaccinated subjects, including the prevention of genital warts and anal cancer, and an indirect benefit for females through herd immunity.[14] However, in Europe and many countries including India, HPV vaccine is only recommended for girls.

Current status of adolescent's immunization

In India, routine immunization given to young children is dismally low. National Family Health Survey 3 shows that only 43.5% children aged 12–23 months are fully immunized. There is also tremendous heterogeneity in state and district level immunization coverage in India with immunization coverage as low as 30% in Uttar Pradesh[15]. It is thus likely that many children reaches adolescent period with no or partial immunization. A large number of adolescents thus are at greater risk of vaccine preventable diseases as they are more exposed to infection due to greater mobility.

Considering that teenage pregnancy rate is very high in the country, catch up vaccination program of adolescents especially girls not only will protect them but will have a direct role in protecting young infants from diseases like pertussis. IAP recommendations for catch-up immunization in adolescents are given in Table 2 and Figure 1. There are also special circumstances for adolescents and vaccination schedule for these situations is given in Table 3. For adolescents going abroad, information on travellers vaccination can be obtained at CDC website at following link: http://wwwnc.cdc.gov/travel/.

Table 2: IAP recommendations for catch–up immunization in adolescents

Vaccine	Schedule
MMR	2 doses at 4–8 weeks interval@
Hepatitis B	3 doses at 0, 1 and 6 months#
Hepatitis A	2 doses at 0, 6 months (prior check for anti-HAV IgG may be cost effective)##
Typhoid	1 dose every 3 years**
Varicella	2 doses at 4–8 weeks interval

@ one dose if previously vaccinated with one dose
#, ## Combination of hepatitis B and hepatitis A may be used in 0, 1, 6 schedule
** A minimum interval of 3 years should be observed between 2 doses of typhoid vaccine

Table 3: IAP recommendations for adolescent immunization in special circumstances

Vaccine	Age recommended
Influenza vaccine	One dose every year
Japanese Encephalitis vaccine	Catch up up to 15 years@
PPSV23 (Pneumococcal) vaccine	2 doses 5 years apart*
Rabies vaccine 0, 3, 7, 14, 28 day	As soon as possible after exposure

@ Only in endemic area as catch up; * Maximum number of doses — Two

What is needed?

Getting adolescents vaccinated, however, is not an easy job who undergo great emotional and psychological development at this stage. A few adolescents seek medical care and that too from diverse set of medical specialties. Even in countries with well-established vaccination program, it has been difficult to implement 2nd dose MMR vaccine older children and adolescents leading to outbreak of measles.[16] For a successful adolescent vaccine program, there is need to sensitize medical professionals, health workers, parents and importantly adolescents. Currently, USA is the only country to issue recommendations for adolescent immunization which is regularly prepared and annually updated since 2005. These recommendations highlight the importance of catch-up strategies for adolescents who did not regularly complete their childhood immunizations as well as the need of vaccination in adolescents high-risk groups because of underlying chronic disease.[17]

Age ▶ Vaccine ▼	7–10 years	11–12 years	13–18 years
Tdap	1 dose (if indicated)	1 dose	1 dose (if indicated)
HPV1	See footnote 1	3 doses	Complete 3-dose series
MMR	Complete 2-dose series		
Varicella	Complete 2-dose series		
Hepatitis B	Complete 3-dose series		
Hepatitis A	Complete 2-dose series		
Typhoid	1 dose every 3 years		
Influenza vaccine	One dose every year		
Japanese Encephalitis vaccine	Catch-up up to 15 years		
Pneumococcal vaccine 2	See footnote 2		
Meningococcal vaccine3	See footnote 3		

	Range of recommended ages for all children
	Range of recommended ages for catch-up immunization
	Range of recommended ages for certain high-risk groups

Figure 1: IAP ACVIP recommended immunization schedule for adolescents, 2013 (with range)

Any dose not administered at the recommended age should be administered at a subsequent visit, when indicated and feasible. The use of a combination vaccine generally is preferred over separate injections of its equivalent component vaccines.

Footnotes:

1. Human papillomavirus (HPV) vaccines

Routine vaccination:

- Minimum age: 9 years
- HPV4 [Gardasil] and HPV2 [Cervarix] are licensed and available.
- Either HPV4 (0, 2, 6 months) or HPV2 (0, 1, 6 months) is recommended in a 3-dose series for females aged 11 or 12 years.

- HPV4 can also be given in a 3-dose series for males aged 11 or 12 years, but not yet licensed for use in males in India.
- The vaccine series can be started beginning at age 9 years.
- Administer the second dose 1 to 2 months after the first dose and the third dose 6 months after the first dose (at least 24 weeks after the first dose).

Catch-up vaccination:

- Administer the vaccine series to females (either HPV2 or HPV4) at age 13 through 45 years if not previously vaccinated.
- Use recommended routine dosing intervals (see above) for vaccine series catch-up.

2. Pneumococcal Vaccines

- Pneumococcal conjugate vaccine [PCV] and pneumococcal polysaccharide vaccine [PPSV] both are used in certain high-risk group of children.
- A single dose of PCV may be administered to children aged 6 through 18 years who have anatomic/functional asplenia, HIV infection or other immunocompromising condition, cochlear implant, or cerebral spinal fluid leak.
- Administer PPSV at least 8 weeks after the last dose of PCV to children aged 2 years or older with certain underlying medical conditions, including a cochlear implant.
- A single re-vaccination (with PPSV) should be administered after 5 years to children with anatomic/ functional asplenia or an immunocompromising condition.

3. Meningococcal vaccine

- Recommended only for certain high risk group of children, during outbreaks, and international travellers, including students going for study abroad and travellers to Hajj and sub-Saharan Africa.
- Both meningococcal conjugate vaccines (Quadrivalent MenACWY-D, Menactra® by Sanofi Pasteur and monovalent group A, PsA–TT, MenAfriVac® by Serum Institute of India) and polysaccharide vaccines (bi- and quadrivalent) are licensed in India. PsA–TT is not freely available in market.

References

1. Hinman AR, Orenstein WA, Schuchat A. Vaccine-preventable diseases, immunizations, and the Epidemic Intelligence Service. Am J Epidemiol 2011; 174 (11Suppl.): S16–22. [5]

2. Pichichero ME. Booster vaccinations: can immunologic memory outpace disease pathogenesis. Pediatrics 2009; 124: 1633–1641.

3. Schiller JT, Castellsagué X, Garland SM. A review of clinical trials of human papillomavirus prophylactic vaccines. Vaccine 2012; 30 Suppl. 5: F123–138.

4. Tartof SY, Lewis M, Kenyon C, White K, Osborn A, Liko J. Waning immunity to pertussis following 5 doses of DTaP. Pediatrics 2013; 131: e1047–1052.

5. Esposito S, Agliardi T, Giammanco A, Faldella G, Cascio A, Bosis S, et al. Long-term pertussis-specific immunity after primary vaccination with a combined diphtheria, tetanus, tricomponent acellular pertussis, and hepatitis B vaccine in comparison with that after natural infection. Infect Immun 2001; 69: 4516–4520.

6. Clark TA, Messonnier NE, Hadler SC. Pertussis control: time for something new.Trends Microbiol 2012; 20: 211–213.

7. Cherry JD. Epidemic pertussis in 2012—the resurgence of a vaccine preventabledisease. N Engl J Med 2012; 367: 785–787.

8. Skoff TH, Cohn AC, Clark TA, Messonnier NE, Martin SW. Early impact of the US Tdap vaccination program on pertussis trends. Arch Pediatr Adolesc Med 2012; 166: 344–349.

9. Quinn HE, McIntyre PB. The impact of adolescent pertussis immunization, 2004–2009: lessons from Australia. Bull World Health Organ 2011; 89: 666–674.

10. Hay JW, Ward JI. Economic considerations for pertussis booster vaccination in adolescents. Pediatr Infect Dis J 2005; 24 (6 Suppl.): S127–133.

11. Vashishtha VM, Bansal CP, Gupta SG. Pertussis Vaccines: Position Paper of Indian Academy of Pediatrics (IAP). Indian Pediatr 2013; 50: 1001–1009.

12. Forman D, de Martel C, Lacey CJ, Soerjomataram I, Lortet-Tieulent J, Bruni L, et al. Global burden of human papillomavirus and related diseases. Vaccine2012; 30 (Suppl. 5): F12–23.

13. Lehtinen M, Dillner J. Clinical trials of human papillomavirus vaccines and beyond. Nat Rev Clin Oncol 2013, http://dx.doi.org/10.1038/nrclinonc. 2013. 84

14. American Academy of Pediatrics. Policy Statement. HPV vaccine recommendations. Pediatrics 2012;129:602–606.

15. DLHS Policy Brief: http://www.rchiips.org/pdf/rch3plocy-brief.pdf

16. Cottrell S, Roberts RJ. Measles outbreak in Europe. BMJ 2011; 342: d3724.

17. Capua T, Katz JA, Bocchini Jr JA. Update on adolescent immunizations: selected review of US recommendations and literature. Curr Opin Pediatr 2013; 25: 397–406.

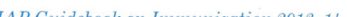

IMMUNIZATION IN SPECIAL SITUATIONS

Reviewed by
Panna Choudhury, Vipin M. Vashishtha

Immunization in the immunocompromised

The immunocompromised are in greater need for vaccines as they are more susceptible to infections. But at the same time the immunogenicity/ efficacy is lower and risk of adverse effects with live vaccines is higher. However, vaccination in an immunocompromised is rather safe than often perceived. General principles for vaccination of the immunocompromised are:[1-3]

- All inactivated vaccines can be given but immunogenicity and efficacy may be lower.

- In severe immunodeficiency, all live vaccines are contraindicated. In mild / moderate immunodeficiency, live vaccines may be given if benefits outweigh the risks. Patients administered live vaccines inadvertently prior to diagnosis of immunodeficiency should be watched for vaccine related adverse effects.

- Ideally, antibody titers should be checked post-immunization on regular basis, and regular boosters may be administered if needed.

- Higher doses, greater number of doses should be given if indicated (hepatitis B), antibody titers should be checked post immunization/ regular basis and regular boosters administered, if needed. For major/ contaminated wounds tetanus immunoglobulin is required in addition to TT even if 3 or more doses of TT have been received in the past.

- Household contacts of immunocompromised should not receive transmissible vaccines such as OPV but can safely receive other non-transmissible live vaccines such as MMR and varicella. All household contacts should be fully immunized including varicella and influenza to reduce risk of transmission to the immuncompromised.

- Some vaccines including pneumococcal, varicella (depending on degree of immunocompromise and in 2 doses 4–12 weeks apart), hepatitis A, inactivated influenza vaccines should be given if resources permit. There is at present insufficient data on the safety and efficacy of the rotavirus vaccine in the immunocompromised.

An international panel of experts prepared an evidenced-based guideline for vaccination of immunocompromised adults and children. These guidelines are intended for use by primary care and subspecialty providers who care for immunocompromised patients.[4]

HIV infection

Children infected by HIV are vulnerable to severe, recurrent, or unusual infections by vaccine preventable pathogens. The efficacy and safety of vaccines depends on the degree of immunodeficiency. Generally, CD4+ counts less than 200 cells/cumm is known to elicit minimal or no host response. Even if there is a better antibody response, such antibody response may wane at a faster rate in HIV infected person. Antiretroviral therapy can improve immune responses to vaccine but not to the levels of an uninfected subject. Live viral and bacterial vaccines pose an enhanced risk for uncontrolled replication of the vaccine strains.

Vaccination is usually safe and effective early in infancy before HIV infection causes severe immune suppression. The duration of protection may be compromised as there is impairment of memory response with immune attrition. In older HIV1 infected children and adults, the immune response to primary immunization may be less but protective immunity to vaccines received prior to the infection is usually maintained. However, immunity to measles, tetanus and hepatitis B wanes faster than other antigens.[5]

IAP, WHO, AAP, ACIP, and CDC recommend all the live vaccines in asymptomatic HIV1 infected children except BCG and OPV. However, in a symptomatic child all live vaccines are forbidden, but at times measles/MMR/varicella vaccines may be considered on individual merit. Yellow fever vaccine is contraindicated in both symptomatic and asymptomatic. For killed vaccines in an HIV infected child, ideally post-vaccination regular monitoring of seroconversion are desirable. In an HIV-infected child, there is a multifold enhanced risk of diseases like tuberculosis, hepatitis (A and B), measles, influenza, varicella, pneumococcal and meningococcal disease, hence in such situations a judicious and intelligent decision of the physician is warranted. Table 1 summarizes IAP recommendations for vaccination of HIV-infected children.

Table 1: IAP recommendations for immunization of HIV-infected children

Vaccine	Asymptomatic	Symptomatic
BCG	Yes (at birth)	No
DTwP/DTaP/ TT/Td/TdaP	Yes, as per routine schedule at 6, 10, 14 wks. 18 mo and 5 yrs	
Polio vaccines	IPV at 6, 10, 14 wks,12–18 mo and 5 yrs If indicated IPV to household contacts If IPV is not affordable, OPV should be given	
Measles	Yes, at 9 mo	Yes, if CD4+ count > 15%
MMR	Yes, at 15 mo and 5 yrs	Yes, if CD4+ count > 15%
Hepatitis B	Yes, at 0,1 and 6 mo	Yes, four doses, double dose, check for seroconversion and give regular boosters
Hib	Yes, as per routine schedule at 6 w, 10 w, 14 w and 12–18 mo	
Pneumococcal vaccines (PCV and PPSV23)	PCV: Yes, as per routine schedule at 6 w, 10 w, 14 w and 12–15 mo PPSV23: One dose 2 mo after PCV, 2nd dose five years after first dose (not more than two doses)	
Inactivated influenza vaccine	Yes, as per routine schedule beginning at 6 mo, revaccination every year	
Rotavirus vaccine	Insufficient data to recommend	
Hepatitis A vaccine	Yes	Yes, check for seroconversion, boosters if needed
Varicella vaccine	Yes, two doses at 4–12 wks interval	Yes, if CD4 count ≥ 15% Two doses at 4–12 wks apart
Vi-typhoid/ Vi-conjugate vaccine	Yes, as per routine schedule	
HPV vaccine	Yes (females only), as per routine schedule of 3 doses at 0, 1–2 and 6 months starting at 10 yrs of age	

Corticosteroids / other immunosuppressive therapy

Children receiving oral corticosteroids in high doses (prednisolone > 2 mg/kg/day or for those weighing more than 10 kg, 20 mg/day or its equivalent) for > 2 weeks should not receive live virus vaccines until the steroids have been discontinued for at least one month. Killed vaccines are safe but may be less efficacious. Children on lesser dose of steroids or those on inhaled or topical therapy may be safely and effectively given their age appropriate vaccines. Children on immunosuppressive therapy other than corticosteroids should avoid live vaccines during therapy unless benefits outweigh risks.[6]

Cancer cases on chemotherapy/ radiotherapy

Influence of cancer per se on immune function is minimal and does not contribute to a major extent in inducing immunocompromised state. Total immunoglobulin concentrations, specific antibody concentrations to already given vaccines are normal at the time of diagnosis indicating that the effect of the cancer on the adaptive immune system is likely to be small.[7] However, chemotherapy for cancer causes major secondary immunodeficiency. The effects of radiotherapy on immune function are likely to be small in comparison to chemotherapy. Vaccination requirements for cancer cases need special consideration as described below.[4]

- Patients aged ≥ 6 months with hematological malignancies or solid tumor malignancies except those receiving anti-B-cell antibodies or intensive chemotherapy, such as for induction or consolidation chemotherapy for acute leukemia should receive inactive influenza vaccine (IIV) annually.

- Pneumococcal conjugated vaccine (PCV) should be administered to newly diagnosed adults and children with hematological or solid malignancies. PPSV23 should be administered to adults and children aged ≥ 2 years at least 8 weeks after PCV.

- Inactivated vaccines (other than IIV) recommended for immunocompetent children can be considered for children who are receiving maintenance chemotherapy. However, vaccines administered during cancer chemotherapy should not be considered valid doses unless there is documentation of a protective antibody level.

IAP Guidebook on Immunization 2013–14

- Live viral vaccines should not be administered during chemotherapy.
- Three months after cancer chemotherapy, patients should be vaccinated with inactivated vaccines and the live vaccines for varicella, MMR as per schedule that is routinely indicated for immunocompetent persons. In regimens that included anti-B-cell antibodies, vaccinations should be delayed at least 6 months.

Quality of evidence and the grade of recommendation of vaccines for use in cancer cases based on Grading of Recommendations Assessment, Development and Evaluation (GRADE) system are given in Table 2.

Transplant Recipients

Hematopoietic Stem Cell Transplants (HSCT)

Recipients of HSCT are like the unimmunized as they have lost all memory responses during marrow ablation. Vaccination requirements for recipients of HSCT cases need special consideration as described below.[4]

- Three doses of tetanus/diphtheria-containing vaccine should be administered 6 months after HSCT. For patients aged ≥ 7 years, a dose of Tdap vaccine may be administered followed by 2 doses of Td vaccine.

- Three doses of IPV, Hib, hepatitis B vaccine should be administered 6–12 months after HSCT. If a post-vaccination anti-HBs concentration of ≥ 10 mIU/mL is not attained, hepatitis B vaccine course can be repeated.

- Three doses of PCV should be administered to adults and children starting at age 3–6 months after HSCT. At 12 months after HSCT, 1 dose of PPSV23 should be given provided the patient does not have chronic GVHD. For patients with chronic GVHD, a fourth dose of PCV can be given at 12 months after HSCT.

- One dose of influenza (IIV) should be administered annually to persons aged ≥ 6 months starting 6 months after HSCT and starting 4 months after if there is a community outbreak of influenza. For children aged 6 months–8 years, who are

Table 2: Immunization of patients with cancer in children (adapted and for details see Ref 4).

Vaccine	Prior to or during chemotherapy		Starting >3 mo post chemotherapy and >6 mo post anti-B-cell antibodies	
	Recommendation	Strength, evidence of quality	Recommendation	Strength, evidence of quality
DT, TT, aP, Td, Tdap	U	Weak, low	U	Strong, moderate
Hepatitis B	U	Weak, low	U	Strong, moderate
Hepatitis A	U	Weak, low	U	Strong, very low
Hib	U	Weak, low	U	Strong, moderate
PCV 13	R	Strong, low, very low	U	Strong, low
PPSV 23	R > 2 yrs	Strong, low	U	Strong, low
IIV	U	Strong-low-to mod	U	Strong, moderate
IPV	U	Weak, low	U	Strong, low
Meningo. Conj.	U	Weak, low	U	Strong, low
MMR-live*	X	Strong, moderate	Starting 3 mo: U	Strong, low
Varicella-live*	X	Strong, moderate	Starting 3 mo: U	Weak, very low
Rotavirus-live*	X	Strong, very low	Not applicable	

Note:

i. *Abbreviations: R, recommended—administer if not previously administered or not current; such patients may be at increased risk for this vaccine-preventable infection; U, usual—administer if patient not current with recommendations for dose(s) of vaccine for immunocompetent persons in risk and age categories; X, contraindicated.*

ii. ** These live vaccines should not be administered unless the vaccine is otherwise indicated as per updated recommendations AND the patient is not immunosuppressed AND there will be an interval of > 4 weeks prior to initiation of chemotherapy.*

iii. *Quality of evidence and the grade of recommendation are based on Grading of Recommendations Assessment, Development and Evaluation (GRADE) system.*

receiving influenza vaccine for the first time, 2 doses should be administered.

- Two doses of meningococcal conjugate vaccine (MCV4) should be administered 6–12 months after HSCT, if the risk of meningococcal disease is high.

- Three doses of HPV vaccine 6–12 months after HSCT for female patients aged 11–26 years may be considered.

- Live vaccines should not be administered to HSCT patients with active GVHD or ongoing immunosuppression.

Quality of evidence and the grade of recommendation of vaccines for use in hematopoietic stem cell transplant cases based on Grading of Recommendations Assessment, Development and Evaluation (GRADE) system are given in Table 3.

Solid organ transplants

The need for immunization in solid organ transplant (SOT) recipients can arise from three factors, each causing a suppression of the immune system: The immunosuppressive activity of the underlying disease (e.g., chronic renal failure), rejection of the organ graft, and the immunosuppressive therapy given after transplantation. Immunizations can be given to candidates awaiting transplantation because the immune response then is more likely to be less suppressed and the patient more likely to respond, after transplantation, or both.[8] Many of the conditions for which patients undergo organ transplantation are at least to some extent immunosuppressive, and vaccinations should be considered early during the disease. In general, standard vaccine series should be given to children awaiting SOT. Recipients of SOTs should complete all immunizations prior to transplant in accelerated schedules if needed. Vaccination with live vaccines should be completed at least 2 weeks prior to transplant. It is desirable that seroconversion be documented.

The optimal time to begin vaccine administration after transplantation is not defined. Immunosuppressive therapy is often most intense during the first couple of months and might influence the effect of vaccination. In the post-transplant period, all live vaccines are contraindicated. In patients where immunization has not been completed prior to transplant,

Table 3: Immunization of patients with hematopoietic stem cell transplant (HSCT) in children (adapted and for details see Ref. 4)

Vaccine	Post-HSCT		Post-HSCT	
	Recommendation	Strength, evidence of quality	Recommendation	Strength, evidence of quality
DT, TT, aP, Td, Tdap	U	Strong, low	R; < 7 yrs DTaP; 6 mo; 3 doses	Strong, low
DTaP, DT, Td, Tdap	U	U	R; > 7 yrs; 1 dose Tdap, then 2 doses Td; 6 mo	Weak, low
Hepatitis B	U	Strong, very low	R; 6 mo; 3 doses	Strong, moderate
Hepatitis A	U	Weak, low	R; 6 mo; 2 doses	Weak, low
Hib	U	Strong, moderate	R; 3 mo; 3 doses	Strong, moderate
PCV 13	R	Strong, low	R; 3 mo; 3 doses	Strong , low
PPSV 23	R	Strong, very low	R; > 12 mo post if no GVHD	Strong , low
IIV	U	Strong, low	R; 4 mo	Strong, moderate
IPV	U	Strong, very low	R; 3 mo; 3 doses	Strong, moderate
Meningo. Conj.	U	Strong, very low	R; 6 mo; 2 doses	Strong, low
MMR-live*	U	Strong, very low	X	Strong, low
Varicella-live*	U	Strong, low	X	Strong, low
Rotavirus-live	X	Weak, very low	X	Weak, very low

Note:

i.   *Abbreviations: R, recommended—administer if not previously administered or not current; such patients may be at increased risk for this vaccine-preventable infection; U, usual-administer if patient not current with recommendations for dose(s) of vaccine for immunocompetent persons in risk and age categories; X, contraindicated.*

ii. ** These live vaccines should not be administered unless the vaccine is otherwise indicated as per updated recommendations AND the patient is not immunosuppressed AND there will be an interval of > 4 weeks prior to initiation of chemotherapy.*

iii. *Quality of evidence and the grade of recommendation are based on Grading of Recommendations Assessment, Development and Evaluation (GRADE) system.*

vaccination with inactivated vaccines can recommence 6 months post-transplant when immunosuppression has been lowered. Boosters for inactivated vaccines should be given as per schedule/ when antibody levels wane (hepatitis A and B) starting 6 months post transplant. Annual influenza vaccination is recommended. All household and health care workers (HCW) contacts should be immunized against influenza and varicella. For details on strength of recommendation and quality of vaccines used in solid organ transplant cases see Table 4.

Asplenia or hyposplenia

Aslenia or hyposplenia may result from sickle cell disease or radiation therapy involving spleen. Children with asplenia/ hyposplenia are at high risk of serious infections with encapsulated organisms. Vaccination with pneumococcal (both conjugate and polysaccharide), Hib, meningococcal and typhoid vaccines is indicated in addition to all routine vaccines. In patients with planned splenectomy, vaccination should be initiated at least 2 weeks prior to splenectomy for achieving a superior immunologic response. In those who have undergone emergency splenectomy, studies indicate that vaccination done 2 weeks after splenectomy is associated with a superior functional antibody response as compared to vaccination immediately following surgery. All live vaccines may be safely given.[9, 10]

Congenital immunodeficiency

In patients with severe B cell immunodeficiency (X linked agammaglobulinemia) live vaccines including OPV, BCG, oral typhoid, and live attenuated influenza are contraindicated. Measles and varicella vaccines may be given but may be ineffective due to concomitant immunoglobulin therapy. Inactivated vaccines may be given but are ineffective. In less severe B cell deficiencies such as IgA and IgG subclass deficiency only OPV is contraindicated.

In patients with severe T cell immunodeficiencies (SCID) all live vaccines are contraindicated and all vaccines are ineffective. Patients who have received live vaccines especially BCG prior to diagnosis face an increased risk of complications including disseminated BCG disease. For patients with combined immunodeficiencies such as Di George syndrome, Wiskott Aldrich

Table 4: Vaccinations prior to or after solid organ transplant (adapted and for details see Ref. 4)

Vaccine	Post-HSCT		Post-HSCT	
	Recommendation	Strength, evidence of quality	Recommendation	Strength, evidence of quality
DTaP, Tdap	U	Strong, moderate	U, if not completed pre-transplant	Strong, moderate
Hepatitis B	U: Age 1–18 y R: ≥ 18 y	Strong, moderate Strong, moderate	R, if not completed pre-transplant*	Strong, moderate
Hepatitis A	U: Age 12–23 mo R: ≥ 2 y	Strong, moderate Strong, moderate	R, if not completed pre-transplant	Strong, moderate
Hib	U	Strong, moderate	U	Strong, moderate
PCV	U: Age ≤ 5 y R: Age ≥ 6 y**	Strong, moderate Strong, very low	U: Age 2–5 y R: Age ≥ 6 y if not administered pre-transplant**	Strong, moderate Strong , very low
PPSV 23	R: Age ≥ 2 y	Strong, moderate	R: Age ≥ 2 y, if not administered pre-transplant	Strong, moderate
Influenza (IIV)	U	Strong, moderate	U***	Strong, moderate
Polio-IPV	U	Strong, moderate	U	Strong, moderate
HPV	U: Females 11–26 y	Strong, moderate	U: Females 11–26 y	Strong, moderate
MMR- live	R^: 6–11 mo U^^: Age ≥ 12 mo	Weak, very low Strong, moderate	X	Strong, low
Varicella-live	R#: 6–11 mo U^^	Weak, very low Strong, low	X##	Strong, low
Rotavirus-live	U#	Strong, moderate	X	Strong, low

Abbreviations:

R, recommended—administer if not previously administered or not current; such patients may be at increased risk for this vaccine-preventable

infection; U, usual—administer if patient not current with annually updated IAP recommendations for inmuno-competent individuals; X, contraindicated.

*Consider hepatitis B vaccine for hepatitis B-infected liver transplant patients (weak, low).

**For patients aged ≥19 years who have received PPSV23, PCV13 should be administered after an interval of ≥1 year after the last PPSV23 dose (weak, low).

***Inactivated influenza vaccine may be administered to solid organ transplant recipients despite intensive immunosuppression (e.g., during the immediate post-transplant period) (weak, low).

^ Administer only if patient is not immunosuppressed and the timing is ≥4 weeks prior to transplant.

^^ Administer only if patient is non-immune, not severely immunosuppressed, and the timing is ≥4 weeks prior to transplant.

#Administer only if patient is not immunosuppressed and the timing is ≥4 weeks prior to transplant.

Selected seronegative patients with renal or liver transplant have been safely vaccinated.

and ataxia telangiectasia, inactivated vaccines may be given but live vaccines are contraindicated.

In complement deficiencies, all vaccines may be safely given; pneumococcal, Hib and meningococcal vaccines are particularly indicated.

In patients with phagocyte defects such as chronic granulomatous disease, only live bacterial vaccines are contraindicated, other vaccines may be safely and effectively given.[11]

Chronic diseases

Children with chronic neurologic, endocrinologic (diabetes), liver, renal, hematologic, cardiac, pulmonary and gastrointestinal disease are at increased risk of infections and serious infections. Live vaccines may be given safely in these children. These children should be offered pneumococcal, hepatitis A, varicella, influenza and rotavirus vaccines. The immunogenicity, efficacy and duration of protection of vaccines are lower than healthy children and hence if indicated higher antigen content/ more doses (hepatitis B), assessment for antibody response and frequent boosters (hepatitis A and B) are recommended. It is important to stress the role of hepatitis A vaccine in patients with liver disease, pertussis boosting in those with stable neurologic disease. Children with severe cardiac and pulmonary diseases should receive pneumococcal and annual influenza vaccines.[11]

Immunization in children with history of allergy

First time immunization with any vaccine is contraindicated in children with history of serious hypersensitivity/ anaphylaxis to any of vaccine components. The package label should always be checked for vaccine constituents which in addition to antigen include stabilizers/ buffers, preservatives, antibiotics and residue from the manufacturing process. Children with history of serious egg allergy should not receive influenza and yellow fever vaccines but can safely receive other vaccines including measles and MMR vaccines. Children with history of any hypersensitivity are at increased risk for allergic reactions with inactivated mouse brain Japanese Encephalitis vaccines and thus should be monitored carefully. Children who have had a serious hypersensitivity reaction/ anaphylaxis to a particular vaccine must never receive it again. A mild reaction is not a contraindication to vaccination. In any case all children should be watched for at least 15 minutes after vaccination for allergy and resuscitation equipment should be kept standby.[11]

Immunization in relation to antibody containing products (whole blood, packed red cells, plasma, immunoglobulin)

Live vaccines

Blood (e.g., whole blood, packed red blood cells, and plasma) and other antibody-containing blood products (e.g., immune globulin, hyperimmune globulin, and IGIV) can inhibit the immune response to live vaccines such as, measles and rubella vaccines for ≥3 months. The effect of blood and immune globulin preparations on the response to mumps and varicella vaccines is unknown; however, commercial immune globulin preparations contain antibodies to these viruses. Other live vaccines like Ty21a typhoid, rotavirus, yellow fever, LAIV, and zoster vaccines may be administered at any time before, concurrent with, or after administration of any immune globulin, hyperimmune globulin, or intravenous immune globulin (IGIV).[11] The length of time that interference with injectable live-virus vaccine can persist after the antibody-containing product depends upon the amount of antigen-specific antibody contained in the product. Therefore, after an antibody-containing product is received, live vaccines (other than oral Ty21a typhoid, LAIV, rotavirus zoster, and yellow fever) should be delayed until the passive antibody has degraded (Table 5).

If a dose of injectable live-virus vaccine (other than yellow fever and zoster) is administered after an antibody-containing product but at an interval shorter than recommended (Table 5), the vaccine dose should be repeated unless serologic testing is feasible and indicates a response to the vaccine. The repeat dose or serologic testing should be performed after the interval indicated for the antibody-containing product (Table 6). Although passively acquired antibodies can interfere with the response to rubella vaccine, the low dose of anti-Rho(D) globulin administered to postpartum women has not been demonstrated to reduce the response to the rubella vaccine.[11] Because of the importance of

Table 5: Guidelines for administering antibody-containing products* and vaccines [11]

Type of administration	Products administered	Recommended minimum interval between doses	
Simultaneous (during the same office visit)	Antibody-containing products and inactivated antigen	Can be administered simultaneously at different anatomic sites or at any time interval between doses	
	Antibody-containing products and live antigen	Should not be administered simultaneously.[†] If simultaneous administration of measles-containing vaccine or varicella vaccine is unavoidable, administer at different sites and revaccinate or test for seroconversion after the recommended interval (see Table 6)	
Non-simultaneous	Administered first	Administered second	
	Antibody-containing products	Inactivated antigen	No interval necessary
	Inactivated antigen	Antibody-containing products	No interval necessary
	Antibody-containing products	Live antigen	Dose related[†,§]
	Live antigen	Antibody-containing products	2 weeks[†]

* Blood products containing substantial amounts of immune globulin include intramuscular and intravenous immune globulin, specific hyperimmune globulin (e.g., hepatitis B immune globulin, tetanus immune globulin, varicella zoster immune globulin, and rabies immune globulin), whole blood, packed red blood cells, plasma, and platelet products.

† Yellow fever vaccine; rotavirus vaccine; oral Ty21a typhoid vaccine; live, attenuated influenza vaccine; and zoster vaccine are exceptions to these recommendations. These live, attenuated vaccines can be administered at any time before or after or simultaneously with an antibody-containing product.

§ The duration of interference of antibody-containing products with the immune response to the measles component of measles-containing vaccine, and possibly varicella vaccine, is dose related (see Table 6).

rubella and varicella immunity among women of child-bearing age, the postpartum vaccination of women without evidence of immunity to rubella or varicella with MMR or varicella vaccines should not be delayed because of receipt of anti-Rho(D) globulin or any other blood product during the last trimester of pregnancy or at delivery. These women should be vaccinated immediately after giving birth and, if possible, tested ≥ 3 months later to ensure immunity to rubella and measles.[11]

Interference might occur if administration of an antibody-containing product becomes necessary after administration of MMR or varicella vaccines. Usually, vaccine virus replication and stimulation of immunity occurs 1–2 weeks after vaccination. If the

Table 6. Recommended intervals between administration of antibody-containing products and measles- or varicella-containing vaccine, by product and indication for vaccination.[11]

Product/Indication	Dose (mg IgG/kg)	Route*	Recommended interval before measles-or varicella-containing vaccine† administration (months)
Tetanus IG	250 units (10 mg IgG/kg)	IM	3
Hepatitis A IG	0.02-0.06 mL/kg (3.3–10 mg IgG/kg)	IM	3
Hepatitis B IG	0.06 mL/kg (10 mg IgG/kg)	IM	3
Rabies IG	20 IU/kg (22 mg IgG/kg)	IM	4
Varicella IG	125 units/10 kg (60–200 mg IgG/kg) maximum 625 units	IM	5
Measles prophylaxis IG		IM	
Standard	0.25 mL/kg (40 mg IgG/kg)		5
Immunocompromised	0.50 mL/kg (80 mg IgG/kg)		6
Blood transfusion		IV	
RBCs, washed	10 mL/kg, negligible IgG/kg		None
RBCs, adenine-saline added	10 mL/kg (10 mg IgG/kg)		3
Packed RBCs (hematocrit 65%)§	10 mL/kg (60 mg IgG/kg)		6
Whole blood (hematocrit 35–50%)§	10 mL/kg (80–100 mg IgG/kg)		6
Plasma/platelet products	10 mL/kg (160 mg IgG/kg)		7
IVIG		IV	
Replacement therapy for immune deficiencies¶	300–400 mg/kg ¶		8
Immune thrombocytopenic purpura treatment	400 mg/kg		8
Postexposure varicella prophylaxis**	400 mg/kg		8
Immune thrombocytopenic purpura treatment	1000 mg/kg		10
Kawasaki disease	2 g/kg		11
Monoclonal antibody to respiratory syncytial virus [MedImmune]††	15 mg/kg	IM	None
Cytomegalovirus IGIV	150 mg/kg maximum	IV	6

Abbreviations:

HIV = human immunodeficiency virus; IG = immune globulin; IgG = immune globulin G; IGIV = intravenous immune globulin; mg IgG/kg = milligrams of immune globulin G per kilogram of body weight; IM = intramuscular; IV = intravenous; RBCs = red blood cells.

*   This table is not intended for determining the correct indications and dosages for using antibody-containing products. Unvaccinated persons might not be protected fully against measles during the entire recommended interval, and additional doses of IG or measles vaccine might be indicated after measles exposure. Concentrations of measles antibody in an IG preparation can vary by manufacturer's lot. Rates of antibody clearance after receipt of an IG preparation also might vary. Recommended intervals are extrapolated from an estimated half-life of 30 days for passively acquired antibody and an observed interference with the immune response to measles vaccine for 5 months after a dose of 80 mg IgG/kg.

†   Does not include zoster vaccine. Zoster vaccine may be given with antibody-containing blood products.

§   Assumes a serum IgG concentration of 16 mg/mL.

¶   Measles and varicella vaccinations are recommended for children with asymptomatic or mildly symptomatic HIV infection but are contraindicated for persons with severe immunosuppression from HIV or any other immunosuppressive disorder.

**   The investigational VariZIG, similar to licensed varicella-zoster IG (VZIG), is a purified human IG preparation made from plasma containing high levels of antivaricella antibodies (IgG). The interval between VariZIG and varicella vaccine is 5 months.

††   Contains antibody only to respiratory syncytial virus

---

interval between administration of any of these vaccines and subsequent administration of an antibody-containing product is < 14 days, vaccination should be repeated after the recommended interval (Tables 5 and 6) unless serologic testing indicates a protective antibody response.[11]

Inactivated Vaccines

Antibody-containing products interact less with inactivated vaccines, toxoids, recombinant subunit, and polysaccharide vaccines than with live vaccines. Therefore, administering inactivated vaccines and toxoids either simultaneously with or at any interval before or after receipt of an antibody-containing product should not substantially impair development of a protective antibody response (exception administration of RIG 7 days after rabies vaccine). The vaccine or toxoid and antibody preparation should be administered at different sites using the standard recommended dose. Increasing the vaccine dose volume or number of vaccinations is not indicated or recommended.[11]

Immunization during illness

Immunization during acute illness may lead to lower immunogenicity or vaccine failure. Hence, vaccination should be postponed in a moderate or severe acute illness and parents instructed to return for vaccination when the illness resolves. Vaccination is also postponed to avoid superimposing vaccine reaction on the underlying illness and to mistakenly attribute a manifestation of underlying illness to vaccination. However, vaccination opportunity should not be missed during minor illnesses like upper respiratory tract infections, mild diarrhea and otitis media.[11]

Immunization of children with bleeding disorders or those receiving anticoagulants

Persons with bleeding disorders such as hemophilia and persons receiving anticoagulant therapy are at increased risk for bleeding after intramuscular injection. When vaccines recommended to be given only by the IM route are to be given, vaccination can be scheduled shortly after administration of clotting factor replacement.

A 23 gauge or smaller needle should be used for the vaccination and firm pressure without rubbing should be applied to the site for at least 5–10 minutes. Alternately, vaccines recommended for intramuscular injection could be administered subcutaneously to persons with a bleeding disorder if the immune response and clinical reaction to these vaccines are expected to be comparable by either route of injection, such as Hib conjugate vaccine, IPV, pneumococcal polysaccharide vaccine, etc.[11]

Immunization in Pregnancy

Live vaccines are generally contraindicated in pregnant women. The yellow fever vaccine should be avoided in pregnant women as far as possible. However, if travel is unavoidable, the vaccine should be given as the risks of infection outweigh the risks of vaccination (preferably in the 1st trimester).[12] Measles, MMR and varicella vaccines are contraindicated in pregnancy and pregnancy should be avoided for 4 weeks after vaccination. However, routine testing for pregnancy prior to immunizing with these vaccines is not recommended. If the vaccine is inadvertently given during pregnancy or pregnancy occurs within 4 weeks of vaccination, termination of pregnancy is not warranted. Small cohort studies show no increased rates of congenital abnormalities in infants born to mothers inadvertently vaccinated in pregnancy. measles, MMR and varicella vaccines can be safely given to contacts of pregnant women as these vaccines do not spread from vaccine to contacts.

Smallpox vaccine is the only vaccine known to be harmful to the fetus.

All inactivated vaccines may be safely given during pregnancy and readers are referred to the chapters on individual vaccines for recommendations. Important are Td/ TT/Tdap vaccines. The IAP ACVIP and CDC ACIP have recommended immunization with Tdap in every pregnancy preferably in the 3rd trimester to reduce the burden of pertussis in young infants.[13, 14] Influenza and hepatitis B are other vaccines of importance in pregnant women. Rabies vaccine should be administered to pregnant women if indicated and is safe.

Passive immunization with immunoglobulin containing preparations is safe in pregnancy. All pregnant women should be evaluated for immunity to rubella, varicella and hepatitis B and those found susceptible should be vaccinated immediately after delivery. All pregnant women should be tested for HbsAg and if found HBsAg-positive should be followed carefully to ensure that the infant receives HBIG and begins the hepatitis B vaccine series no later than 12 hours after birth and completes the recommended hepatitis B vaccine series on schedule.

Immunization in Lactation

All inactivated vaccines whether conjugated, toxoid, or subunit vaccines are safe in breast feeding women and pose no harm to the babies. Although live vaccines multiply in the body of the mother, most pose no harm to the babies as they are generally not excreted in breast milk. Rubella vaccine may be excreted in milk but does not infect the baby or if it all causes mild asymptomatic infection. The only exception to live vaccine use is yellow fever vaccine. Transmission of the yellow fever vaccine virus through breast milk and resulting in infantile meningoencephalitis has been described. Hence, yellow fever vaccine should be avoided in breast feeding mothers. If mandatory, then breast feeding should be interrupted for the 10 day post-vaccination viremic period.[12]

Immunization in preterm/low birth weight infants

In principle, all vaccines may be administered as per schedule according to the chronological age irrespective of birth weight or period of gestation. BCG and birth dose of OPV can be safely and effectively given to low birth weight and preterm babies after stabilization and preferably at the time of discharge.[15, 16] Studies have shown that the take of BCG as assessed by induration following Mantoux test and lymphocyte migration inhibition test (LMIT) is similar in preterm/low birth weight babies whether given at discharge or later.[17] The birth dose of hepatitis B vaccine can be administered at any time after birth in babies weighing > 2 kg. However, in babies less than 2 kg that immunogenicity of the birth dose of the vaccine has been shown to be suboptimal in some studies.[15] Hence the birth dose of hepatitis B vaccine in these babies should be delayed till the age of 1 month. Alternatively, these babies may also be given the first dose of the vaccine at the time of discharge if consistent weight gain is achieved. In babies less than 2 kg born to a hepatitis B positive mother, hepatitis B vaccine should be given along with HBIG within 12 hours of birth and 3 more doses at 1, 2 and 6 months are recommended. All other childhood vaccines may be given as per chronologic age and have acceptable safety, immunogenicity and efficacy. Full dose of the vaccines should be used. Since preterm and LBW babies may have low muscle mass, the use of needles with lengths of 5/8 inch or less is appropriate to ensure effective, safe, and deep anterolateral thigh intramuscular administration. As preterm, low birth weight babies have increased susceptibility to infections, vaccines such as pneumococcal conjugate vaccines, rotavirus and influenza should be offered if resources permit.

Lapsed immunization/ preponed immunization/ unknown immunization status

There is no need to restart a vaccine series regardless of the time that has elapsed between individual doses due to immune memory. Immunizations should be given at the next visit as if the usual interval had elapsed and the immunization scheduled should be completed at the next available opportunity. Doses should not be given 4 or less days from the minimum interval. If inadvertently given 5 or more days from the minimum interval, the dose should not be counted. In case of unknown immunization status, the child should be considered unimmunized and vaccinated accordingly. Self-reported doses should not be accepted in the absence of documentation with the exception of influenza and PPSV vaccines. Serologic testing is also an option in patients with uncertain status but is usually not cost effective, may reduce compliance and may result in missed opportunities for vaccination.[11]

Interchangeability of brands

There is sufficient data that brands of Hib, hepatitis B and hepatitis A may be safely interchanged with no compromise on immunogenicity and efficacy. However, robust data for immunogenicity of vaccination with different brands of DTaP is lacking. Hence, vaccination with DTaP should be completed with the same brand. However, if previous brand is not known or no longer available, any brand may be used and vaccination should not be delayed or cancelled.

Catch-up Immunization

Vaccination catch up regimens should preferably be individualized. The basic principles are discussed. Any number of vaccines live/ inactivated may be given on the same day either singly or as combination vaccines maintaining a gap of 5 cm between different vaccines. Inactivated vaccines can be given at any time in relation to any other live/ inactivated vaccines. If not given on the same day, a gap of 4 weeks should be maintained between two live injectable vaccines, especially MMR and varicella and also yellow fever and live attenuated influenza vaccines. However OPV, rotavirus and oral typhoid vaccines may be given at any time in relation to any live/ inactivated vaccine. For catch-up immunization, doses should preferably be given at the minimum possible interval to entail early protection.[11]

References

1. Casswall TH, Fischler B. Vaccination of the immunocompromised child. Expert Rev Vaccines. 2005; 4: 725–738.

2. McFarland E. Immunizations for the immunocompromised child. Pediatr Ann 1999; 28: 487–496.

3. Canadian Immunization Guide. General recommendations and Principles. Available from http://www.phac-aspc.gc.ca/publicat/cig-gci/p03-07-eng.php#a7. (Accessed on Dec 17, 2013)

4. Rubin GL, Levin MJ, Ljungman P, Davies EG, Avery R, Tomblyn M et al. 2013 Clinical practice guidelines for vaccination of the immunocompromised host. Clin Infect Dis. 2013 Dec 4. [Epub ahead of print]

5. Moss W, Halsey N. Vaccination of Human immunodeficiency virus-infected persons. In: PlotkinS , Orenstein W, Offit P , editors. Vaccines. 5th ed. US: Saunders Elsevier Publishers & Distributors; 2008.p.1417–1430.

6. American Academy of Pediatrics. Immunization in special clinical circumstances. In: Pickering LK, Baker CJ, Kimberlin DW, Long SS. eds. Red Book: 2009 Report of the Committee on Infectious Diseases. 28th ed. Elk Grove Village, IL: American Academy of Pediatrics; 2009.

7. Martín Ibáñez I, Arce Casas A, Cruz Martínez O, Estella Aguado J, Martín Mateos MA. Humoral immunity in pediatric patients with acute lymphoblastic leukaemia. Allergol Immunopathol (Madr). 2003; 31: 303–310.

8. Danzinger-Isakov L., Kumar D.: Guidelines for vaccination of solid organ transplant candidates and recipients. Am J Transplant 2009; 9(suppl 4): S258–S262.

9. Shatz DV, Schinsky MF, Pais LB, Romero-Steiner S, Kirton OC, Carlone GM. Immune responses of splenectomized trauma patients to the 23-valent pneumococcal polysaccharide vaccine at 1 versus 7 versus 14 days after splenectomy. J Trauma 1998; 44: 760–765.

10. Price VE, Blanchette VS, Ford-Jones EL. The prevention and management of infections in children with asplenia or hyposplenia. Infect Dis Clin North Am 2007; 21: 697–710.

11. CDC. General Recommendations on Immunization. Recommendations of the Advisory Committee on Immunization Practices (ACIP). MMWR 2011; 60: 1–61.

12. Imbert P, Moulin F, Mornand P, Méchaï F, Rapp C. Should yellow fever vaccination be recommended during pregnancy or breastfeeding? Med Trop (Mars). 2010; 70: 321–324.

13. Updated Recommendations for Use of Tetanus Toxoid, Reduced Diphtheria Toxoid, and Acellular Pertussis Vaccine (Tdap) in Pregnant Women - Advisory Committee on Immunization Practices (ACIP), 2012.MMWR Morb Mortal Wkly Rep. 2013; 62: 131–135.

14. Vashishtha VM, Kalra A, Bose A, Choudhury P, Yewale VN, Bansal CP et al. Indian Academy of Pediatrics (IAP) Recommended Immunization Schedule for Children Aged 0 through 18 years — India, 2013 and Updates on Immunization. Indian Pediatr 2013; 50: 1095–1108.

15. Saari TN. American Academy of Pediatrics Committee on Infectious Diseases. Immunization of Preterm and Low Birth Weight Infants. Pediatrics 2003; 112: 193–198.

16. Thayyil-Sudhan S, Singh M, Broor S, Xess I, Paul VK, Deorari AK. Is zero dose oral polio vaccine effective in preterm babies? Ann Trop Paediatr. 1998; 18: 321–324.

17. Thayyil-Sudhan S, Kumar A, Singh M, Paul VK, Deorari AK. Safety and effectiveness of BCG vaccination in preterm babies. Arch Dis Child Fetal Neonatal Ed. 1999; 8: F64–66.

■ ■ ■ ■ ■ ■

VACCINATION STRATEGIES FOR TRAVELLERS

4.3

Reviewed by
Digant Shastri, Panna Choudhury

For travellers, vaccination offers the possibility of avoiding a number of diseases that may be encountered while international travel. While evaluating the need for vaccination in travellers, it is important to consider not only the incidence rate but also the impact of the respective infection.[1] Immunized travellers will also be less likely to contaminate other travellers or the local population with a number of potentially serious diseases.

Travellers in most countries rarely seek health advice before travel. From a cross sectional survey in Europe, it is noticed that only 52.1% of responders had sought travel health advice.[2] The travellers need to know about prevalence of diseases in destination country, magnitude and risk of acquiring the diseases and means to prevent illness. The risk to a traveller of acquiring a disease also depends on age, immunization status and current health state of traveller, travel itinerary, duration and style of travel. Based on these factors, health care professional has to decide about need for immunizations and/or preventive medication (prophylaxis) and provide advice. Regardless of administration of vaccine/ medications traveller should always follow all possible precautions against infection for avoiding disease.

Vaccination Schedule

There cannot be single schedule for the administration of immunizing agents which may be applicable to all travellers. With considering individual traveller's immunization history, the countries to be visited, the type and duration of travel, and the availability of time for vaccination before departure a tailored made schedule should be suggested to travellers.

Timing of vaccination

Traveller should consult health care provider sufficiently in advance before departure about the need of immunization. The time period may vary depending on type of vaccine and number of doses required for immunity to develop. At times usual vaccination schedule may have to vary marginally to meet the requirement of the travellers. If full vaccination is not possible, partial vaccination may be done with advice to complete the schedule after reaching the destination country. If multiple live vaccines are to be given, they should be simultaneously at multiple sites, as otherwise inoculation of two live virus vaccines should be separated by at least 4 weeks.

Combination vaccines offer important advantages of compliance because of reduced number of injection and visits.

Choice of vaccines

Vaccines for travellers include: (1) basic vaccines used in routine immunization programmes, in all age groups; (2) vaccines that may be advised before travel to countries or areas at risk of these diseases. As per International Health Regulations vaccination to

Table 1: Vaccines for travellers

Routine vaccination	• Diphtheria • Hepatitis B • *Haemophilus influenzae* type b • Seasonal influenza • Measles • Mumps • Pertussis • Rubella • Pneumococcal disease • Poliomyelitis (Polio) • Rotavirus • Tuberculosis (TB) • Tetanus • Varicella
Selective use for travellers	• Hepatitis A • Typhoid fever • Rabies • Cholera • Japanese encephalitis • Tick-borne encephalitis • Meningococcal disease • Yellow fever

prevent yellow fever and meningococcal diseases are required for visiting certain countries.[3] The vaccines that may be recommended or considered for travellers are summarized in Table 1.

Routine vaccination

Travellers need to have undergone routine immunizations or have a change in the routine immunization schedule as it applies to travellers.[3,4]

BCG Vaccine

BCG immunization may be considered for travellers planning extended stays in areas of high tuberculosis prevalence and where tuberculin skin testing and appropriate chemoprophylaxis may not be feasible or where primary isoniazide resistance of *Mycobacterium tuberculosis* is high.

DTwP/DTaP/Tdap and its combination Vaccine

For infants embarking on travel, the primary vaccination series with diphtheria, tetanus, whole cell/acellular pertussis, polio, *Haemophilus influenzae* type b can be accelerated and can started at 6 weeks of age. For adults who have not previously received a dose of pertussis vaccine, it is recommended that they are offered Tdap vaccine rather than the tetanus and diphtheria booster dose (Td).

Measles and MMR Vaccine

Pan-American Health Organization (PAHO)/WHO recommends vaccination against measles and rubella for all travellers visiting countries in the Americas. PAHO also recommends that any resident of the Americas planning to travel to other regions of the world should be protected against measles and rubella prior to departing on their trip. Two doses of measles-containing vaccine (MMR) are recommended for all unimmunized adult travellers who were born in or after 1957 and who are en route to a measles-endemic area, unless there is serologic proof of immunity or physician documentation of prior measles. Infants aged 6–11 months should have at least 1 MCV dose. Infants vaccinated before age 12 months must be revaccinated on or after the first birthday with 2 doses of MCV separated by ≥ 28 days. Preschool children aged ≥12 months should have 2 MCV doses separated by ≥28 days and school-age children should have 2 MCV doses separated by ≥28 days.[3,5]

Hepatitis B Vaccine

Travellers including children who will be visiting areas with high levels of endemic hepatitis B infection and are likely to have contact with blood or blood products are recommended pre-travel hepatitis B vaccination.

Selective use for travellers

Meningococcal Disease

Invasive meningococcal disease, in both endemic and epidemic forms is the cause of significant morbidity and mortality worldwide. Among the different serogroups of *N. meningitidis*, serogroups A, B, and C account for up to 90% of the disease.[6] In the last few years, there has been a shift in the epidemic pattern of meningococcal disease during the Hajj (pilgrimage) season, with predominance of *Neisseria meningitidis* serogroup W135.

The recommendation for meningococcal vaccine for travellers mainly relates to: (i) Travellers to areas with current outbreaks; (ii) Travellers particularly < 30 years age who is travelling to the sub-Saharan meningitis belt during the dry season (December–June); (iii) All pilgrims arriving to Saudi Arabia for purposes of umra and Hajj[7]; (iv) Refugee settings with overcrowding, and persons who travel to work in these settings; (v) Individuals with underlying health problems recognized to increase the risk of acquiring meningococcal disease, e.g. functional or anatomic asplenia, terminal complement deficiency, or any other immune-suppressing conditions.

The quadrivalent meningococcal vaccine is already mandatory for Hajj pilgrims. For travellers or pilgrims who have received prior bivalent meningococcal vaccine, crossover vaccination with the quadrivalent meningococcal vaccine may be justified in view of the seriousness of the W135 problem. Travellers who have already received the conjugate C vaccine need to additionally receive the quadrivalent meningococcal vaccine, if travelling to countries where serogroups other than serogroup C are prevalent.

Yellow Fever

Yellow fever occurs in sub-Saharan Africa and tropical South America, where it is endemic and intermittently epidemic. In rural West Africa yellow fever virus transmission is seasonal, (usually July–October) while that in South America is highest during the rainy season (January–May).[8] Vaccination is required for travellers to countries and areas with risk of yellow fever transmission and when required by countries. The 17D live attenuated yellow fever vaccine is the only commercially available vaccine and has been widely acknowledged as one of the most effective vaccine in use.[9] Yellow fever vaccine is contraindicated for infants aged < 6 months, those with h/o hypersensitivity and for people with AIDS. A single subcutaneous (or intramuscular) injection of live, attenuated vaccine should be administered 10 days before the travel date. The period of validity of the International Vaccination Certificate for yellow fever is 10 years, beginning 10 days after primary vaccination and immediately after re-vaccination.[10]

Hepatitis A

Protection against hepatitis A is highly recommended for all non-immune travellers to areas or with inadequate sanitary facilities in countries where the disease is endemic. As the hepatitis A virus has long incubation period even if the inactivated vaccine is administered on the day of departure will be protective. One dose of monovalent hepatitis A vaccine administered at any time before departure can provide adequate protection for most healthy people aged ≤40 years. For adults aged >40 years, immunocompromised people, and people with chronic liver disease or other chronic medical conditions planning to depart to an area in <2 weeks should receive the initial dose of vaccine along with immunoglobulin in dose of 0.02 mL/kg.[11] For infants < 1 year of age protection may be provided by immune globulin. Since immune globulin provides protection for only 3 to 5 months it should be given immediately before departure and would provide protection for only 3 to 5 months.

Rabies

Countries are categorized as 1 (no risk) to 4 (high risk). In countries or areas belonging to categories 2–4, pre-exposure immunization against rabies is recommended for travellers.

Modern rabies vaccines-cell-culture or embryonated-egg origin are safer and more effective. Pre-exposure immunization should be considered for: (i) travellers intending to live or work in areas where rabies is enzootic and rabies control programs for domestic animals are inadequate; (ii) travel to area where adequate and safe post-exposure management is not available; (iii) travellers with extensive outdoor exposure in rural areas—such as might occur while running, bicycling, hiking, camping, etc. irrespective of the travel duration; (iv) individuals travelling to countries or areas where modern rabies vaccines are in short supply.

A course of three intramuscular injections of modern vaccines of cell-culture vaccine should be administered in schedule of one on each of days 0, 7 and 21 or 28.

Japanese Encephalitis

Japanese encephalitis (JE) occurs in many Asian countries. The risk varies according to season, destination, duration of travel and activities. The recommendations for JE vaccine for travellers is for: (i) Travellers who plan to spend ≥1 month in endemic areas during the JEV transmission season; (ii) Expatriates who will be based in urban areas but are likely to visit endemic rural or agricultural areas during a high-risk period of JEV transmission; (iii) Short-term (< 1 month) travellers to endemic areas during the JEV transmission season for travellers with extensive outdoor exposure (camping, hiking, working, etc.); (iv) Travellers to an area with an ongoing JE outbreak.[12]

The live attenuated SA 14-14-2 vaccine is widely used in China and in an increasing number of countries within the Asian region, including India, the Republic of Korea, Sri Lanka, and Thailand. A Vero cell-derived, inactivated JE vaccine was approved in 2009 in North America, Australia and various European countries. The vaccine is based on the attenuated SA 14-14-2 JE viral strain, inactivated and alum-adjuvanted. The immunization series should be completed at least 1 week before potential exposure to JEV. For the pre-travel prophylaxis two doses are administered 4 weeks apart.

Typhoid Fever

Vaccine should be recommend to those travelling to destinations where the risk of typhoid fever is high, especially individuals staying in endemic areas for >1 month and/or in locations where antibiotic resistant strains of *S. typhi* are prevalent. The vaccination should be given one week before departure. Travellers should be informed that typhoid immunization is not 100% effective and other hygienic measure should be undertaken.

Cholera

Cholera vaccination is not required as a condition of entry to any country. The vaccine should be consider for travellers visiting endemic areas and who are at high risk, e.g. emergency or relief workers. In India, killed bivalent oral O1 and O139 is available. Two doses are given 14 days apart for individuals aged ≥ 1 year. One booster dose is recommended after 2 years. Whenever to be used the 1st dose should be administered at least 2 weeks before the departure and for the effective protection ideally the full course of two doses should be completed before departure.

Vaccination for immunocompromised travellers

Immunocompromised hosts travelling overseas are at risk for exposure to endemic pathogens. In general, the vaccine response rate in these patients is diminished and they may be more likely to have adverse effects from vaccines containing live attenuated virus. In addition, vaccines are immunomodulatory and may impact immunologic conditions. Immunocompromised hosts planning to travel overseas should be evaluated by a travel medicine specialist familiar with the patient's immuno-compromised state and medications.[13,14]

The traveller's immune status is particularly relevant to immunizations. Overall considerations for vaccine recommendations, such as destination and the likely risk of exposure to disease, are the same for immunocompromised travellers as for other travellers. The risk of a severe outcome from a vaccine-preventable disease must be weighed against potential adverse events from administering a live vaccine to an immunocompromised patient. In some complex cases when travellers cannot tolerate recommended immunizations or prophylaxis, the traveller should consider changing the itinerary, altering the activities planned during travel, or deferring the trip.[15]

The travellers who has been on corticosteroid therapy for > 2 weeks at a dose equivalent to > 20 mg per day of prednisone, should be considered analogous to patients with HIV infection with a CD4 cell count < 200 cells/mm³ and decision of administration of live vaccines should be taken accordingly. Patients receiving other immunosuppressive drugs should be advised on a case-by-case basis depending on the degree of immune suppression as judged by the prescribing physician.

Asplenic patients and persons with terminal complement deficiencies are susceptible to overwhelming sepsis with encapsulated bacterial pathogens. These groups of people should be immunized with the meningococcal A/C/Y/W-135 conjugate vaccine.[6]

Patients with limited immune deficits or asymptomatic HIV going to yellow fever endemic areas may be offered yellow fever vaccine and monitored closely for possible adverse effects. As vaccine response may be suboptimal, such vaccinees are candidates for serologic testing 1 month after vaccination. Travellers with severe immune compromise should not be vaccinated with yellow fever vaccine and should be strongly discouraged from travel to destinations that put them at risk for yellow fever.

Vaccination for pregnant travellers

No evidence exists of risk from vaccinating pregnant women with inactivated virus, bacterial vaccines, or toxoids. The benefits of vaccinating pregnant women usually outweigh potential risks when the likelihood of disease exposure is high, infection would pose a risk to the mother or foetus, and the vaccine is unlikely to cause harm. Pregnant travellers may visit areas of the world where diseases eliminated by routine vaccination in their native country are still endemic, and therefore may require immunizations before travel. If the pregnant traveller is at risk for influenza on this trip (high season), she should be advised to be vaccinated with inactivated whole virus or subunit influenza vaccine.

Vaccination Document

Travellers should be provided with a written record of all vaccines administered preferably using the international vaccination certificate. This certificate must be signed by the clinician or authorized health worker. The certificate must also bear the official stamp of the administering centre, however. The certificate should be either in English or in French. However, in addition to these two languages the certificate may also be completed in another language on the same document. The traveller should be advised to carry copy of the certificate. As a proof of yellow fever vaccination, traveller must carry the original International Certificate of Vaccination.

References

1. Steffen R, Connor BA. Vaccines in travel health: From risk assessment to priorities. J Travel Med 2005; 12: 26–35

2. Van Herck K, Van Damme P, Castelli F, Zuckerman J, Nothdurft H, Dahlgren AL, et al, Knowledge, Attitudes and Practices in Travel-related Infectious Diseases: The European Airport Survey. J Travel Med. 2004; 11: 3–8.

3. Vaccine preventable diseases and vaccines- International travel and health. Available from http://whqlibdoc.who.int/publications/2007/9789241580397_6_eng.pdf. (Accessed on Dec 14, 2013)

4. CDC. Traveller's Health. Available from http: // wwwnc. cdc. gov/travel/destinations/list. (Accessed on Dec 14, 2013)

5. Epidemiological Alert: PAHO recommendations to travellers to preserve America without measles or rubella (28/04/2011). Available from http:// www.who.int / immunization / GIN _ June_2011.pdf. (Accessed on Dec 14, 2013)

6. World Health Organization (WHO). Control of epidemic meningococcal disease: WHO practical guidelines. 2nd ed. WHO/EMC/BAC/98.3: 1. Geneva: WHO, 1998.

7. Steffen R, Connor BA. Vaccines in travel health: from risk assessment to priorities. J Travel Med 2005; 12: 26–35. Ministry of Hajj. Kingdom of Saudi Arabia. Important notices. Visas. 2010. Available at: http://www.hajinformation.com/main/t1510.htm. (Accessed on Dec 14, 2013)

8. Monath TP, Cetron MS. Prevention of yellow fever in people travelling to the tropics. Clin Infect Dis. 2002; 34: 1369–1378.

9. Monath TP, Nichols R, Archambault WT, Moore L, Marchesani R, Tian J, et al. Comparative safety and immunogenicity of two yellow fever 17D vaccines (ARILVAX and YF-VAX) in a phase III multicenter, double-blind clinical trial. Am J Trop Med Hyg. 2002; 66: 533–541.

10. Yellow fever vaccine. WHO Position Paper. Wkly Epidemiol Rec 2003; 78: 349–359.

11. CDC. Update: Prevention of hepatitis A after exposure to hepatitis A virus and in international travellers. Updated recommendations of the Advisory

Committee on Immunization Practices (ACIP). MMWR Morb Mortal Wkly Rep. 2007; 56: 1080–1084.

12. Fischer M, Lindsey N, Staples JE, Hills S. Japanese encephalitis vaccines: Recommendations of the Advisory Committee on Immunization Practices (ACIP). MMWR Recomm Rep. 2010; 59(RR-1): 1–27.

13. Boggild AK, Sano M, Humar A. Travel patterns and risk behavior in solid organ transplant recipients. J Travel Med 2004; 11: 37–43.

14. Roukens AH, van Dissel JT, de Fijter JW, Visser LG. Health preparations and travel-related morbidity of kidney transplant recipients travelling to developing countries. Clin Transplant 2007; 21: 567–570.

15. CDC. Immunocompromised Travellers. Available from http://wwwnc.cdc.gov/travel/yellowbook/2014/chapter-8-advising-travelers-with-specific-needs / immunocompromised - travelers. (Accessed on Dec 14, 2013)

■ ■ ■ ■ ■ ■

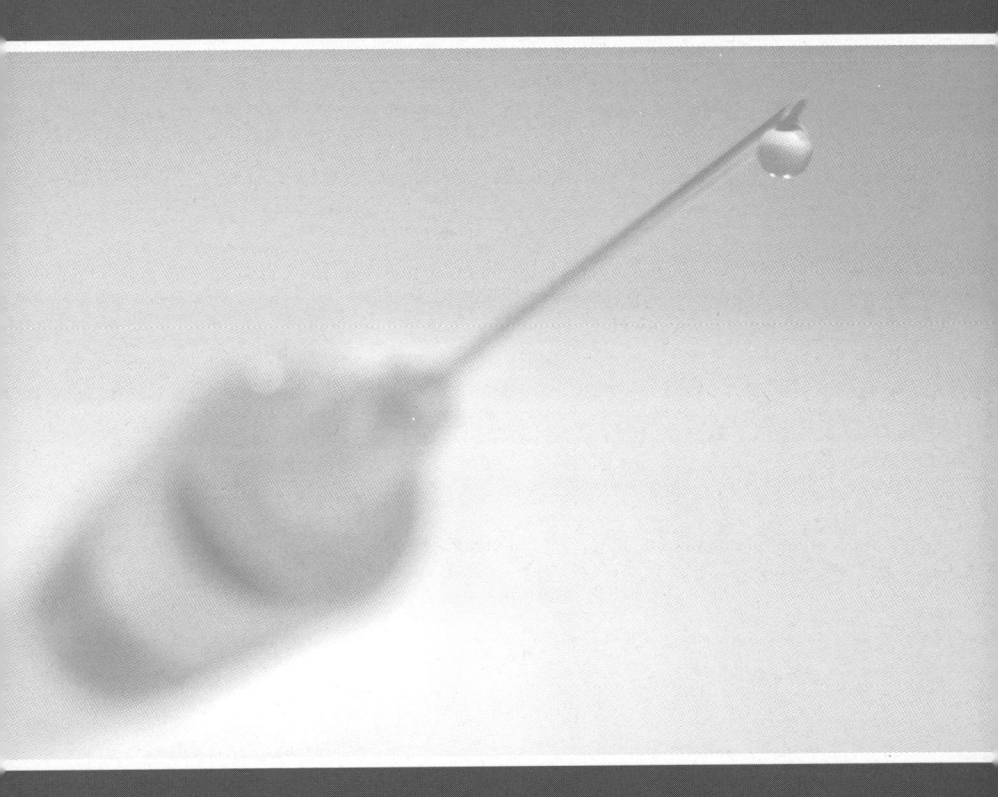

Annexure

Annexure I: IAP Immunization Schedule 2013

IAP Recommended Immunization Schedule 2013 for Children Aged 0–18 years (with range)

Age / Vaccine	Birth	6 wk	10 wk	14 wk	18 wk	6 mo	9 mo	12 mo	15 mo	18 mo	19–23 mo	2–3 yr	4–6 yr	7–10 yr	11–12 yr	13–18 yr
BCG	BCG															
Hep B	Hep B1	Hep B2				Hep B3										
Polio	OPV 0	IPV 1	IPV 2	IPV 3		OPV 1	OPV 2		IPV B1				OPV 3			
DTP		DTP 1	DTP 2	DTP 3					DTP B1				DTP B2			
Tdap															Tdap	
Hib		Hib 1	Hib 2	Hib 3					Hib Booster							
Pneumococcal		PCV 1	PCV 2	PCV 3					PCV Booster						PCV	
PPSV23														PPSV		
Rotavirus		RV 1	RV 2	RV 3												
Measles							Measles									
MMR									MMR 1				MMR 2			
Varicella										VAR 1			VAR 2			
Hep A									Hep A1 & Hep A2							
Typhoid												Typhoid				
Influenza						Influenza (yearly)										
HPV															HPV 1–3	
Meningococcal												Meningococcal				
Cholera												Cholera 1 & 2				
JE											Japanese encephalitis					

Legend:
- Range of recommended ages for all children
- Range of recommended ages for catch-up immunization
- Range of recommended ages for certain high-risk groups
- Not routinely recommended

- This schedule includes recommendations in effect as of November 2013.
- These recommendations must be read with the footnotes that follow. For those who fall behind or start late, provide catch-up vaccination at the earliest opportunity as indicated by the green bars in Figure 1.

Annexure II: Self Declaration on Conflicts of Interest Issues

DECLARATION OF CONFLICT OF INTERESTS FOR
ADVISORY COMMITTEE ON VACCINE AND IMMUNIZATION PRACTICES (ACVIP)
MEMBERS/EXPERTS OF INDIAN ACADEMY OF PEDIATRICS (2013)

Name:

Institution:

Retired/Private practice/ Others (Please specify):

Email:

Date and title of meeting/ work:

Description of your role:

Your current designation (in ACVIP):

DECLARATION OF CONFLICT OF INTEREST

IAP Advisory Committee on Vaccines & Immunization Practices (ACVIP) has been mandated to frame recommendations for our own members about the usage of available licensed vaccines in the country. Apart from this primary responsibility, as a professional organization, we are also entrusted with the responsibility to serve as a source of evidence-based information pertaining to vaccination in children for the public at large. This unique responsibility demands that ACVIP members have integrity of the highest order, particularly those members who are empowered with the right of voting for important decisions made by ACVIP, which have far reaching consequences and impact on child health. In order to ensure professional integrity and public confidence in the activities and recommendations made by ACVIP, it is imperative that each member voluntarily declare any potential conflict of interest (i.e. any interest that may effect, or may reasonably be perceived to effect, the member's objectivity, independence and judgment) while discharging his/her professional duties as a member. The potential conflict of interest also includes relevant interest of the immediate family members of ACVIP member.

All the potentially significant interests will be disclosed to the ACVIP Secretariat at least one month before the meeting and updated for any recent change/ endorsed before the start of the meeting.

Self declaration forms of each member, submitted at least one month before the meeting, will be scrutinized by a sub-committee constituted by ACVIP. The declaration forms will be scrutinized based on the information provided by the members. However, if it is discovered later on that the declaration was incorrect or some facts have been suppressed, ACVIP Secretariat will have the option of banning the member from the committee for three years.

If any member discloses a conflict of interest or is unable or unwilling to disclose the details of an interest that may pose a real or perceived conflict in member's objectivity, independence or judgment, the ACVIP Secretariat may decide to ask him/her to totally recluse from the meeting.

IAP Guidebook on Immunization 2013–14

FORM A: DECLARATION OF INTERESTS

Please answer each of the questions below. If the answer to any of the questions is "yes", briefly describe the circumstances In FORM B.

The term "you" refers to yourself, your employer and your immediate family members (i.e., spouse/ partner with whom you have a similar close personal relationship, and your minor children). "Commercial entity" includes—aside from any commercial business — an industry association, research institution or other enterprise whose funding is significantly derived from commercial sources having an interest related to the subject of the meeting or work. "Meeting" includes a series or cycle of meetings.

1. **EMPLOYMENT, CONSULTING and FAVORS**

    1a   Within the past 4 years, have you received remuneration/ honorarium from a commercial entity with an interest related to the subject of the meeting or work? Please also report any application or negotiation for future work. **Yes | No**

    1b   Within the past 4 years, have you received any travel grant from a commercial entity with an interest related to the subject of the meeting or work? Please also report any travel grant or favor in near future from a commercial entity. **Yes | No**

2. **RESEARCH SUPPORT**

    Within the past 4 years, have you or your department or research unit received support or funding from a commercial entity or other organization with an interest related to the subject of the meeting or work? Please also report any application or award for future research support.

    2a   Research support, including grants, collaborations, sponsorships, and other funding **Yes | No**

    2b   Non-monetary support valued at more than Rs. 25,000 overall (include equipment, facilities, research assistants, paid travel to meetings, etc.) **Yes | No**

3. **INVESTMENT INTERESTS**

    Do you have current investments (valued at more than Rs. 1,00,000 overall) in a commercial entity with an interest related to the subject of the meeting or work? Please also include indirect investments such as a trust or holding company.

    3a   Stocks, bonds, stock options, other securities (e.g. short sales) **Yes | No**

    3b   Commercial business interests (e.g. proprietorships, partnerships, joint ventures) **Yes | No**

4. **INTELLECTUAL PROPERTY**

    Do you have any current intellectual property rights that might be enhanced or diminished by the outcome of the meeting or work?

4a   Patents, trademarks, or copyrights (also include pending applications)
Yes | No

4b   Proprietary know-how in a substance, technology or process **Yes | No**

5.   PUBLIC STATEMENTS AND POSITIONS (within the past one year)

5a   As part of a regulatory, legislative or judicial process, have you provided an expert opinion or testimony, related to the subject of the meeting or work, for a commercial entity?   **Yes | No**

5b   Are you holding an office or other position, where you may be expected to represent interests or defend a position related to the subject of the meeting or work?   **Yes | No**

6.   ADDITIONAL INFORMATION

6a   If not already disclosed above, have you worked for the competitor of a product which is the subject of the meeting or work, or will your participation in the meeting or work enable you to obtain access to a competitor's confidential proprietary information, or create for you a financial or commercial competitive advantage?   **Yes | No**

6b   To your knowledge, would the outcome of the meeting or work benefit or adversely affect interests of others with whom you have substantial common personal, financial or professional interests (such as your adult children or siblings, close professional colleagues, administrative unit or department)?   **Yes | No**

6c   Is there any other aspect of your background or present circumstances not addressed above that might be affecting your objectivity or independence?   **Yes | No**

FORM B: EXPLANATION OF "YES" RESPONSES

If the answer to any of the above questions is "yes", check above and briefly describe the circumstances on this page. If you do not provide, the amount or value of the interest, where requested, it will be assumed to be significant.

Nos. 1 – 4 Type of interest, question number and category (e.g. Intellectual Property 4.a copyrights) and basic descriptive details.	Name of company, organization, or institution	Belongs to you, a family member, employer, research unit or other?	Amount of income or value of interest (if not disclosed, is assumed to be significant)	Current interest
Nos. 5 – 6: Describe the subject, specific circumstances, parties involved, time frame and other relevant details				

Date:

Place:

                                Signature

Annexure III: Internet Resources on Immunization Information

S. No.	Organization/ sponsor	Web address	Salient contents
1	National Library of Medicine	www.pubmed.com	Abstracts and full texts of vaccine related articles published in indexed journals
2	IAPCOI	www.iapcoi.com	Electronic copy of guidebook, Q & A facility
3	WHO	www.who.int/immunization/en/index.html	WHO position papers
4	Centers for Disease Control (CDC)	www. cdc.gov/vaccines/	ACIP vaccine recommendations, travel immunization
5	Immunization Action Coalition	www.immunize.org/	Educational material for parents
6	National Network for Immunization Information	www.immunizationinfo.org	Separate sections for parents, listserv that gives updated information
7	Children's Hospital Philadelphia	www.vaccine.chop.edu/	Info for parents, vaccine safety
8	GAVI	www.gavialliance.org	Info on GAVI policy and funding
9	PATH	www. path.org/ vaccineresources/index.php	Vaccine resource library
10	Vaccine manufacturers (in alphabetical order)	www.bharatbiotech.com www.biomed.co.in www.biologicale.com www.gskvaccines.com www.indimmune.com www.merckvaccines.com www.novartisvaccines.com www. panacea-biotec.com www.sanofipasteur.com www.shanthabiotech.com www.seruminstitute.com www.wyeth.com/vaccines	Prescribing information for various vaccines
11	Miscellaneous	*Vaccines:* www.sciencedirect.com/ science/journal/0264410X *Expert Review of Vaccines:* www.expert reviews.com/loi/erv *PneumoAdip:* http://pneumoadip.org/ *ADVAC :* www.advac.org *Infectious Diseases in Children:* www.pediatricsupersite.com/ issue.aspx?pubid=idc	Information, presentations, and journal articles on vaccines and immunization practices

Annexure IV: Ready Reckoner for Vaccines Currently Available in India

Vaccine	Content/dose	Nature and diluent	Storage	Dose, route, site	Schedule	Protective efficacy	Major adverse effects	Contraindications
BCG (LAV)	0.1 billion to 0.4 million viable bovine mycobacteria	Lyophilized, normal saline	Freezer/ 2 to 8°C, Protect from light	0.1 ml ID, left deltoid	Single dose at birth or first contact below 5 years	0–80%	Axillary lymphadenilis	Cellular immunodeficiency. Should not be given with measles/MMR
OPV (LAV)	Sabin strain Type 1- 10^6 CC ID_{50} Type 2- 10^6 CC ID_{50} Type 3- 10^6 CC ID_{50}	Liquid vaccine	Freezer/ 2 to 8°C	2 drops oral	Birth, 6, 10, 14 weeks, 15–18 months, 5 years, NID's, SNID's	10–15% per dose (India), 30% per dose (world)	Rarely VAPP	Immunodeficient patients and household contacts
IPV (Inactiv- ated)	Salk strain Type 1 - 40 units Type 2 - 8 units Type 3 - 32 units	Liquid vaccine	2 to 8°C	0.5 mL IM or SC, thigh*/ deltoid	6, 10, 14 weeks, booster at 15–18 months	95–100%	None	Serious hypersensitivity
DTwp/ DTap	Diphtheria toxoid 20–30 Lf, tetanus toxoid 5–25 Lf, wP 4 IU/ aP 3 µg to 25 µg of 2 to 5 purified pertussis antigens	Liquid vaccine	2 to 8°C Protect DTaP from light	0.5 mL IM thigh/ deltoid	6, 10, 14 weeks, booster at 15–18 months, 5 years Not recommended above 7 years	95–100% for diphtheria/ tetanus and 70–90% for pertussis	Rare, More with D TwP High fever, excessive crying, seizures, HHE, encephalopathy	Serious hypersensitivity, encephalopathy following previous dose
DT	Same as above with no pertussis	Liquid vaccine	2 to 8°C	0.5 mL IM thigh/ Deltoid	Replacement for DTwP/ DTaP in those with contraindications for pertussis vaccination, not recommended above 7 years			

Vaccine	Content/dose	Nature and diluent	Storage	Dose, route, site	Schedule	Protective efficacy	Major adverse effects	Contraindications
TT	Tetanus toxoid 5 Lf	Liquid vaccine	2 to 8°C	0.5 mL IM thigh/ deltoid	As routine at 10 years and every 10 years thereafter, pregnancy, wound management (Td/T dap preferred to TT)			
Td	Tetanus toxoid 5 Lf, Diphtheria 2 Lf	Liquid vaccine	2 to 8°C	0.5 mL IM thigh/ deltoid	As replacement for DTwp / D TaP / DT for catch-up vaccination in those aged above 7 years (along with Tdap), and as replacement for TT at all ages			
Tdap	Tetanus toxoid 5 Lf, Diphtheria toxoid 2 Lf, 2.5 to 8 µg of three pertussis antigens	Liquid vaccine	2 to 8°C	0.5 mL IM thigh/ deltoid	Single dose at 10–12 years	90%	None	As for DTwP/DTaP
Measles (LAV)	1000 CCID$_{50}$ of Edmonston Zagreb strain of measles virus	Lyophilized, diluent sterile water	Freezer/ 2 to 8°C Protect from light	0.5 mL SC thigh/ deltoid	Single dose at 9 months	80%	Mild measles like illness in < 5%, Rarely/thrombocy-topenicpurpura	Severely immuno-compromised, pregnancy
Rubella (LAV)	5000 CCID$_{50}$ of RA 27/3 strain of rubella virus	Lyophilized, diluent sterile water	Freezer/ 2 to 8°C	0.5 mL SC thigh/ deltoid	As for MMR, MMR preferred	95%	Mild rubella like illness in < 5%, rarely arthritis, ITP	Severely immuno-compromised, pregnancy
MMR (LAV)	Measles and rubella as above; Mumps 5000 CCID$_{50}$ of Jeryl Lynn/Urate strain	Lyophilized, diluent sterile water	Freezer/ 2 to 8°C Protect from light	0.5 mL SC thigh/ deltoid	Two doses at 15–18 months and 5 years	95%	Same as measles and rubella, high fever, rarely parotid swelling aseptic meningitis	Severely immuno-compromised, pregnancy

Vaccine	Content/dose	Nature and diluent	Storage	Dose, route, site	Schedule	Protective efficacy	Major adverse effects	Contraindications
Hep B	20 µg/mL of HBsAg antigen	Liquid vaccine	2 to 8°C	<18 year 0.5 mL, > 18 year 1 m IM deltoid/ thigh	Birth, 6 14 weeks OR 6, 10, 14 weeks OR 0, 1, 6 months	> 90%	None	Serious hypersensitivity
Hib	10 µg of PRP- T or HbOC	Liquid or Lyophilized, (diluent sterile water)	2 to 8°C	0.5 mL IM thigh/ deltoid	6, 10, 14 weeks, booster at 15–18 months	> 90%	None	Serious hypersensitivity
DTwP+ Hib	As for DTwp and Hib	Liquid vaccine or lyophilized Hib reconstituted with liquid DTwP	2 to 8°C	0.5 mL IM thigh/ deltoid	6,10,14 weeks booster at 15–18 months	As for DTwP and Hib		
DTwP+ Hep B	As for DTwP and 10 µg of Hep B	Liquid vaccine	2 to 8°C	0.5 mL IM thigh/ deltoid	6, 10, 14 weeks,	As for DTwP and Hep B		
DTwP+ Hib+ Hep B	As for DTwP, Hib, 10 µg of Hep B	Liquid vaccine or lyophilized Hib reconstituted with liquid DTwP+Hep B	2 to 8°C	0.5 mL IM thigh/ deltoid	6 ± 10, 14 weeks	As for DTwP, Hib and Hep B		
DTaP+ Hib	As for DTaP and Hib	Lyophilized Hib reconstituted with liquid DTap	2 to 8°C	0.5 mL IM thigh/ deltoid	6, 10, 14 weeks and booster at 15–18 months	As for DTaP and Hib		

Vaccine	Content/dose	Nature and diluent	Storage	Dose, route, site	Schedule	Protective efficacy	Major adverse effects	Contraindications
DTaP+ Hib+IPV	DTaP (two component), IPV and Hib	Liquid vaccine	2 to 8°C	0.5 mL IM thigh/ deltoid	6, 10, 14 weeks and booster at 15–18 months	As for DTaP, IPV and Hib		
Vi typhoid Poly-saccharide	25–30 µg of Vi polysaccharide	Liquid vaccine	2 to 8°C	0.5 mL IM thigh/ deltoid	Above 2 years, single dose, revaccination every 3 years	60%	None	Serious hypersensitivity
Vi-PS-TT Conjugate Typhoid	25 µg of Vi-polysaccharide conjugated to tetanus toxoid per 0.5 mL	Liquid vaccine	2 to 8°C	0.5 mL IM deltoid/ thigh	Single dose at ≥ 6 months, booster after 3 years	> 90% sero-conversion in > 6 months–45 years	None, only minor systemic & local side effects	Severe hypersensitivity to any constituent -Pregnant & lactating mother
HPV quadri-valent	L1 protein of serotypes 6, 11, 16, 18	Liquid vaccine	2 to 8°C	0.5 mL IM thigh/ deltoid	10–12 years 0, 2, 6 months	> 90% against serotype specific cervical cancer	None	Serious hypersensitivity pregnancy
HPV bivalent	L1 protein of serotypes 16, 18				10–12 years 0, 1, 6 months			
PCV	Capsular polysaccharide of serotypes 4, 6B, 9V, 14, 18C, 19F, 23, 1, 5, 6A, 7F, 3 linked to CRM 197	Liquid vaccine	2 to 8°C	0.5 mL IM thigh/ deltoid	6, 10, 14 weeks, booster at 15–18 months	95% against serotype specific invasive disease	None	Serious hypersensitivity

Vaccine	Content/dose	Nature and diluent	Storage	Dose, route, site	Schedule	Protective efficacy	Major adverse effects	Contraindications
PPSV23	Capsular	Liquid vaccine	2 to 8°C	0.5 mL SC/ IM thigh/ deltoid	Single dose at ≥ years Revaccination only once after 3–5 years	70% against invasive disease in high risk children	None	Serious hypersensitivity
In-activated Hep A	HM 175 strain Composition varies with brands/age	Liquid vaccine	2 to 8°C	Below 15–18 years (as per brand) 0.5 mL IM deltoid/ thigh	Two doses 6 months apart, 18 months onwards	> 95%	None	Serious hypersensitivity
Hep A & Hep B	Composition varies with age	Liquid vaccine	2 to 8°C	Below 18 years 0.5 mL	0, 1 and 6 months, 18 months onwards	> 95%	None	Serious hypersensitivity
Live attenuated Hep A	6.5 log particles of H2 strain	Lyophilized, sterile water	2 to 8°C	1 mL SC deltoid/ thigh	Two doses 6 months apart 18 months onwards till 15 years	> 95%	None	Immunodeficient patients
Varicella	≥ 1000 PFU of Oka strain	Lyophilized, sterile water	2 to 8°C Protect from light	0.5 mL SC deltoid/ thigh	>13 years 2 doses, at 16 months & 5 years ≥ 13 years two doses 4–8 weeks apart	70–90% with one dose > 95% with 2 doses	Varicella like rash in 5%	Pregnancy, severely immuno-compromised

Vaccine	Content/dose	Nature and diluent	Storage	Dose, route, Site	Schedule	Protective efficacy	Major adverse effects	Contraindications
Rotavirus (monov- alent) LAV	Human rotavirus strain 89-12 (G1P8)	Lyophilized, sterile water based specific liquid diluent	2 to 8° C Protect from light	1 mL orally	2 doses, first dose at 6–15 weeks, second to be completed by 32 weeks and not to be initiated after 15 weeks	85–98% against severe rotavirus diarrhea	None	Acute gastroenteritis, beyond 6 months
Human Bovine Pentava- lent vaccine	5 rotavirus reassortant strains G1, G2, G3, G4 and P1A (8)	Liquid vaccine	2 to 8° C	2 mL orally	3 doses, 1st dose at 6–15 weeks and then at 4 weeks interval schedule to be completed by 32 weeks	85–98% against severe rotavirus diarrhea	None	Beyond 32 weeks age
Inactivated Kolar strain JE vaccine (JENVAC)	Inactivated, Kolar strain, 821564XY JE vaccine 5.0 µg per 0.5 mL	Liquid vaccine	2 to 8°C	0.5 mL Intramuscular deltoid/ thigh	Two doses at 4 weeks interval from 1 year of age & onwards (up to 50 years) Booster may be needed	> 90% sero- conversion & seropr- otection after one dose in 1–50 years	None, only fever & local side effects	Severe hypersensitivity to any constituent

Vaccine	Content/dose	Nature and diluent	Storage	Dose, route, site	Schedule	Protective efficacy	Major adverse effects	Contraindications
Inactivated SA-14-14-2 strain JE vaccine (JEEV)	6 µg per 0.5 mL of Inactivated Vero cell culture-derived SA 14-14-2 JE vaccine	Liquid vaccine	2 to 8°C	1–3 years: 0.25 mL; 3–18 yrs: 0.5 mL IM ; deltoid/ thigh	2 doses at 4 weeks interval; Booster may be needed	> 90% sero-conversion	None, only fever & local side effects	Severe hypersensitivity to any constituent
Live JE vaccine, SA-14-14-2	5.4 log PFU of SA 14-14-2 strain of JE virus	Liquid vaccine	2 to 8°C	0.5 mL SC thigh/ deltoid	Single dose at ≥ 9 months	> 90%	None	Immunodeficient patients and their household contacts
MPSV	Bivalent (A + C) Quadrivalent (A + C + Y + W135)	Lyophilized, diluent sterile water	2 to 8°C	0.5 mL SC or thigh/ deltoid	If indicated, single dose above 2 years revaccination once after 3–5 years	90%	None	Serious hypersensitivity
MCV4 Quadri-valent	4 µg of Meningococcal group A,C,Y & W0135 polysaccharides conjugated to 48 µg of diphtheria toxoid	Liquid vaccine	2 to 8° C	0.5 mL IM deltoid	Single dose from > 2–55 years	Effectiveness: 80– 85%	None, no extra risk of GBS amongst vaccine	Severe hypersensitivity to any constituent

Vaccine	Content/dose	Nature and diluent	Storage	Dose, route, site	Schedule	Protective efficacy	Major adverse effects	Contraindications
Yellow fever vaccine	17 D strain of yellow fever virus	Lyophilized, sterile diluent	2 to 8°C	0.5 mL SC thigh/ deltoid	Single dose, revaccination every 10 years if needed	> 90%	Rarely neurologic/ visoerotropic disease	Below 6 months, serious egg allergy severe immunodeficiency, thymus disease
Cholera	–	Liquid vaccine	2 to 8°C	1.5 mL po	Two doses above 1 years & weeks apart	60%	None	None

Annexure V: IAP Immunization Timetable 2016

I. IAP recommended vaccines for routine use

Age (completed weeks/ months/years)	Vaccines	Comments
Birth	BCG OPV 0 Hep B$_1$	Administer these vaccines to all newborns before hospital discharge
6 weeks	DTwP 1 IPV 1 Hep B$_2$ Hib 1 Rotavirus 1 PCV 1	**DTP:** • DTaP vaccine/combinations should preferably be avoided for the primary series • DTaP vaccine/combinations should be preferred in certain specific circumstances/conditions only • No need of repeating/giving additional doses of whole-cell pertussis (wP) vaccine to a child who has earlier completed their primary schedule with acellular pertussis (aP) vaccine-containing products **Polio:** • All doses of IPV may be replaced with OPV if administration of the former is unfeasible • Additional doses of OPV on all supplementary immunization activities (SIAs) • Two doses of IPV instead of 3 for primary series if started at 8 weeks, and 8 weeks interval between the doses • No child should leave the facility without polio immunization (IPV or OPV), if indicated by the schedule

		• See footnotes under figure titled IAP recommended immuniza-tion schedule (with range) for recommendations on intra-dermal IPV
		Rotavirus: • 2 doses of RV1 and 3 doses of RV5 and RV116E • RV1 should be employed in 10- and 14-week schedule, 10- and 14-week schedule of RV1 is found to be more immunogenic than 6- and 10-week schedule
10 weeks	DTwP 2 IPV 2 Hib 2 Rotavirus 2 PCV 2	**Rotavirus:** If RV1 is chosen, the first dose should be given at 10 weeks
14 weeks	DTwP 3 IPV 3 Hib 3 Rotavirus 3 PCV 3	**Rotavirus:** • Only 2 doses of RV1 are recommended • If RV1 is chosen, the 2nd dose should be given at 14 weeks
6 months	OPV 1 Hep B$_3$	**Hepatitis B:** The final (3rd or 4th) dose in the Hep B vaccine series should be administered no earlier than age 24 weeks and at least 16 weeks after the first dose
9 months	OPV 2 MMR 1	**MMR:** • Measles-containing vaccine ideally should not be adminis-tered before completing 270 days or 9 months of life • The 2nd dose must follow in 2nd year of life • No need to give stand alone measles vaccine

9–12 months	Typhoid conjugate vaccine	• Currently, two typhoid conjugate vaccines, Typbar-TCV® and PedaTyph® available in Indian market; either can be used • An interval of at least 4 weeks with the MMR vaccine should be maintained while administering this vaccine
12 months	Hep A$_1$	**Hepatitis A:** • Single dose for live attenuated H2 strain Hep A vaccine • Two doses for all inactivated Hep A vaccines are recommended
15 months	MMR 2 Varicella 1 PCV booster	**MMR:** • The 2nd dose must follow in 2nd year of life • However, it can be given at anytime 4–8 weeks after the 1st dose **Varicella:** The risk of break-through varicella is lower if given 15 months onwards
16 to 18 months	DTwP B$_1$/DTaP B$_1$ IPV B$_1$ Hib B1	The first booster (4th dose) may be administered as early as age 12 months, provided at least 6 months have elapsed since the third dose **DTP:** • 1st and 2nd boosters should preferably be of DTwP • Considering a higher reacto-genicity of DTwP, DTaP can be considered for the boosters
18 months	Hep A 2	**Hepatitis A:** 2nd dose for inactivated vaccines only

2 years	Booster of typhoid conjugate vaccine	• A booster dose of typhoid conjugate vaccine (TCV), if primary dose is given at 9–12 months • A dose of typhoid Vi-polysaccharide (Vi-PS) vaccine can be given if conjugate vaccine is not available or feasible • Revaccination every 3 years with Vi-polysaccharide vaccine • Typhoid conjugate vaccine should be preferred over Vi-PS vaccine
4 to 6 years	DTwP B$_2$/DTaP B$_2$ OPV 3 Varicella 2 MMR 3	**Varicella:** The 2nd dose can be given at anytime 3 months after the 1st dose **MMR:** The 3rd dose is recommended at 4–6 years of age
10 to 12 years	Tdap/Td HPV	**Tdap:** It is preferred to Td followed by Td every 10 years **HPV:** • Only 2 doses of either of the two HPV vaccines for adolescent/preadolescent girls aged 9–14 years • For girls 15 years and older, and immunocompromised individuals 3 doses are recommended • For 2-dose schedule, the minimum interval between doses should be 6 months • For 3-dose schedule, the doses can be administered at 0, 1–2 (depending on brand) and 6 months